Anton Krige • Michael J. P. Scott
Editors

Analgesia in Major Abdominal Surgery

Springer

Editors
Anton Krige
Department of Anaesthetics
and Critical Care
Royal Blackburn Hospital
Blackburn, Lancashire
United Kingdom

Michael J. P. Scott
Department of Anesthesiology
and Critical Care
Virginia Commonwealth University
Hospital
Richmond, VA
USA

ISBN 978-3-030-06860-8 ISBN 978-3-319-94482-1 (eBook)
https://doi.org/10.1007/978-3-319-94482-1

This Springer imprint is published by the registered company Springer Nature Switzerland AG
The registered company address is: Gewerbestrasse 11, 6330 Cham, Switzerland

Analgesia in Major Abdominal Surgery

Foreword

Enhanced post-operative recovery programmes were developed about 20 years ago, initially in minor abdominal procedures but rapidly followed by major abdominal procedures. The clinical and economic benefits of these programmes have been repeatedly confirmed by centres around the world and later including programmes from all other surgical specialties.

A prerequisite for enhanced recovery is provision of "dynamic pain relief", meaning that patients are comfortable and able to mobilize. During the last decade, several developments of new analgesic techniques and drugs have been available, making it difficult for the practical clinician to make evidence-based procedure-specific choices. Consequently, this book which reviews the many different possibilities to optimize analgesia in major surgery is an important step forward to help clinicians to achieve further improvement in their enhanced recovery pathways. The authors are to be congratulated for their efforts to put this knowledge together, which deserves widespread interest and distribution.

Henrik Kehlet
Section for Surgical Pathophysiology 7621
Rigshospitalet
Copenhagen, Denmark

Introduction

This millennium has seen dramatic changes in how major abdominal surgery is performed with rapid increases in the use of minimally invasive surgical techniques, utilizing laparoscopic or robotic assistance. The result is a reduction in abdominal wound site and visceral injury, which has in turn led to a different approach to analgesia management as pain is often controlled with oral multimodal analgesia within 24–36 h post-operatively.

Surgical technique and newer surgical instruments (such as the harmonic scalpel) have also led to a reduction in the amount of tissue damage and blood loss during surgery, regardless of whether a minimally invasive or open approach is used. The result has been surgery with less primary injury and reduction in blood loss enabling patients to recover more rapidly after surgery.

The development of accelerated peri-operative care pathways (so-called enhanced recovery programmes), originally described by Kehlet in the 1990s, which enable patients to recover faster after open colorectal surgery, has also changed the approach to analgesia in patients undergoing all major abdominal surgery globally. This emphasizes early mobilization after surgery to reduce complications and insulin resistance, in order to improve outcomes, and dynamic analgesic techniques are pivotal in achieving these goals.

Analgesic techniques that reduce mobilization, or encumber the patient, are therefore problematic even before they have been commenced. The avoidance of high doses of opiates is also imperative to reduce their unwanted side effects, which include nausea, vomiting, sedation, lethargy, confusion and delirium. There is also an increased risk of ileus and constipation with opiate use. The recognition that early oral feeding is beneficial and without risk, compared to long periods of starvation with a nasogastric tube in situ, has led to the acceptance of early feeding as a standard clinical practice in both upper and lower GI surgery across Europe. Although the timing, initial quantity and increase in buildup of feeds differ between specialties, the era of not feeding the gut for many days after surgery is over. This has presented the opportunity for administering medication orally, thereby reducing the need for complex pumps, which in turn reduce mobility and create psychological dependence. These changes jointly lead to greater simplicity in delivering effective analgesia.

The development and availability of new technology has not been limited to surgery. The advent of highly sophisticated portable ultrasound machines has enabled anaesthetists to perform ultrasound-guided nerve blocks at the bedside or in the operating room environment. Ultrasound is useful for both single-shot and catheter placement for paravertebral blocks and abdominal wall blocks, e.g. TAP, QLB and rectus sheath blocks, as well as increasingly used in difficult spinal or epidural catheter placement in patients with high body mass index. The result has been the increased safety and efficacy of nerve blocks as anatomy can be accurately targeted and vascular structures identified and avoided. Chapters 9–12 comprehensively cover this range of nerve blocks with continuous wound infusions covered in Chap. 13.

Whilst all these newer techniques are challenging the position long held by thoracic epidural analgesia, Dr. Antrobus devotes Chap. 8 to the discussion of what is still considered the gold standard by many. The other neuraxial block, the spinal blockade using intrathecal opiate, has found a new niche as an effective postoperative analgesic option and is ably discussed by Dr. Dhillon.

It is imperative that surgeons and anaesthetists have knowledge of anatomy of the abdominal wall and nerve distribution to ensure appropriate selection, safety and efficacy of these techniques depending on the surgical approach and patient factors. In Chap. 1, Professor Timothy Rockall outlines the anatomy and approach of different techniques that provide a solid foundation for the regional techniques that follow.

This era has also seen advancements in pharmacology and the introduction of newer analgesic drugs. The release of older drugs in newer formulations has also improved efficacy of analgesia during the peri-operative period when there is gut dysfunction or when the patient is not able to ingest enteral medication.

Paracetamol (acetaminophen) is one such drug. It is now available in intravenous form enabling delivery of up to 4 g a day providing good blood concentrations of the drug as the backbone to peri-operative multimodal opioid-sparing analgesia. Many NSAIDs (including COX2) are available in intravenous form as another addition to paracetamol in multimodal analgesia. Dr. Baldini in Chap. 2 covers simple multimodal analgesia as well as systemic opiate in Chap. 3, which although minimized is still frequently required at lower dosage for control of visceral pain or as a step down from the more potent regional techniques.

Although gabapentinoids (gabapentin, pregabalin) have been used for many years for chronic pain, these drugs are being increasingly used as an adjunct to multimodal opioid-sparing analgesia, and they are expertly dissected by Dr. Jeremy Cashman in Chap. 4.

Other exciting non-opioid adjuvants discussed in detail are ketamine and intravenous lidocaine infusions by Dr. Naveen Eipe in Chaps. 5 and 6. Both drugs have been in use for many decades but have only recently been identified as safe and useful opioid-sparing options, along with other benefits involving inflammation in the case of ketamine and inflammation and gut function in the case of lidocaine. Although a plethora of other non-opioid molecules with varying degrees of analgesic effect has been identified and is used in research settings or by pain experts, for example, beta adrenergic blockers, glucocorticoids, alpha-2 agonists, magnesium, epinephrine, antidepressants, cholinomimetics, antihistamines, nitroglycerine and calcium channel blockers, we have chosen to confine this book to the aforementioned agents as these have the greatest evidence of efficacy and safety and have already been incorporated as standard items in the analgesic package of many enhanced recovery programmes.

Pain is multifactorial in nature and has large inter-individual variation. Indeed the final chapter by Dr. Searle deals with the challenging task of managing of acute pain in patients with pre-existing chronic pain. There is increased awareness that treating the pain score alone, without addressing the consequences of the analgesic method, can worsen outcomes after surgery. Examples are the patient who is rendered immobile with a thoracic epidural due to motor block or a patient who is obtunded or confused as a result of liberal opioid use.

Therefore, the concept of "effective analgesia" is a key principle to keep in mind when reading this book and choosing combinations of techniques to suit your practice and institution.

Multimodal analgesia, including simple analgesia (Chap. 2) along with non-opioid adjuvants (Chaps. 4–6) delivered in a standardized package to reduce the need for opiates and their related side effects, is the backbone of analgesia for enhanced recovery pathways. A major analgesic modality, the so-called primary technique (usually one of regional techniques described in Chaps. 7–13), is needed to achieve this during surgery and the immediate post-operative period. The duration of this depends on the type of surgery, surgical approach and patient factors. The role of systemic opiates ideally remains low dose as rescue.

The primary technique should provide adequate pain relief for early mobilization, enable early return of gut function and have minimal adverse effects (in particular hypotension and excessive motor block which prohibit mobilization). Importantly, the techniques that fulfil all of these attributes, and are therefore the most effective choices, are not always the option with the best pain scores initially. The key to success of any analgesic strategy is patient education and setting of appropriate goals and expectations. Dr. Rockett in Chap. 14 highlights fascinating emerging research surrounding such non-pharmacological adjuncts to analgesia.

It is important for hospitals to have several different approaches for analgesia in case one is inappropriate, contraindicated or in the case of failure. Other factors to consider in choice of technique are the healthcare time involved in managing the interventions, the skill set required for insertion (ideally use interventions with rapid learning curves or already existing skill sets thus enabling rapid system-wide implementation), and portability of infusion devices (ideally use techniques that are single shot thus not requiring infusions or long-acting transdermal patches which do not rely on administration compliance). Finally, many analgesic methods need troubleshooting to ensure efficacy so constant monitoring of pain scores, patient function and vital signs are necessary.

The emphasis for optimal analgesia in modern surgery is therefore multifaceted:

1. A basis of patient education with realistic setting of their expectations and psychological preparation which improves analgesia throughout the peri-operative pathway including after discharge to home. This is an often overlooked component.
2. An overall aim to reduce opioid use and their associated side effects of sedation, nausea and vomiting, pruritus, confusion and ileus.

3. Some form of local anaesthetic block, either central neuraxial, truncal or wound infusions, to reduce opiate consumption in the immediate peri-operative period.
4. Early commencement of multimodal analgesia.
5. Reduction of opiates using other pharmacological methods (gabapentinoids, ketamine, lidocaine). This may include non-pharmacological techniques.
6. Recognition of the chronic pain patient presenting for surgery and those at risk of developing chronic postsurgical pain and developing a robust peri-operative analgesic plan incorporating acute pain team involvement proactively.

The selection of analgesic techniques used in many hospitals around the world is still often based on that which was used during a physician's period in training or what has been historically used in a hospital based on studies from 10 to 20 years ago. This book aims to give the reader an up-to-date evidence-based guide of the analgesic choices available for patients undergoing major abdominal surgery, along with the practical knowledge and tips of the experts to enable you to implement these interventions into your practice and across your wider institutions.

When compiling the chapter list, we engaged some of the world's most eminent authority on each subject. We hope you enjoy reading it and find the contents relevant to your clinical practice.

Blackburn, UK Anton Krige, MBChB, DIMC, FRCA, FFICM
Guildford, UK Michael J. P. Scott, MBChB, FRCP, FRCA, FFICM

Abbreviations

ACC	Anterior cingulate cortex
AMPA	α-Amino-3-hydroxy-5-methyl-4-isoxazolepropionic acid
AMPAR	α-Amino-3-hydroxy-5-methyl-4-isoxazolepropionic acid receptor
ASIS	Anterior superior iliac spine
BD	Bilateral dual
CBT	Cognitive behavioural therapy
CI	Confidence interval
CNB	Central neuraxial blockade
CNCP	Chronic non-cancer pain
CNS	Central nervous system
COX	Cyclooxygenase
CT	Computed tomography
CTL	Costotransverse ligament
CWI	Continuous wound infusion
CWIC	Continuous wound infusion catheter
DNIC	Diffuse noxious inhibitory control
DRG	Dorsal root ganglion
EO	External oblique
ER	Extended release
ERAS	Enhanced recovery after surgery
EREM	Extended-release epidural morphine
ES	Erector spinae muscles
ESRA	European Society of Regional Anaesthesia & Pain Therapy
FDA	United States Food and Drug Administration
FLK	FentaKetaCaine
fMRI	Functional magnetic resonance imaging
GABA	γ-Aminobutyric acid
GI	Gastrointestinal
GP	General practitioner
IASP	International Association for the Study of Pain
IBW	Ideal body weight
ICB	Intercostal block
ICBG	Iliac crest bone grafting
IHN	Iliohypogastric nerve

IIN	Ilioinguinal nerve
IO	Internal oblique
IL	Interleukin
ILO	Ivor-Lewis oesophagectomy
IM	Intramuscular
IV	Intravenous
L4	Vertebral body of L4
LA	Local anaesthetic
LAST	Local anaesthetic systemic toxicity
LAT	L-Amino acid transporter
LOS	Length of stay
MAC	Minimum alveolar concentration
MCID	Minimal clinically important difference
MCT-1	Monocarboxylate transporter-1
MIO	Minimally invasive oesophagectomy
NAP	National Audit Project
NF-κB	Nuclear factor-kappa B
NMDA	N-methyl-D-aspartate
NNH	Number needed to harm
NNT	Number needed to treat
NSAID	Nonsteroidal anti-inflammatory drug
OFA	Opioid-free anaesthesia
OIH	Opioid-induced hyperalgesia
OR	Odds ratio
PACU	Post-anaesthetic care unit
PAG	Periaqueductal grey
PCA	Patient-controlled analgesia
PCEA	Patient-controlled epidural analgesia
PCP	Phencyclidine
PCTS	Patient-controlled transdermal fentanyl
PO	Per os
POCD	Post-operative cognitive dysfunction
PONV	Post-operative nausea and vomiting
PVB	Paravertebral blockade
RSB	Rectus sheath block
RSC	Rectus sheath catheter
QL	Quadratus lumborum
QLB	Quadratus lumborum block
QST	Quantitative sensory testing
PSU	Presurgical unit
PVS	Paravertebral space
RA	Rectus abdominis
RCT	Randomized controlled trial
RFA	Radiofrequency ablation
RSB	Rectus sheath block

RSC	Rectus sheath catheter
RSS	Rectus sheath space
SC	Subcutaneous
SD	Standard deviation
TA	Transversus abdominis
TAP	Transversus abdominis plane
TCI	Target-controlled infusion
TEA	Thoracic epidural analgesia
TERSC	Thoracic Epidural versus Rectus Sheath Catheter study
TFP	Transversalis fascia plane
TLO	Thoracoscopic-laparoscopic oesophagectomy
TP	Transverse process
TPBV	Thoracic paravertebral block
TQL	Transmuscular quadratus lumborum block
UA	Ultrasound assisted
USG	Ultrasound guided
VDCC	Voltage-dependent calcium channel
VPL	Ventral posterolateral
VR	Virtual reality
WHO	World Health Organization
WMD	Weighted mean difference

Contents

Contributors

Jonathan Antrobus, MD Department of Anesthesia, Borders General Hospital, Melrose, Roxburgshire, UK

Gabriele Baldini, MD, MSc Department of Anesthesiology, McGill University Health Centre, Montreal General Hospital, Montreal, QC, Canada

Rafael Blanco, MB, BS, FRCA, DEAA Department of Anaesthesia & Intensive Care Medicine, King's College Hospital, Dubai, UAE

Jens Børglum, MD, PhD Department of Anesthesiology & Intensive Care Medicine, Zealand University Hospital, University of Copenhagen, Roskilde, Denmark

Jeremy Cashman, BSc, MB, BS, BA, MD, FRCA Department of Anaesthetics, St. George's Hospital, London, UK

Mark Daugherty, MBChB, FRCA Department of Anaesthesia, Royal Devon and Exeter Hospitals, Exeter, UK

Sabrina Dhillon, MD Virginia Commonwealth University Health System, Richmond, VA, USA

Naveen Eipe, MD Department of Anesthesiology and Pain Medicine, The Ottawa Hospital, University of Ottawa, Ottawa, ON, Canada

Kevin King, DO Department of Anesthesiology, University of Pittsburgh Medical Center, Passavant Hospital, Pittsburgh, PA, USA

Anton Krige, MBChB, DIMC, FRCA, FFICM Department of Anaesthesia & Critical Care, Royal Blackburn Teaching Hospital, East Lancashire Hospitals NHS Trust, Blackburn, UK

Nicholas Marshall, MBBS, FRCA Department of Anaesthesia, Royal Cornwall Hospital, Truro, Cornwall, UK

Aisling McMahon, FCAI, FJFICMI Department of Anesthesia, Clinical Sciences Institute, National University of Ireland, Galway, Ireland

John G. McDonnell, MD, FCARCSI Department of Anaesthesia and Intensive Care Medicine, Galway University Hospitals, Galway, Ireland

Giuliano Michelagnoli Department of Anesthesia, McGill University Health Centre, Montreal General Hospital, Montreal, QC, Canada

Oana Predescu, MD, MSc, PhD Department of Anesthesiology, McGill University Health Centre, Montreal General Hospital, Montreal, QC, Canada

Timothy A. Rockall, MB, BS, FRCS, MD Royal Surrey County Hospital NHS Trust, Guildford, Surrey, UK

Clinical Research Facility, Galway University Hospitals, Galway, Ireland

Mark Rockett, BSc, MB ChB, PhD, MRCP, FRCA Department of Anaesthesia, Intensive Care and Pain Medicine, Derriford Hospital, Plymouth, UK

Michael J. P. Scott, MB, ChB, FRCP, FRCA, FFICM Department of Anesthesiology, Virginia Commonwealth University Health System, Richmond, VA, USA

Robert Searle, MBChB, MD Department of Anaesthesia, Royal Cornwall HospitalTruro, Cornwall, UK

Nicholas T. Ventham, MRCS(Eng), MBBS Department of Colorectal Surgery, Western General Hospital, Edinburgh, UK

Illustrations in Chapter 1 courtesy of Anna Scott - ALScottUK@gmail.com

Anatomy of the Innervation of the Abdomen

1

Timothy A. Rockall

Key Points

1. Somatic pain from abdominal wall trauma is the major component following abdominal surgery.
2. Visceral pain is the lesser component, although initially intense, is of shorter duration.
3. The somatic component receives innervations from the T7 to T12 spinal nerves.
4. Regional techniques can target nerve blockade anywhere from the subarachnoid space to the terminal nerve endings of T7 to T12 to achieve somatic analgesia.
5. The central neuraxial techniques will simultaneously achieve blockade of the autonomic nerve supply to the abdomen and therefore the visceral pain component. Other regional techniques will require additional analgesia for this component.

Introduction

Pain is an important indicator of abdominal pathology and the site and nature of the pain is an important indicator of the likely cause. Pain is also an inevitable consequence of operating in the abdomen. The major cause of post-operative pain is the trauma to the abdominal wall required to access the pathology of the peritoneal cavity, but pain may also originate from the abdominal organs (visceral pain) and the peritoneum. For many surgical procedures the advent of minimally invasive techniques has dramatically reduced the component of post-operative pain originating from the abdominal wall without necessarily impacting on the lesser visceral component.

T. A. Rockall
Royal Surrey County Hospital NHS Trust,
Minimal Access Therapy Training Unit (mattu),
Guildford, Surrey, UK

A. Krige, M. J. P. Scott (eds.), *Analgesia in Major Abdominal Surgery*,
https://doi.org/10.1007/978-3-319-94482-1_1

An array of local and regional anaesthetic techniques are used to control post-operative pain either as a sole method or as an opiate sparing adjunct to systemic analgesia. The technique used is a reflection of the type of abdominal surgery being performed and the site and size of the abdominal wound(s). However, it also reflects the expertise and preference of the anaesthetist and surgeon involved.

This chapter deals with the anatomy of the abdominal musculature, the spinal canal and the sensory nervous system as it relates to methods of pain control following major abdominal surgery. Knowledge of the anatomy is pertinent to the practice of all the different local and regional anaesthetic techniques that can be used to control pain. The specifics of each technique as well as the advantages and disadvantages and relative merits will be discussed in detail in subsequent chapters.

Innervation of The Abdomen

The abdominal wall can be divided into myotomes and dermatomes each being supplied by the spinal nerve originating in the thoracic column. Classically the abdominal wall is described as being innervated by the T7–T12 spinal nerves. In reality the xiphisternum is within the T5 distribution and the pubic bone within the L1 distribution (Fig. 1.1). This is because of the crossover of innervation between

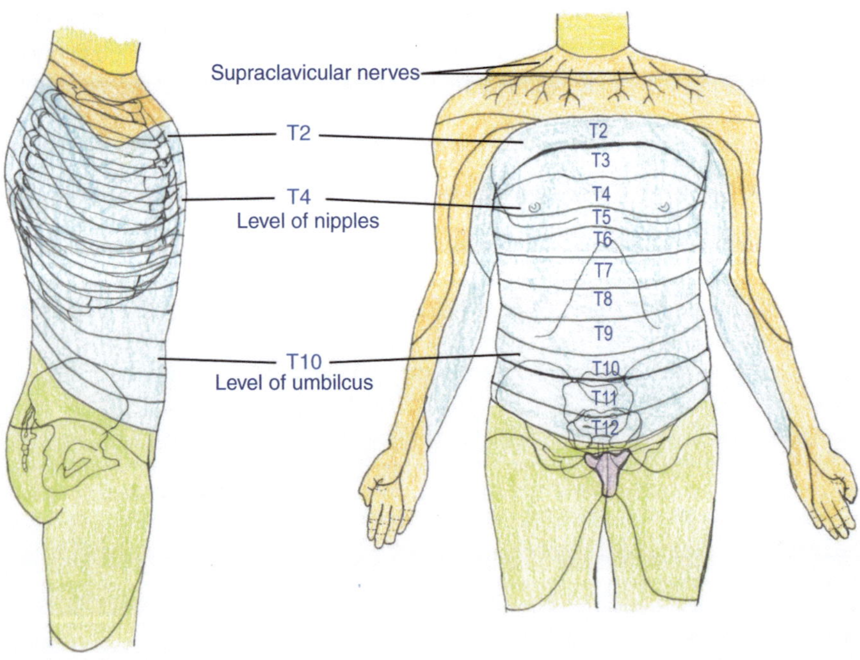

Fig. 1.1 Dermatomes of the thorax and abdomen. Illustration courtesy of A.L. Scott

dermatomes. Branches of the spinal nerves also supply the parietal peritoneum but the intra-abdominal organs are innervated by the autonomic nervous system. The sympathetic supply is via the splanchnic nerves and the parasympathetic via the vagus nerve and sacral parasympathetic outflow.

The Spinal Column

An understanding of the anatomy of the spinal column is critical to successful access to the dural and epidural space and to avoiding the complications that may arise. Equally an understanding of the anatomy of the vertebrae and paravertebral muscles is critical to the application of regional blocks and catheters in relation to the psoas muscle, the quadratus lumborum muscle and the paravertebral space.

Sensory nerves arise from the dorsal root and motor nerves from the ventral root of the spinal column. The dorsal and ventral roots combine to form 31 pairs of spinal nerves. Each spinal nerve divides into a dorsal ramus and a ventral ramus. It is the ventral ramus that supplies motor and sensory fibres to the anterior abdominal wall. Each spinal nerve communicates with the sympathetic trunk via grey and white rami communicantes (Fig. 1.2). The spinal nerves supply motor fibres in a distribution called a myotome and sensory fibres to the skin in a distribution called a dermatome.

The spinal cord which gives rise to the dorsal and ventral roots is surrounded by the spinal meninges (Pia mater, Arachnoid mater and Dura mater). The Dura

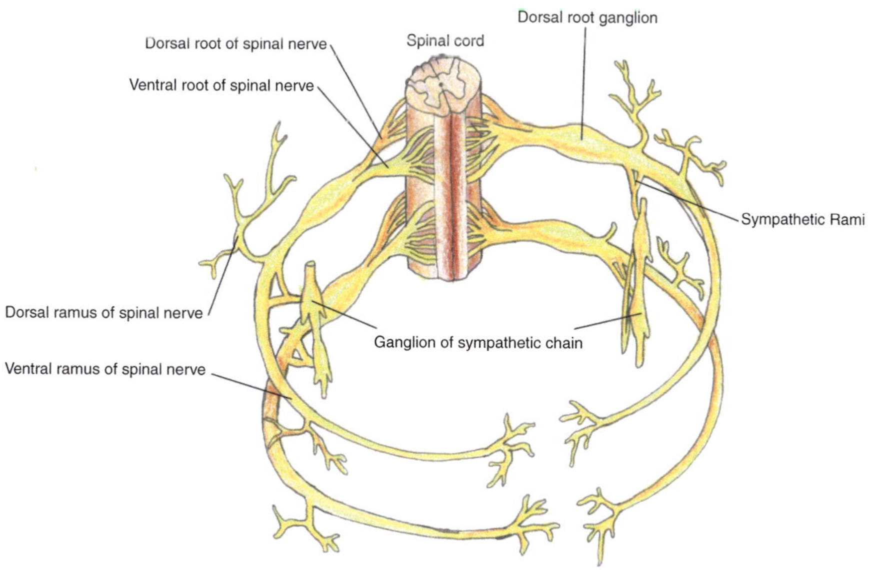

Fig. 1.2 Anatomy of the spinal nerve. Illustration courtesy of A.L. Scott

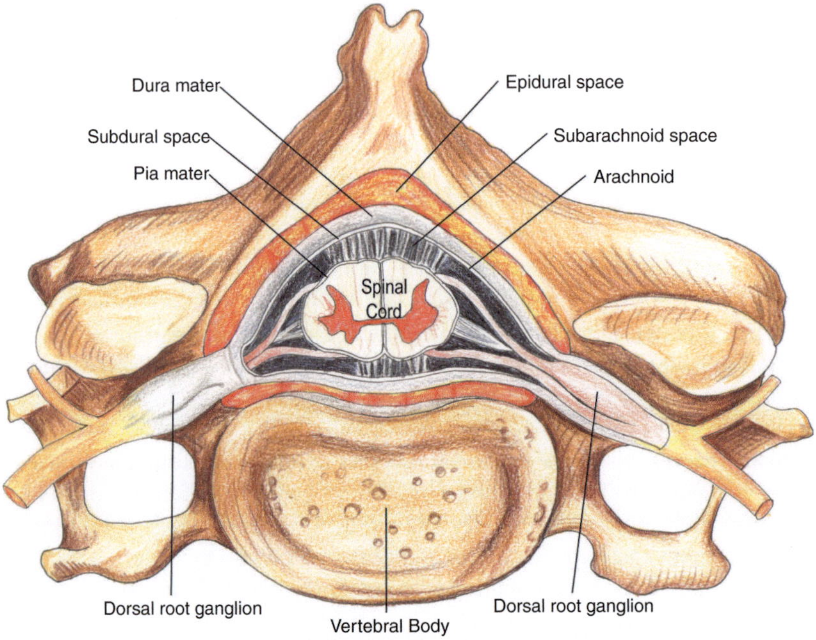

Fig. 1.3 Cross-section of the spinal column. Illustration courtesy of A.L. Scott

mater is also referred to as the Dural sheath. These three layers give rise to two potential spaces known as the sub-arachnoid and sub-dural spaces. Outside of this is the Epidural space, which contains fat and blood vessels. Within the Dural sheath the spinal cord is bathed in cerebrospinal fluid that is continuous with the cerebrospinal fluid surrounding the brain (Fig. 1.3). The spinal column gives way to the corda equina in its lower part at the level of approximately the first lumbar vertebra (Fig. 1.4).

The spinal column is protected by the vertebral bones that articulate and provide a gap between the vertebra called the intervertebral foramen through which the fused dorsal and ventral roots (dorsal root ganglion) pass (Fig. 1.5). After the dorsal root (spinal) ganglion it becomes known as the spinal nerve which then gives off a dorsal ramus supplying motor and sensory fibres to the back and ventral ramus which for the thoracic nerves is also known as the intercostal nerve (Subcostal for T12).

Anteriorly the vertebrae and intervertebral discs and the posterior longitudinal ligament protect the spinal column. Posteriorly the spinal cord is protected by the bony vertebral arches, and in-between the arches by the supraspinous ligament, interspinous ligament and ligamentum flavum (Fig. 1.6). Access to the subarachnoid or epidural space is through these ligaments. Vascularity is least in the midline.

Strong muscles encased in a tough thoracolumbar fascia support the vertebral column. The thoracic spinal nerves travel initially in the space between the internal intercostal membrane (formed by the fusion of the external and internal

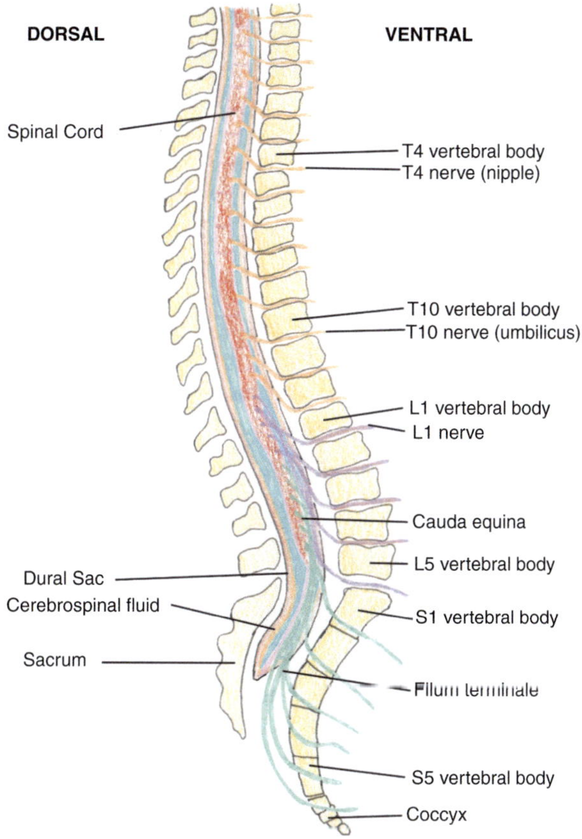

Fig. 1.4 Sagittal section of the spinal cord. Illustration courtesy of A.L. Scott

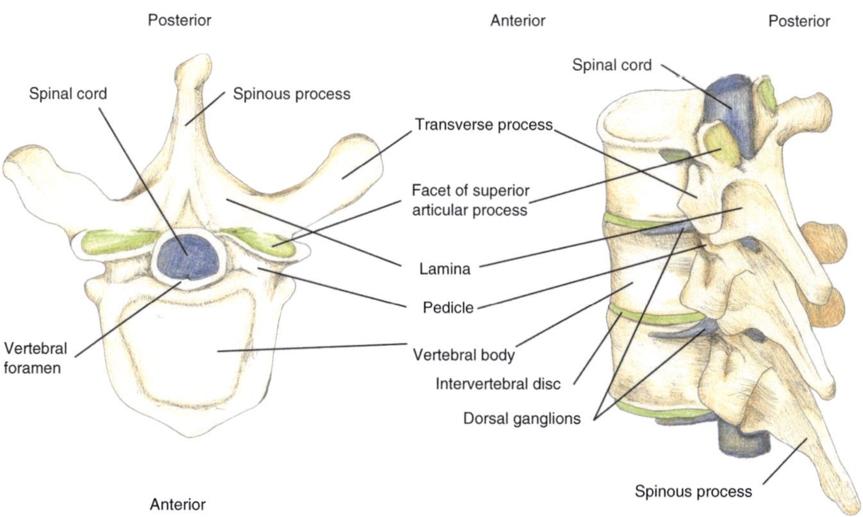

Fig. 1.5 Bony anatomy of the vertebral column. Illustration courtesy of A.L. Scott

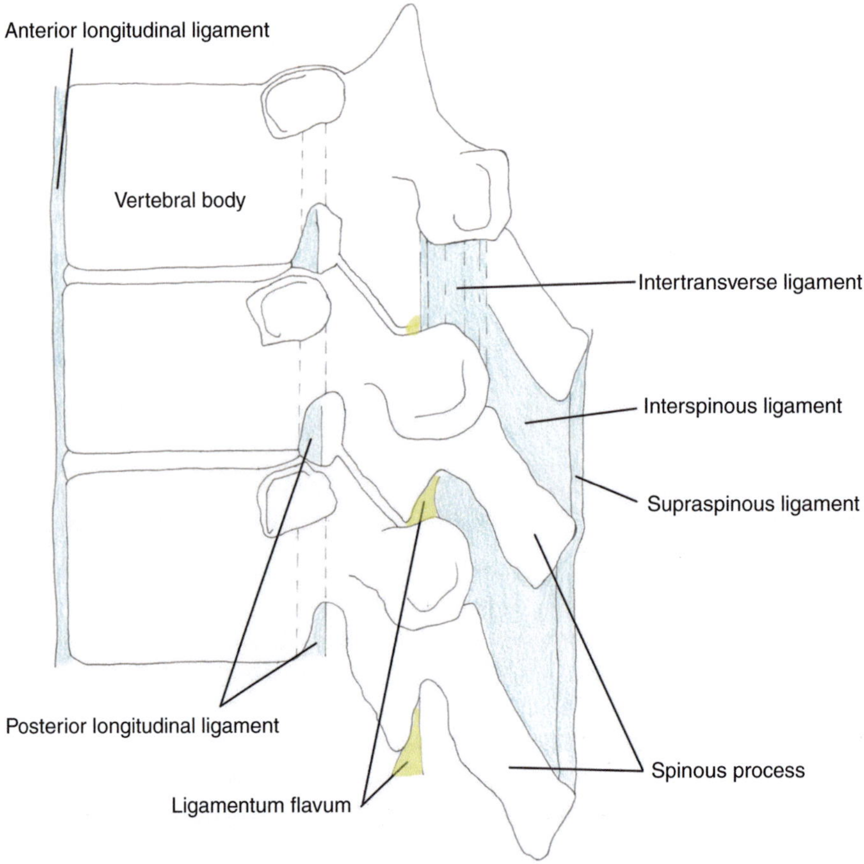

Fig. 1.6 Ligaments of the vertebrae. Illustration courtesy of A.L. Scott

intercostal muscles attached to the transverse process) and the endothoracic fascia. Deep to the endothoracic fascia is the parietal pleura (Fig. 1.7). For this reason, one of the complications of paravertebral blocks is a pneumothorax. More laterally the intercostal nerves enter the plane between the innermost intercostal and internal intercostal muscles. As they travel anteriorly they will enter the plane between the internal and external oblique muscles of the anterior abdominal wall.

The Anterior Abdominal Wall

The motor and sensory fibres from the intercostal (T7–T11) and subcostal (T12) nerves, which arise from the ventral rami of the thoracic nerve root (Fig. 1.8), innervate the peritoneum, abdominal musculature and the overlying skin. Each nerve is connected to the sympathetic trunk by grey and white rami communicantes. T7–T12 supply the thoracic and abdominal wall. T12 supplies the abdominal wall as

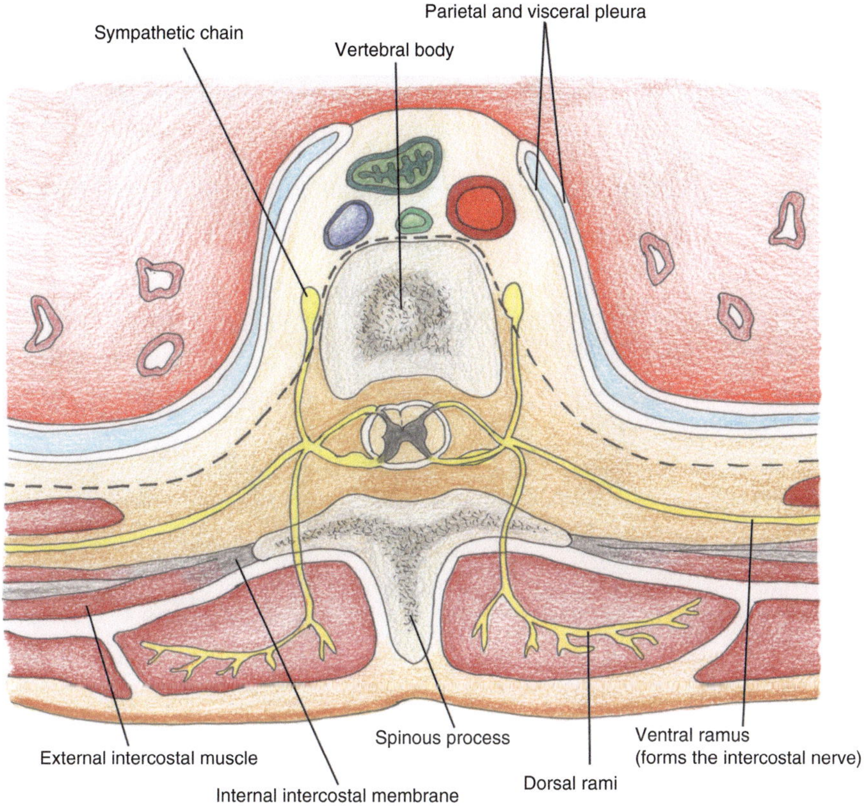

Fig. 1.7 Fascial and pleural relationships. Illustration courtesy of A.L. Scott

well as the gluteal skin. The fibres of T7–12 communicate freely as they traverse the abdomen resulting in overlap of sensory distribution in the dermatomes.

T7–T12 ventral rami continue from the intercostal spaces in which they travel into the abdominal wall. T7 and T8 exit the anterior end of the intercostal space and travel between the digitations of the transversus abdominis muscle. They then pierce the internal oblique aponeurosis to lie posterior to the rectus abdominis. They supply the rectus muscle and then pierce the anterior rectus sheath near its lateral border to supply the skin. Anatomically T7 and T8 cross the costal margin medial to the lateral border of rectus abdominis.

T9–T11 pass between the digitations of the diaphragm and transversus abdominis muscle to lie between transversus abdominis and internal oblique. At the lateral edge of rectus abdominis they pierce the internal oblique aponeurosis to pass behind the rectus muscle similar to T7/T8. T10 supplies the skin at the level of the umbilicus.

Motor fibres of the thoracic nerves supply the intercostal, subcostal and abdominal wall muscles. Sensory fibres supply the costal part of the diaphragm and related parietal pleura and peritoneum and give rise to collateral, lateral and anterior branches that supply the skin.

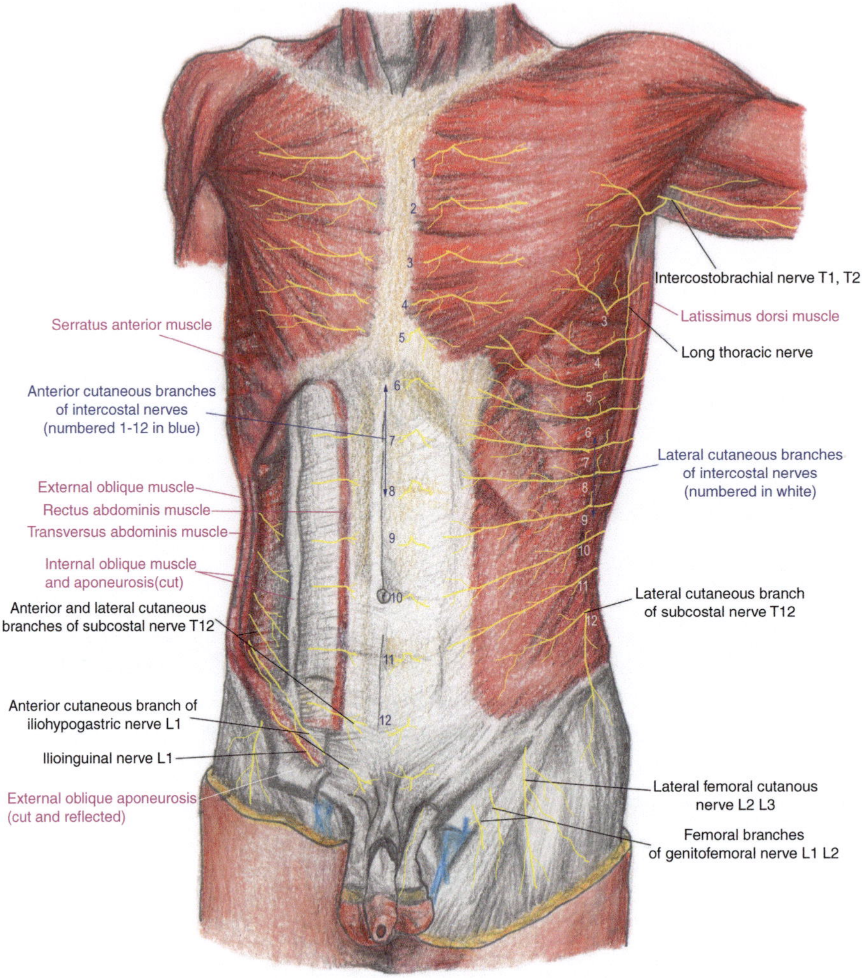

Fig. 1.8 Nerves of the anterior abdominal wall. Illustration courtesy of A.L. Scott

The T12 ventral rami are larger than the other thoracic rami and communicate with the L1 rami. The nerve communicates with the Iliohypogastric nerve and gives motor branches to the pyramidalis muscle.

Peritoneum

The parietal peritoneum is innervated differently to the visceral peritoneum. Branches of the somatic nerves innervate the parietal peritoneum and the sensors respond to a number of stimuli that are perceived as localised pain which is often exacerbated by movement. Sympathetic fibres carried via the splanchnic nerves innervate the visceral peritoneum, and when stimulated cause the patient to perceive poorly localised, often midline, pain. Pain may be generated by ischaemia, spasm, distension and capsular tension rather than direct trauma.

Viscera and Visceral Peritoneum

Autonomic nerve fibres from the coeliac and hypogastric plexae supply the abdominal viscera. The coeliac plexus is situated at the level of T12/L1 vertebra and has two large ganglia. The plexus surrounds the coeliac trunk and the root of the superior mesenteric artery. The plexae are formed by branches of the greater and lesser splanchnic nerves, and some fibres from the vagus nerve. Secondary plexae form in the distribution of the major named arteries of the abdominal cavity.

Sympathetic nerve fibres to the small intestine are motor to the ileo-caecal valve but inhibitory to gut smooth muscle generally and also stimulate vasoconstriction. The sympathetic system is inhibitory and the parasympathetic is motor to the colon. The parasympathetic fibres originate from sacral nerves in the lower gut and via the vagus in the foregut and mid-gut.

Afferent autonomic fibres are responsible for initiating autonomic reflexes but are also the route through which visceral pain is sensed, such as abdominal colic due to muscle spasm and stretching stimuli.

Approaches to Blocking the Sensory Innervation of the Abdominal Wall, Peritoneum and Viscera

Sensory innervation can be blocked at a number of accessible sites along the somatic nerve pathway using a local anaesthetic agent. Nerve blockade can be achieved by a single bolus injection, which has a limited duration, or by continuous infusion via a catheter. This is true of all spaces other than the subarachnoid space where infusion catheters are not used routinely.

For a spinal anaesthetic (*see* Chap. 7). the **Subarachnoid space** can be accessed at any vertebral level but to avoid spinal cord injury is accessed at a space below the termination of the spinal cord (L2/3). The approach is through the intervertebral ligaments in the midline and is accessed by puncturing the skin, the ligamentum flavum and the dura. Access to the correct space is confirmed by the flow of cerebrospinal fluid. Bleeding is least likely by maintaining the midline position. The **Epidural space** (*see* Chap. 5) is accessed by the same route but stopping short of the dural sheath (Fig. 1.9).

The **Paravertebral space** (*see* Chap. 7) is accessed by injecting lateral to the midline, traversing the skin, thoraco-lumbar fascia, erector spinae muscle and intercostal membrane to enter the space between the intercostal membrane and the endothoracic fascia (Fig. 1.10). Deep to the endothoracic fascia is the parietal pleura.

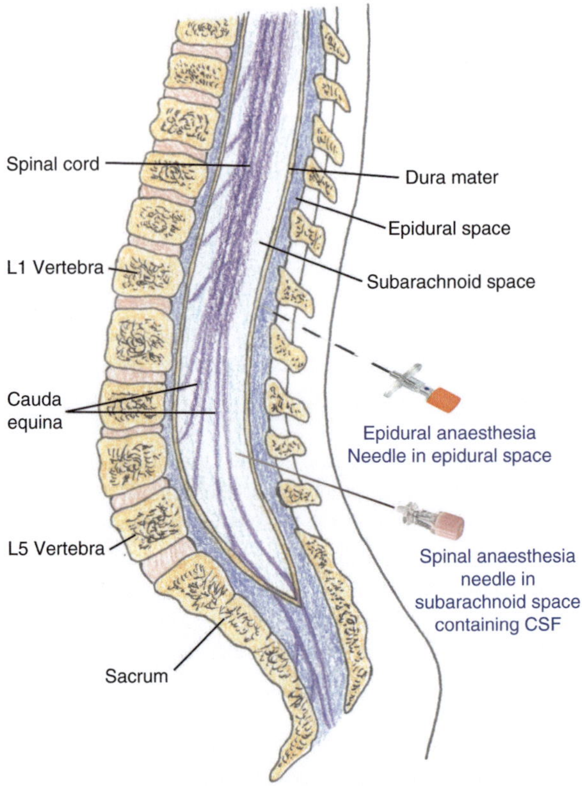

Fig. 1.9 Spinal and epidural spaces. Illustration courtesy of A.L. Scott

The **Intercostal space** is accessed just below each rib. The neuro-vascular bundle travels in the intercostal groove between the inner and innermost intercostal muscles. The pleura lies just deep to the innermost intercostal muscle (Fig. 1.11).

The transversis abdominis plane (TAP) (*see* Chap. 9) lies between the internal oblique and transversus abdominis muscles. Ultrasound of the abdominal wall clearly show the three layers of the abdominal wall laterally so that the space can be accessed by passing a needle through external and internal oblique muscles. A common site for accessing this plane is through the triangle of Petit which is bordered by the Iliac crest below, the latissimus dorsi posteriorly and the external oblique anteriorly. T10–T12 are most readily blocked through this approach (Fig. 1.12).

The rectus sheath space (*see* Chap. 10) can be accessed indirectly by ultrasound guidance or directly by the surgeon. The rectus sheath in the upper two thirds encases the rectus muscle. The posterior sheath is deficient in its lower third and the lower edge of the rectus sheath is called the arcuate ligament. Below the level of the

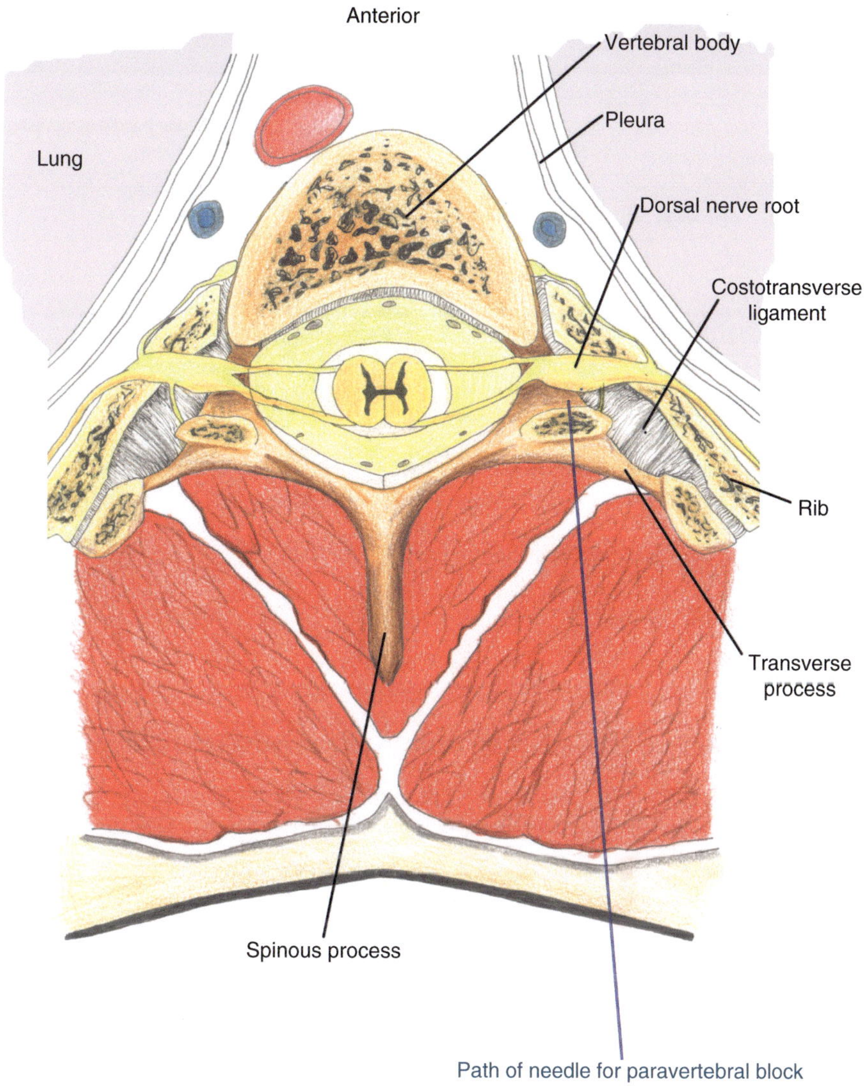

Fig. 1.10 Paravertebral approach. Illustration courtesy of A.L. Scott

arcuate ligament the peritoneum lies deep to the rectus muscle. Where the recti meet in the midline is called the linea alba and the lateral edge of the rectus sheath is the linea semilunaris. Large blood vessels travel along the posterior aspect of the rectus muscle. The superior epigastric artery from above and the inferior epigastric artery from below.

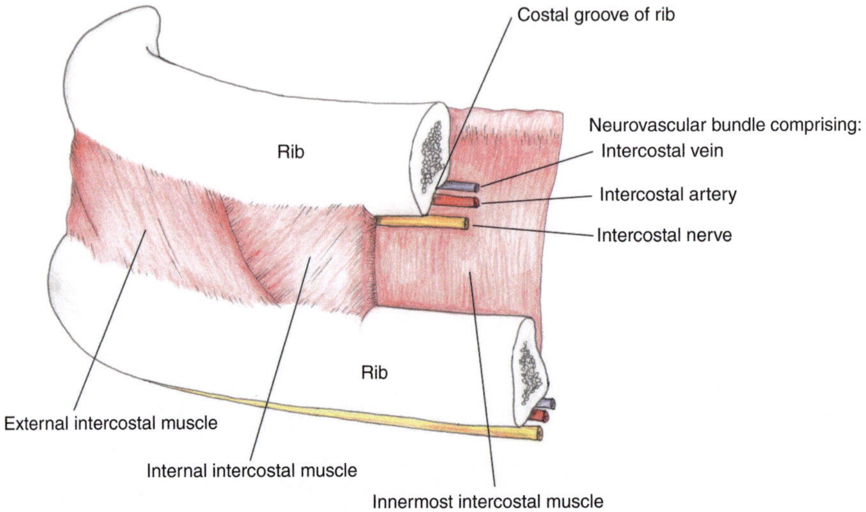

Fig. 1.11 Intercostal anatomy. Illustration courtesy of A.L. Scott

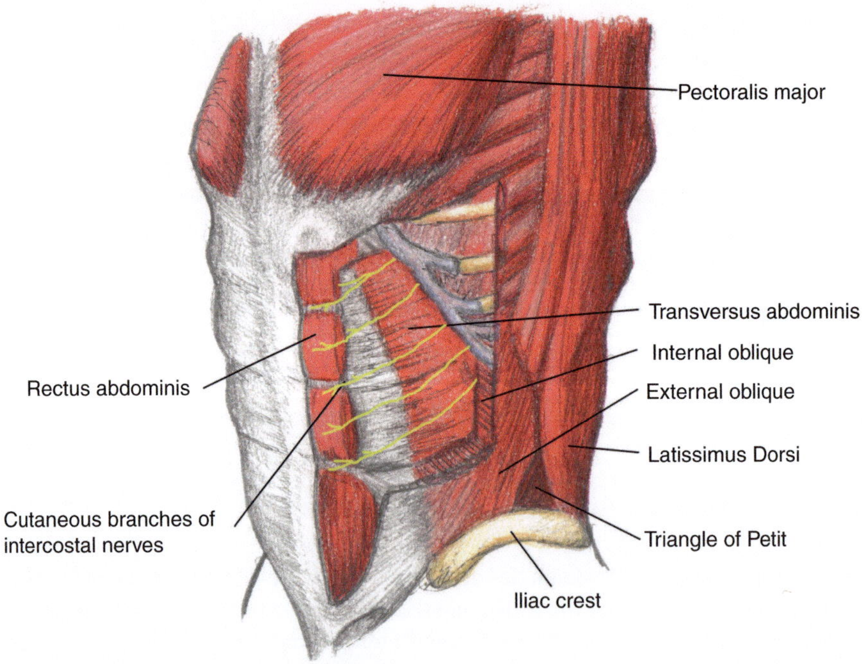

Fig. 1.12 Triangle of Petit. Illustration courtesy of A.L. Scott

Analgesic Techniques in Relation to Common Incisions

As a general principal transverse incisions and lower abdominal incisions are considered less painful than large midline longitudinal incisions.

Kocher's Incision

Classically used for open cholecystectomy but now more frequently for liver resection and can be extended across the midline as a roof-top incision. It is a painful incision and cuts across the nerve fibres of T7–T11 or 12.

Midline Incisions

This incision is the one most commonly deployed in major open abdominal surgery and T7–T12 dermatomes are involved.

Para-Median Incisions

These are less commonly used but have the potential advantage of lateralising the pain stimulus to one side as well as to reduce the midline wound complication rate. The same dermatomes are involved as a median incision albeit only one sides dermatomes although there is some contralateral cross-over of sensory innervation.

Pfannenstiel Incisions

These are commonly used in gynaecology and obstetrics. A short Pfannenstiel incision is commonly used for specimen extraction and bowel exteriorisation in a range of laparoscopic colorectal procedures, particularly involving the left colon and rectum. Laparoscopic-assisted procedures involving the right colon or small bowel more commonly utilise a peri-umbilical incision.

Multimodal Simple Analgesia

2

Giuliano Michelagnoli and Gabriele Baldini

Key Points

1. Multimodal analgesia relies on the principle of administering different types of analgesic medications, which through an additive or synergistic effect can improve post-operative pain control.
2. This allows a reduction in systemic opioid requirements and their associated adverse effects, with the ultimate goal of facilitating early feeding and post-operative mobilization in patients undergoing abdominal surgery.
3. Such a protocol should be procedure-specific and include non-opioid analgesics administered regularly, with systemic opioids to treat moderate–severe break-through pain, and regional anaesthesia techniques for certain surgical procedures.

Introduction

Despite improvements in understanding the pathophysiologic mechanisms leading to post-operative pain, data from three different surveys published in the last 20 years have shown that 86% of patients experience pain after surgery, with three quarters of these reported as moderate-to-extreme intensity [1].

Uncontrolled surgical pain is not only an unpleasant experience, but it also induces autonomic and endocrine-metabolic changes, and behavioural responses that can significantly affect post-operative outcomes. Moreover, poor pain control

G. Michelagnoli
Department of Anesthesia, McGill University Health Centre,
Montreal General Hospital, Montreal, QC, Canada

G. Baldini (✉)
Department of Anesthesiology, McGill University Health Centre,
Montreal General Hospital, Montreal, QC, Canada
e-mail: gabriele.baldini@mcgill.ca

A. Krige, M. J. P. Scott (eds.), *Analgesia in Major Abdominal Surgery*,
https://doi.org/10.1007/978-3-319-94482-1_2

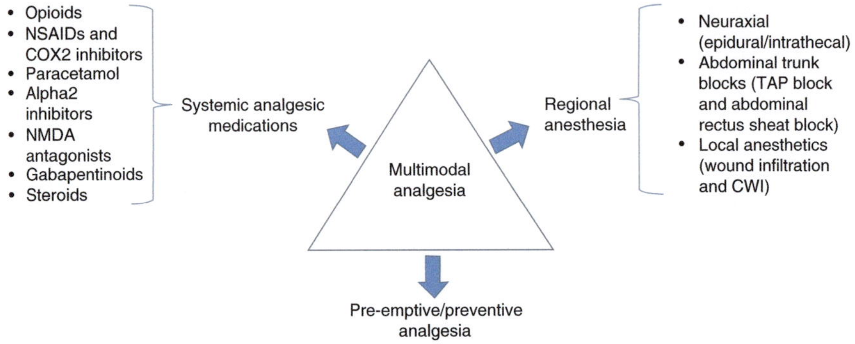

Fig. 2.1 Multimodal analgesia: main components. *COX* cyclooxygenase, *CWI* continuous wound infusion, *NSAIDs* nonsteroidal anti-inflammatory drugs, *TAP* transversus abdominis plane

may lead to peripheral and central neuronal sensitisation with subsequent development of chronic pain syndromes.

Because of the complexity of surgical pain, post-operative pain cannot be adequately treated with a single medication without experiencing significant side effects. Results of several clinical trials have shown that the most effective way to treat pain and prevent the development of chronic pain syndromes is by adopting a multimodal analgesic strategy. This approach includes multiple analgesic interventions with different pharmacological mechanisms to block transmission of painful stimuli to the central nervous system (CNS) at different levels, and on multiple receptors, from the moment the nociceptive stimulus is transmitted to the CNS (Fig. 2.1) (Table 2.1).

Combining different analgesic medications allows a dose reduction of each analgesic drug thereby minimizing the risk of developing medication related side effects. A broader definition of multimodal analgesia also includes regional and non-pharmacological analgesic techniques along with peri-operative strategies aimed at reducing the severity of post-operative pain along with preventing central and peripheral sensitisation and the occurrence of postsurgical chronic pain (Pre-emptive and Preventive Analgesia) [2]. A multimodal analgesic protocol should also be procedure-specific to maximize the clinical impact of post-operative analgesia on surgical outcomes [3].

Although systemic opioids remain the cornerstone of surgical pain management in patients undergoing abdominal surgery, they cause several dose-dependent side-effects that delay surgical recovery [4]. Moreover, experimental trials have demonstrated that opioids, mainly morphine, might also facilitate cancer progression and its recurrence, by negatively modulating the immune response induced by surgery [5]. A multimodal analgesic approach would allow a reduction in opioid requirements and side-effects thereby facilitating surgical recovery, especially in the context of Enhanced Recovery After Surgery (ERAS) Programmes [6].

Analgesic medications used to reduce opioids requirements include paracetamol and/or selective and non-selective cyclo-oxygenase (COX) inhibitors. Other

Table 2.1 Type of intervention, sites and mechanisms of action, and side effects of various analgesics

Type of intervention	Site of action	Mechanism of action	Effect	Clinically relevant side-effects
Opioids • Systemic • Intrathecal	Opioid receptors • Spinal (dorsal horn) • Supraspinal	Hyperpolarization of sensory neurons decreased neuron excitability	Inhibition of neural transmission	• PONV • Constipation • Urinary retention • Cognitive impairment
Local anaesthetics • Epidural • Spinal	Spinal nerve roots	Activation of Na^+ channels		• Hypotension • Urinary retention • Local anaesthetic toxicity
Local anaesthetics (wound infiltration/TAP block)	Nerves endings (nociceptors)	Activation of Na^+ channels		
Intravenous lidocaine	Systemic	↓ IL-6, IL1R ↓ CD11b/CD18 expression	Anti-inflammatory	Local anaesthetic toxicity
NSAIDs	Systemic	COX-1 and COX-2 inhibition		• Bleeding • Gastrointestinal ulcer • ↓ Renal function • Cardiovascular complications • Anastomotic leakage (?)
Paracetamol	Systemic	Uncertain (neural COX-3 inhibition)	Uncertain	Hepatotoxicity
Gabapentinoid	Systemic	↓ Glutamate, substance P	Inhibition of neuronal excitability	Dizziness, sedation
Dexamethasone	Systemic	Uncertain	Anti-inflammatory	Hyperglycemia, immune modulation (long term therapy)

analgesics include gabapentinoids (*see* Chap. 4), such as gabapentin and pregabalin, α_2-agonists, and *N*-methyl-D-aspartic acid receptor antagonists (NMDA) (e.g. ketamine [*see* Chap. 5] and magnesium). Peri-operative infusion of intravenous lidocaine (*see* Chap. 6) and oral corticosteroids, have also been shown to be useful analgesic adjuvants (Fig. 2.1).

The role of pre-emptive analgesic strategies still remains unclear. However, epidural blockade before surgery seems the only pre-emptive analgesic technique that systematically reduces pain, analgesic consumption and time to rescue analgesia after major surgery [7].

Pathophysiology of Pain After Abdominal Surgery

Nociceptors are widely disseminated in the skin, mucosa, peritoneum (visceral and parietal), blood vessels and in the connective tissue surrounding the abdominal viscera. They consist of free nerve endings (Aδ and C fibers) that represent the more distal part of sensory neurons placed in the dorsal root ganglions (DRGs). Surgical trauma, inflammation, carbon-dioxide, pneumoperitoneum, and deep pelvic dissection activate nociceptors that then transmit nociceptive stimuli from the periphery to the dorsal horns of the spinal cord, and from here to the supraspinal sites. The ventral-posterior-lateral (VPL) nucleus of the thalamus and the somatosensory cortex [8, 9] are the main supraspinal pain centers involved in the perception and transmission of the painful stimuli.

Surgical pain after abdominal surgery has both somatic and visceral components. Somatic pain results from the injury of cutaneous and muscular tissues and from the injury of parietal peritoneum (laparotomy, trocars, drains). Visceral pain results from surgical manipulation, stretching and inflammation of visceral structures (connective sheaths of organs, blood vessels and the diaphragm) and distension of the abdominal cavity induced by pneumoperitoneum during laparoscopic procedures. Deep dissection of pelvic structures may also injure the pelvic plexus and lead to neuropathic pain.

Local Anaesthetics are frequently and successfully administered in patients undergoing abdominal surgery as they block nerve conduction at different sites along the pain pathways. Moreover, they can also be administered systemically due to their analgesic and anti-inflammatory properties [10].

Nonsteroidal anti-inflammatory drugs (NSAIDs) and corticosteroids inhibit the synthesis of pro-inflammatory mediators such as prostaglandin E, serotonin, bradykinin, and histamine, and cytokines that directly activate nociceptors and can sensitize peripheral and central nociceptors during prolonged and intense stimulation [11]. The mechanism of action of paracetamol remains uncertain. Alpha2-adrenoreceptor agonists (clonidine, dexmedetomidine) and NMDA receptor antagonists (ketamine, magnesium) are used as coanalgesic agents, to spare opioids and improve analgesia.

The Major Components of Multimodal Analgesia

By adopting a multimodal analgesic strategy, different pharmacological analgesic agents can be simultaneously used to control surgical pain, either acting on the periphery where painful stimuli are generated, or acting more centrally by blocking the transmission of nociceptive stimuli to the central nervous system (Fig. 2.2). A broader definition of multimodal analgesia also includes the use of regional anaesthesia techniques.

Systemic Opioids

Systemic opioids remain a cornerstone in the treatment of moderate to severe surgical pain. However, independently of the route of administration and of the type of

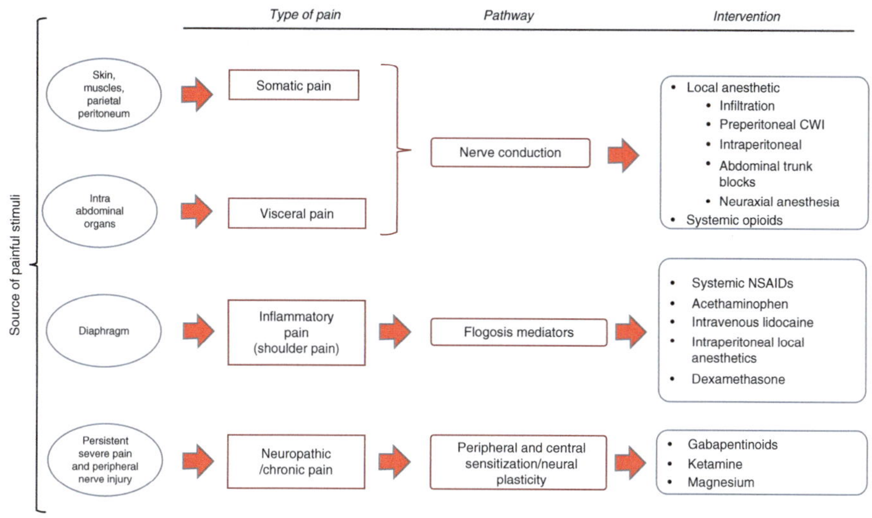

Fig. 2.2 Pathophysiology and treatment of surgical pain after abdominal surgery. *CWI* continuous wound infusion, *NSAIDs* nonsteroidal anti-inflammatory drugs

opioid used, they are associated with many side-effects that are dose-dependent and can significantly impair surgical recovery, especially in the context of an ERAS program [4]. These include respiratory depression, nausea and vomiting, postoperative ileus, pruritus, urinary retention and sedation. The overall aim of multimodal analgesia is to reduce the amount of opioids the patient is administered to avoid these opioid-related side effects. This chapter focuses on these nonopioid options. The use of systemic opioids in patients undergoing abdominal surgery is described in detail in Chap. 3.

Local Anaesthetics

Local anaesthetics block nerve conduction by binding the intracellular portion of sodium voltage channels of the peripheral nerves or at the level of the spinal cord, by preventing the generation of action potentials. They are frequently used in the context of a multimodal analgesic regimen.

1. *Local infiltration analgesia and preperitoneal continuous infusion of local anaesthetic* (*see* Chap. 13): local anaesthetic can be injected around the surgical wound to block the terminal ends of pain fibers, either as local infiltration, or infused continuously after surgery through preperitoneal multi-holed catheters (*see* Chap. 13). Local infiltration analgesia and preperitoneal continuous infusion of local anaesthetic are effective analgesic strategies to reduce opioid consumption [12–16]. Liposomal bupivacaine is a novel local anaesthetic formulation that provides analgesia up to 72 h after surgery. It has successfully provided

optimal analgesia and reduced opioid consumption in patients undergoing open and laparoscopic colorectal surgery [17, 18].

2. *Intraperitoneal administration of local anaesthetic*: local anaesthetic can also be administered in the abdominal cavity either in patients undergoing open abdominal surgery [19] or in patients undergoing laparoscopic abdominal surgery [20, 21]. Nebulization systems can facilitate the spread of local anaesthetics into the abdominal cavity to better control visceral pain [22–26].
3. *Abdominal trunk blocks* (*see* Chaps. 9, 10, 11, and 12): local anaesthetic can be injected to block thoraco-abdominal nerves (*T6-L1*) that innervate the abdominal wall and the parietal peritoneum. Transversus Abdominis Plane Block (TAP Block), Rectus Sheath block and Transversalis Fascia plane block are the most common blocks used in patients undergoing abdominal surgery to attenuate somatic pain. They are considered "*fascial plane blocks*" as they don't target specific nerves, but rely on the distribution of local anaesthetics in a compartment where the distal branches of the thoracoabdominal nerves are located [27, 28].
4. *Neuraxial blockade (Intrathecal or Epidural analgesia)* (*see* Chaps. 7 and 8): local anaesthetics injected in the epidural or subarachnoid space block nerve conduction at the level of the spinal nerve roots. They have been extensively and successfully used in patients undergoing open and laparoscopic abdominal procedures. While thoracic epidural analgesia with a mixture of local anaesthetic and opioids remains the gold standard to treat surgical pain after open abdominal surgery, use in patients undergoing laparoscopic surgery remains controversial. Moreover, recent studies have demonstrated that epidural analgesia in patients undergoing laparoscopic surgery can delay surgical recovery compared to patients receiving systemic opioid or intrathecal analgesia in the context of a multimodal analgesic regimen [29, 30]. In contrast, intrathecal administration of local anaesthetic and diamorphine has shown to provide adequate analgesia and facilitate hospital discharge after laparoscopic colorectal surgery [31].

Nonsteroidal Anti-Inflammatory Drugs (NSAIDs)

NSAIDs are effective analgesic agents that attenuate the local and systemic inflammatory response caused by the surgical insult. NSAIDs block the synthesis of pro-inflammatory mediators, such as prostaglandins and thromboxanes through the inhibition of the Cyclo-oxygenase (COX) enzyme, which exist in two isoforms, type 1 and type 2. While the COX-1 is an enzyme, which is present in most of the tissues (endothelium, kidneys, stomach), COX-2 synthesis and activity are mainly induced by noxious or painful stimuli in injured and inflamed tissues. Non-selective NSAIDs target both COX isoforms, while selective NSAIDs preferentially inhibit COX-2 isoform (COX-2 inhibitors).

When used in combination with systemic opioids in the context of a multimodal analgesic regimen, NSAIDs improve post-operative analgesia, whilst reducing opioid consumption by 30% [32, 33] together with the related side effects of nausea, vomiting and sedation [33]. These benefits can be particularly useful in patients receiving systemic opioids, especially after epidural analgesia or intravenous morphine (or other opioids) patient-controlled analgesia (PCA) discontinuation.

Several NSAIDs have been used in clinical practice at different dosages and with different regimens.

Intravenous (iv) ketorolac has been used at different dosages and regimens as an effective analgesic medication to treat postsurgical pain in patients undergoing abdominal surgery [34–37]. A single dose of 10, 30 or 60 mg of iv ketorolac has been shown to reduce opioid requirements, pain intensity at rest, post-operative nausea and vomiting, facilitate the recovery of bowel function and facilitate ambulation [34, 38]. A single 30 mg dose of iv ketorolac does not provide superior analgesia than 10 mg [35, 36], and preventive analgesia has not been observed at any of these dosages [37]. The analgesic efficacy of a single dose of 30 mg of intramuscular (im) ketorolac was similar to 10 mg administered orally (PO) (number need to treat (NNT) = 3.4 and NNT = 2.6, respectively), as the plasma concentration of ketorolac rises more rapidly after enteral administration than when given im [37, 39]. Compared to iv ketorolac, a greater opioid sparing effect has been observed after im administration, perhaps because of a slower clearance of the active (S) enantiomer [34].

A single post-operative dose of 400 mg ibuprofen PO or 500–550 mg of naproxen PO provides adequate analgesia and an opioid-sparing effect of approximately equivalent to 10 mg of morphine in 24 h [40]. A greater opioid sparing effect has been observed when NSAIDS are administered as continuous infusions or in multiple doses (18.3 and 19.7 mg of morphine in 24 h, respectively) [41]. Caution is required when using these drugs in patients with pre-existing renal disease, history of gastric ulcer and in those with cardiac and cerebrovascular disease because of the increased risk of thrombotic events. However, this risk seems marginal in patients undergoing non-cardiac surgery and receiving NSAIDs for a short period (3–5 days) [42]. Caution should also be used in patients at risk of bleeding. Finally, case series, observational and experimental studies have shown an association between the perioperative use of NSAIDs and the risk of anastomotic leakage after colorectal surgery [43]. Recent meta-analyses of six randomized controlled trials (RCTs) (480 patients) has shown a non-significant increased risk of anastomotic leakage in patients undergoing colorectal surgery and receiving at least one dose of nonselective NSAIDs or COX-2 inhibitors within 48 h of surgery (Peto odds ratio [OR] = 2.16 [95% confidence interval [CI] = 0.85–5.53]). Among different NSAIDs the risk is minimal with COX-2 inhibitors and ketorolac [6, 44]. A recent retrospective cohort study of 13,082 patients undergoing bariatric and colorectal surgery over 5 years at 47 hospitals demonstrated a significant association between anastomotic leakage and the use of NSAIDs in the first 24 h after surgery, but only among patients undergoing emergency colonic resection (anastomotic leakage occurred in 12.3% in the NSAID group and 8.3% in the non-NSAID group, OR = 1.70 [95% CI, 1.11–2.68]) [45]. Balancing these results against their beneficial analgesic effects, further evidence is necessary before completely abandoning the use of NSAIDs in patients undergoing colorectal surgery, as also suggested by the ERAS guidelines for patients undergoing colorectal surgery [6]. However, as the pathogenesis of anastomotic leakage is multifactorial, clinicians should consider avoiding NSAIDS in patients at high-risk of anastomotic leakage due to the presence of other risk factors.

Paracetamol (Acetaminophen)

Paracetamol (called acetaminophen in the USA) is commonly administered in patients undergoing abdominal surgery as part of a multimodal analgesic regimen. It has analgesic and antipyretic properties, but it lacks anti-inflammatory effects. The mechanism of action is not completely understood, as it weakly inhibits COX-1 and COX-2, but selectivity binds COX-3 located in the CNS. It is unclear if it relieves pain via central inhibition of COX-3 or by weakly inhibiting COX-2 enzymatic activity [46].

Oral bioavailability is high, with peak plasma concentrations reached in 30–60 min and with a plasma half-life of 2–4 h at therapeutic plasma levels. Paracetamol is predominantly converted to pharmacologically inactive glucuronide and sulfate conjugates, with a minor fraction being oxidised to a reactive metabolite which is primarily responsible for paracetamol-induced hepatotoxicity [47].

It has been shown to be effective in treating post-operative pain, and reducing opioid consumption by 20% in combination with intravenous PCA using morphine [48]. Most of the studies have shown that paracetamol does not reduce the incidence of opioid-related adverse effects [41]. However, a recent meta-analysis has demonstrated that paracetamol, mainly administered intravenously, also reduced post-operative nausea and vomiting. This antiemetic effect was not attributed to an opioid-sparing effect, but rather to its analgesic efficacy, since the reduction of nausea correlated with the reduction of pain intensity and not with the reduction of post-operative opioid consumption [49]. Pre-emptive analgesic properties were also demonstrated, as the analgesic efficacy of paracetamol was higher if it was administered before surgery, than if administered after surgery [49].

Paracetamol exists in different formulations (PO, per rectum and intravenous), which affects bioavailability, particularly when administered rectally when levels are less predictable. Plasma and effect site concentration after intravenous administration of paracetamol are approximately double the plasma concentration following oral or rectal administration, resulting in greater CNS penetration, which in turn results in better analgesia compared to oral paracetamol. A meta-analysis of five RCTs (726 patients) assessing the analgesic efficacy of paracetamol has shown that patients receiving paracetamol more frequently reported excellent satisfaction than patients receiving placebo (32.3% vs 15.9%, respectively) [50].

Intravenous Lidocaine (See Chap. 6)

Intravenous lidocaine has shown analgesic, antihyperalgesic and anti-inflammatory properties. Several RCTs and meta-analyses have demonstrated that intravenous lidocaine in patients undergoing different types of surgical procedures can significantly improve post-operative pain and facilitate hospital discharge [51]. Although several dosages and regimens have been used, a common approach is administration of a 1.5-mg/kg bolus within 30 min before induction of anaesthesia, followed by a continuous infusion of 1.5–2 mg/kg/hour until the end of surgery. A meta-analysis including 29 studies of patients ($n = 1754$) undergoing abdominal surgery showed that intravenous lidocaine reduced post-operative pain intensity, opioid requirements, improved recovery of bowel function and accelerated hospital discharge with minimal side effects [52]. These results can be partially explained by the anti-inflammatory effects demonstrated by the peri-operative use of intravenous lidocaine, indicated by reduced C-reactive protein, interleukin-6 (IL-6) levels and leukocyte activation. Experimental trials have also indicated that intravenous lidocaine might have an anticancer effect [53].

Many of these benefits seem to be more evident in patients undergoing open surgery and limited to the early post-operative period (within 6 h) with minimal clinical benefits observed 48 h after surgery and in patients undergoing laparoscopic procedures [54]. While some patients experience signs of local anaesthetic toxicity with plasma concentrations below toxic levels (5 μg/mL) for lidocaine, others remain asymptomatic with lidocaine plasma concentrations that exceed toxic thresholds. Moreover, despite the low reported incidence of side effects associated with peri-operative infusion of intravenous lidocaine, it must be acknowledged that only a few studies measured plasma concentrations and systematically screened for adverse events [51].

***N*-Methyl-D-Aspartate Receptor Antagonist: Ketamine and Magnesium** (See Chap. 5)

Stimulation of *N* methyl D-aspartate (NMDA) receptors located in the central and peripheral nervous system contributes to central sensitization and development of chronic pain. NMDA-receptor antagonists, such as ketamine and magnesium, have been used in the peri-operative period as effective analgesic adjuvants, as they have been shown to improve post-operative analgesia and reduce post-operative opioid consumption. Subanaesthetic doses of ketamine have been successfully used as an adjunctive analgesic, especially in patients with chronic pain and opioid tolerance, as it reduces or reverses opioid tolerance [55]. It also has a direct analgesic effect and can prevent central sensitization. Due to its mechanisms of action and beneficial analgesic effects, it is considered a useful analgesic adjuvant to manage acute and severe post-operative pain, neuropathic pain, and possibly prevents opioid induced hyperalgesia [55]. Indeed, a 20–25% reduction of pain intensity and 30–50% reduction of analgesic consumption up to 48 h after surgery have been reported when used in the peri-operative setting [56]. This is independent of the type of opioid used, dose administered and timing of administration [57]. A reduction of post-operative nausea and vomiting (PONV) has been also demonstrated [56]. When administered during general anaesthesia, the major psychotropic side effects (hallucinations, nightmares, sedation, nausea, and vomiting) are not observed. These effects can be present when ketamine is administered as a sedative-analgesic, especially if not combined with benzodiazepines. A recent meta-analysis investigating the analgesic efficacy of ketamine administered with intravenous hydromorphone or morphine PCA, demonstrated that ketamine reduces total opioid consumption 48 h after surgery and significantly decreases PONV, without increasing adverse effects [58]. A loading dose of 0.5 mg/kg followed by a continuous infusion of 10–30 μg/kg/min has been shown to reduce post-operative morphine consumption by 40%, without significant side effects, in patients undergoing abdominal surgery [59]. To prevent chronic pain or central sensitization it is recommended that ketamine infusion is initiated in the intra-operative period [60].

Peri-operative use of low dose of intravenous magnesium has also shown analgesic benefits, but as it also potentiates neuromuscular blockade and may affect cardiac conduction it is not commonly used in clinical practice.

Gabapentinoids (See Chap. 4)

Gabapentinoids, such as gabapentin and pregabalin, prevent central sensitization and reduce the incidence of neuropathic pain by blocking the $\alpha 2\delta$ subunit-containing voltage-dependent calcium channels (VDCCs) of the γ-aminobutyric acid (GABA) receptor. However, they produce weak analgesic effects in patients with normal nociceptive pathways. Pregabalin is about three times more potent than gabapentin and it has a better pharmacokinetic profile, as its oral bioavailability is higher, and duration of action longer. Even if gabapentinoids are more commonly used in patients with chronic and/or neuropathic pain, they are also administered in the peri-operative setting and in the context of multimodal analgesia programmes. Despite a few trials showing that peri-operative gabapentinoids improve post-operative analgesia (they reduce static and dynamic pain scores), decrease post-operative opioid consumption, prevent opioid tolerance, and the occurrence of chronic post surgical pain the evidence supporting the systematic use of gabapentinoids as peri-operative analgesic adjuvants is inconclusive [61, 62]. Moreover, the most effective dose and timing of administration associated with optimal analgesia and minimal side effects still remains to be determined. A single dose of gabapentin has been shown to be superior to placebo but inferior to other commonly used analgesic medication for post-operative surgical pain control [63]. A single dose of 150–300 mg pregabalin administered pre-operatively is frequently used, but side effects such as sedation, dizziness and leg oedema are not infrequent and are more common at higher doses [64, 65].

α_2-Adrenoreceptor Agonists (Clonidine and Dexmedetomidine)

α_2-Adrenoreceptors are involved in the modulation of pain at a supraspinal level (locus coeruleus in the brainstem), and at the level of the lamina II in the dorsal horn of the spinal cord (substantia gelatinosa). Commonly used drugs for targeting these receptors to modulate painful afferents are clonidine and dexmedetomidine. Both selectively stimulate the presynaptic α_2-adrenoreceptor and prevent neuronal firing and local signal propagation, but dexmedetomidine has an eightfold greater affinity for the α_2-adrenoreceptor than clonidine. When administered peri-operatively to control surgical pain, clonidine and dexmedetomidine mildly reduce pain intensity 24 h after surgery (weighted mean difference [WMD] = −0.7 cm, 95% CI = −1.2 to −0.1 cm on a 10-cm visual analog scale, and WMD = −0.6 cm; 95% CI = 0.9 to −0.2 cm, respectively), opioid consumption (WMD = −4.1 mg; 95% CI = −6.0 to −2.2, and WMD = −14.5 mg;

95% CI = −22.1 to −6.8, respectively), early post-operative nausea (number needed to treat [NNT] = 9), without prolonging emergence from anaesthesia [66].

Studies comparing the analgesic efficacy and safety of these two drugs in patients undergoing abdominal surgery are lacking. The most common side effects associated with clonidine is intra-operative and post-operative hypotension (number needed to harm (NNH) = 9; NNH = 20, respectively) and sedation, while post-operative bradycardia is more common after dexmedetomidine administration (NNH = 3.1) [66].

Glucocorticoids

Recent meta-analyses have shown that peri-operative glucocorticoids also have analgesic and mild opioid-sparing properties, in addition to their well-recognized prophylactic antiemetic properties. An intermediate dose of intravenous dexamethasone (0.11–0.2 mg/kg) leads to a 10% reduction in opioid consumption without increasing the risk of infection or delaying wound healing [67, 68]. However, blood glucose levels might temporarily increase and return to normal values within 24 h after surgery. Administration of higher doses of glucocorticoids (e.g., 10 mg of oral dexamethazone, 16 mg IV dexamethazone or 30 mg/kg of intravenous methylprednisolone) in the context of a multimodal analgesic regimen might provide a greater analgesic effect. Glucocorticoids also attenuate the stress response to surgery and improve pulmonary function after colorectal surgery [69]. However, further studies are warranted to establish the efficacy and safety of high-dose glucocorticoids in patients undergoing abdominal surgery.

Pre-Emptive and Preventive Analgesia

Pre-emptive analgesia involves administering an analgesic medication before the painful stimulus has been generated, in order to prevent the synthesis of pain mediators and the transmission of painful stimuli to the central nervous system. This should improve post-operative pain control and prevent postsurgical chronic pain by reducing central and peripheral sensitisation. As a result, the analgesic efficacy of an analgesic intervention initiated before surgery is greater than if administered during surgery or in the post-operative period [70, 71]. It is suggested that the pre-emptive analgesic effect may be maximized if pre-operative analgesic interventions are continued throughout surgery and in the post-operative period [70, 71]. The pre-emptive analgesia of NSAIDs, opioids, NMDA receptor antagonists, epidurals, and peripherally administered local anaesthetics have been extensively studied, but contrasting and inconclusive results are currently available [72]. Epidural analgesia seems the only analgesic technique showing a consistent pre-emptive analgesic effect, as it reduces pain scores, opioid consumption and also time to rescue analgesia [73]. The role of pre-emptive analgesic strategies, such as pre-operative administration of paracetamol, COX-2 inhibitors, NMDA antagonists, and/or gabapentinoids remains unclear for patients undergoing abdominal surgery and in the context of an ERAS program.

Preventive analgesia aims at minimizing peripheral and central sensitization induced by noxious surgical stimuli. An analgesic medication that reduces post-operative pain, or analgesic consumption, for a period of time that outlasts its direct pharmacological effect (longer than 5.5 half-lives) is considered to have a preventive analgesic effect. This effect is independent of the time of administration. Regional anaesthesia techniques have extensively demonstrated preventive analgesic properties as they provide extended post-operative analgesia and reduce the risk of developing persistent post-operative surgical pain [74, 75]. However, it remains to be determined if these analgesic benefits are in part the results of a systemic analgesic effect of local anaesthetics which is well documented following intravenous lidocaine administration [76, 77]. It is also possible that preventive analgesia is due to an opioid sparing effect of regional anaesthesia techniques, as opioids enhance central sensitization and can induce hyperalgesia. Preventive analgesia has been shown after intravenous lidocaine administration [78], but the preventive analgesic effect of ketamine and gabapentinoids remains uncertain [78].

The Impact of Multimodal Analgesia on Nonanalgesic Outcomes

Immunomodulation and Cancer Recurrence

The inflammatory response and the peri-operative immunological changes induced by surgical stress can potentially contribute to cancer progression.

In vitro and *in vivo* studies have shown that, by promoting tumour angiogenesis and by suppression of natural killer (NK)-cell activity [79], opioids might influence cancer recurrence and survival in patients undergoing oncologic surgery [80–82], but recent findings have not confirmed these results [83]. Based on this preliminary and inconclusive evidence systemic opioids still remain a cornerstone in the treatment of moderate-severe surgical pain, and further large clinical trials are warranted to establish the role of peri-operative opioids on oncologic outcomes. A completely multimodal non-opioid regimen is appealing, but further studies are needed to establish the efficacy and safety in patients undergoing surgery.

Peri-operative administration of NSAIDs might also protect against cancer progression, either directly by reducing proangiogenic inflammatory markers (prostaglandin E), as the expression of COX-2 enzymes is upregulated in several cancer tissues [84], or indirectly by reducing opioid consumption. Similar immune-modulatory effects have not been observed after sufentanil, ketamine and clonidine administration [85, 86].

Cognitive Function

With the increasing age of patients requiring and undergoing major surgery, and the coexistence of comorbidities, more patients are at risk of developing post-operative delirium and cognitive dysfunction [87].

Post-operative delirium is described as an acute change in mental status characterized by reduced attention and awareness of the environment and is present in 5–15% of patients after elective surgery. The prevalence is even higher after emergency surgery. Even though it is considered a temporary disturbance it can significantly affect patients' outcome, and lead to increased dependence, mortality, and persistent cognitive impairment [88, 89]. The pathogenesis is multifactorial and inadequate post-operative analgesia contributes to the development of delirium.

Post-operative Cognitive Dysfunction [90] is characterized by reduced cognitive functions such as memory, concentration, learning and speed of mental processing. Similar to post-operative delirium, several risk factors have been identified which include patients greater than 60 years old, patients undergoing prolonged major surgery and those having a lower grade of education. It can occur days or weeks after surgery, with different grades of severity: from a new inability to complete an easily attainable task, to catastrophic loss of cognitive function, risk of dependence and increased risk of mortality [87, 90].

Emerging evidence suggests that multimodal analgesic strategies aiming at reducing opioid consumption can minimize the risk of post-operative delirium and POCD [91], although this is as yet unproven.

References

1. Gan TJ, Habib AS, Miller TE, White W, Apfelbaum JL. Incidence, patient satisfaction, and perceptions of post-surgical pain: results from a US national survey. Curr Med Res Opin. 2014;30(1):149–60.
2. Gritsenko K, Khelemsky Y, Kaye AD, Vadivelu N, Urman RD. Multimodal therapy in perioperative analgesia. Best Pract Res Clin Anaesthesiol. 2014;28(1):59–79.
3. PROcedure SPECific postoperative pain menagemenT (PROSPECT) [PROcedure SPEC postoperative pain managemenT]. Available at: http://www.postoppain.org/.
4. Wheeler M, Oderda GM, Ashburn MA, Lipman AG. Adverse events associated with postoperative opioid analgesia: a systematic review. J Pain. 2002;3(3):159–80.
5. Le-Wendling L, Nin O, Capdevila X. Cancer recurrence and regional anesthesia: the theories, the data, and the future in outcomes. Pain Med. 2016;17(4):756–75.
6. Gustafsson UO, Scott MJ, Schwenk W, Demartines N, Roulin D, Francis N, et al. Guidelines for perioperative care in elective colonic surgery: Enhanced Recovery After Surgery (ERAS®) Society recommendations. World J Surg. 2013;37(2):259–84.
7. Ong CK, Lirk P, Seymour RA, Jenkins BJ. The efficacy of preemptive analgesia for acute postoperative pain management: a meta-analysis. Anesth Analg. 2005;100(3):757–73.
8. Kandel ER. Principles of neural science. 5th ed. New York: McGraw-Hill; 2013.
9. Millan MJ. The induction of pain: an integrative review. Prog Neurobiol. 1999;57(1):1–164.
10. Marret E, Rolin M, Beaussier M, Bonnet F. Meta-analysis of intravenous lidocaine and postoperative recovery after abdominal surgery. Br J Surg. 2008;95(11):1331–8.
11. Fishman S, Ballantyne J, Rathmell JP, Bonica JJ. Bonica's management of pain. 4th ed. Baltimore, MD: Lippincott, Williams & Wilkins; 2010.
12. Dahl JB, Moiniche S. Relief of postoperative pain by local anaesthetic infiltration: efficacy for major abdominal and orthopedic surgery. Pain. 2009;143(1–2):7–11.
13. Moiniche S, Jorgensen H, Wetterslev J, Dahl JB. Local anesthetic infiltration for postoperative pain relief after laparoscopy: a qualitative and quantitative systematic review of intraperitoneal, port-site infiltration and mesosalpinx block. Anesth Analg. 2000;90(4):899–912.

14. Beaussier M, El'Ayoubi H, Schiffer E, Rollin M, Parc Y, Mazoit JX, et al. Continuous preperitoneal infusion of ropivacaine provides effective analgesia and accelerates recovery after colorectal surgery: a randomized, double-blind, placebo-controlled study. Anesthesiology. 2007;107(3):461–8.
15. Jouve P, Bazin JE, Petit A, Minville V, Gerard A, Buc E, et al. Epidural versus continuous preperitoneal analgesia during fast-track open colorectal surgery: a randomized controlled trial. Anesthesiology. 2013;118(3):622–30.
16. Bertoglio S, Fabiani F, Negri PD, Corcione A, Merlo DF, Cafiero F, et al. The postoperative analgesic efficacy of preperitoneal continuous wound infusion compared to epidural continuous infusion with local anesthetics after colorectal cancer surgery: a randomized controlled multicenter study. Anesth Analg. 2012;115(6):1442–50.
17. Cohen SM. Extended pain relief trial utilizing infiltration of Exparel®, a long-acting multivesicular liposome formulation of bupivacaine: a Phase IV health economic trial in adult patients undergoing open colectomy. J Pain Res. 2012;5:567–72.
18. Candiotti KA, Sands LR, Lee E, Bergese SD, Harzman AE, Marcet J, et al. Liposome bupivacaine for postsurgical analgesia in adult patients undergoing laparoscopic colectomy: results from prospective Phase IV sequential cohort studies assessing health economic outcomes. Curr Ther Res Clin Exp. 2014;76:1–6.
19. Kahokehr A, Sammour T, Zargar Shoshtari K, Taylor M, Hill AG. Intraperitoneal local anesthetic improves recovery after colon resection: a double-blinded randomized controlled trial. Ann Surg. 2011;254(1):28–38.
20. Kahokehr A, Sammour T, Srinivasa S, Hill AG. Systematic review and meta-analysis of intraperitoneal local anaesthetic for pain reduction after laparoscopic gastric procedures. Br J Surg. 2011;98(1):29–36.
21. Stuhldreher JM, Adamina M, Konopacka A, Brady K, Delaney CP. Effect of local anesthetics on postoperative pain and opioid consumption in laparoscopic colorectal surgery. Surg Endosc. 2012;26(6):1617–23.
22. Bucciero M, Ingelmo PM, Fumagalli R, Noll E, Garbagnati A, Somaini M, et al. Intraperitoneal ropivacaine nebulization for pain management after laparoscopic cholecystectomy: a comparison with intraperitoneal instillation. Anesth Analg. 2011;113(5):1266–71.
23. Ingelmo PM, Bucciero M, Somaini M, Sahillioglu E, Garbagnati A, Charton A, et al. Intraperitoneal nebulization of ropivacaine for pain control after laparoscopic cholecystectomy: a double-blind, randomized, placebo-controlled trial. Br J Anaesth. 2013;110(5):800–6.
24. Scalia Catenacci S, Lovisari F, Peng S, Allegri M, Somaini M, Ghislanzoni L, et al. Postoperative analgesia after laparoscopic ovarian cyst resection: double-blind multicenter randomized control trial comparing intraperitoneal nebulization and peritoneal instillation of ropivacaine. J Minim Invasive Gynecol. 2015;22(5):759–66.
25. Somaini M, Brambillasca P, Ingelmo PM, Lovisari F, Catenacci SS, Rossini V, et al. Effects of peritoneal ropivacaine nebulization for pain control after laparoscopic gynecologic surgery. J Minim Invasive Gynecol. 2014;21(5):863–9.
26. Bugada D, Scalia Catenacci S, Lovisari F, Bronco A, Sahillioglu E, Minardi C, et al. Intraperitoneal nebulization of local anesthetics for postoperative analgesia: theory, practice and future trends. Abstracts and highlight papers of the 31st annual European Society of Regional Anaesthesia (ESRA) Congress 2012. Reg Anesth Pain Med. 2012;37(5):E161–3.
27. De Oliveira GS Jr, Castro-Alves LJ, Nader A, Kendall MC, McCarthy RJ. Transversus abdominis plane block to ameliorate postoperative pain outcomes after laparoscopic surgery: a meta-analysis of randomized controlled trials. Anesth Analg. 2014;118(2):454–63.
28. Keller DS, Ermlich BO, Schiltz N, Champagne BJ, Reynolds HL Jr, Stein SL, et al. The effect of transversus abdominis plane blocks on postoperative pain in laparoscopic colorectal surgery: a prospective, randomized, double-blind trial. Dis Colon Rectum. 2014;57(11):1290–7.
29. Hubner M, Blanc C, Roulin D, Winiker M, Gander S, Demartines N. Randomized clinical trial on epidural versus patient-controlled analgesia for laparoscopic colorectal surgery within an enhanced recovery pathway. Ann Surg. 2015;261(4):648–53.

30. Levy BF, Scott MJ, Fawcett W, Fry C, Rockall TA. Randomized clinical trial of epidural, spinal or patient-controlled analgesia for patients undergoing laparoscopic colorectal surgery. Br J Surg. 2011;98(8):1068–78.
31. Levy BF, Scott MJ, Fawcett WJ, Rockall TA. 23-Hour-stay laparoscopic colectomy. Dis Colon Rectum. 2009;52(7):1239–43.
32. Dahl JB, Nielsen RV, Wetterslev J, Nikolajsen L, Hamunen K, Kontinen VK, et al. Post-operative analgesic effects of paracetamol, NSAIDs, glucocorticoids, gabapentinoids and their combinations: a topical review. Acta Anaesthesiol Scand. 2014;58(10):1165–81.
33. Marret E, Kurdi O, Zufferey P, Bonnet F. Effects of nonsteroidal antiinflammatory drugs on patient-controlled analgesia morphine side effects: meta-analysis of randomized controlled trials. Anesthesiology. 2005;102(6):1249–60.
34. De Oliveira GS Jr, Agarwal D, Benzon HT. Perioperative single dose ketorolac to prevent postoperative pain: a meta-analysis of randomized trials. Anesth Analg. 2012;114(2):424–33.
35. Brown CR, Moodie JE, Wild VM, Bynum LJ. Comparison of intravenous ketorolac tromethamine and morphine sulfate in the treatment of postoperative pain. Pharmacotherapy. 1990;10(6, Pt 2):116S–21S.
36. Peirce RJ, Fragen RJ, Pemberton DM. Intravenous ketorolac tromethamine versus morphine sulfate in the treatment of immediate postoperative pain. Pharmacotherapy. 1990;10(6, Pt 2):111S–5S.
37. Smith LA, Carroll D, Edwards JE, Moore RA, McQuay HJ. Single-dose ketorolac and pethidine in acute postoperative pain: systematic review with meta-analysis. Br J Anaesth. 2000;84(1):48–58.
38. Gillis JC, Brogden RN. Ketorolac. A reappraisal of its pharmacodynamic and pharmacokinetic properties and therapeutic use in pain management. Drugs. 1997;53:139–88.
39. Tramer MR, Williams JE, Carroll D, Wiffen PJ, Moore RA, McQuay HJ. Comparing analgesic efficacy of non-steroidal anti-inflammatory drugs given by different routes in acute and chronic pain: a qualitative systematic review. Acta Anaesthesiol Scand. 1998;42(1):71–9.
40. McDaid C, Maund E, Rice S, Wright K, Jenkins B, Woolacott N. Paracetamol and selective and non-selective non-steroidal anti-inflammatory drugs (NSAIDs) for the reduction of morphine-related side effects after major surgery: a systematic review. Health Technol Assess. 2010;14(17):1–153.
41. Elia N, Lysakowski C, Tramer MR. Does multimodal analgesia with acetaminophen, nonsteroidal antiinflammatory drugs, or selective cyclooxygenase-2 inhibitors and patient-controlled analgesia morphine offer advantages over morphine alone? Meta-analyses of randomized trials. Anesthesiology. 2005;103(6):1296–304.
42. Nussmeier NA, Whelton AA, Brown MT, Joshi GP, Langford RM, Singla NK, et al. Safety and efficacy of the cyclooxygenase-2 inhibitors parecoxib and valdecoxib after noncardiac surgery. Anesthesiology. 2006;104(3):518–26.
43. Gorissen KJ, Benning D, Berghmans T, Snoeijs MG, Sosef MN, Hulsewe KW, et al. Risk of anastomotic leakage with non-steroidal anti-inflammatory drugs in colorectal surgery. Br J Surg. 2012;99(5):721–7.
44. Bhangu A, Singh P, Fitzgerald JE, Slesser A, Tekkis P. Postoperative nonsteroidal anti-inflammatory drugs and risk of anastomotic leak: meta-analysis of clinical and experimental studies. World J Surg. 2014;38(9):2247–57.
45. Burton TP, Mittal A, Soop M. Nonsteroidal anti-inflammatory drugs and anastomotic dehiscence in bowel surgery: systematic review and meta-analysis of randomized, controlled trials. Dis Colon Rectum. 2013;56(1):126–34.
46. Graham GG, Scott KF. Mechanism of action of paracetamol. Am J Ther. 2005;12(1):46–55.
47. Prescott LF. Paracetamol overdosage. Pharmacological considerations and clinical management. Drugs. 1983;25(3):290–314.
48. Remy C, Marret E, Bonnet F. Effects of acetaminophen on morphine side-effects and consumption after major surgery: meta-analysis of randomized controlled trials. Br J Anaesth. 2005;94(4):505–13.

49. Apfel CC, Turan A, Souza K, Pergolizzi J, Hornuss C. Intravenous acetaminophen reduces postoperative nausea and vomiting: a systematic review and meta-analysis. Pain. 2013;154(5):677–89.
50. Apfel CCSK, Portillo J, Dalal P, Bergese SD. Patient satisfaction with intravenous acetaminophen: a pooled analysis of five randomized, placebo controlled studies in the acute postoperative setting. J Healthc Qual. 2015;37(3):155–62.
51. Swenson BR, Gottschalk A, Wells LT, Rowlingson JC, Thompson PW, Barclay M, et al. Intravenous lidocaine is as effective as epidural bupivacaine in reducing ileus duration, hospital stay, and pain after open colon resection: a randomized clinical trial. Reg Anesth Pain Med. 2010;35:370–6.
52. Vigneault L, Turgeon AF, Cote D, Lauzier F, Zarychanski R, Moore L, et al. Perioperative intravenous lidocaine infusion for postoperative pain control: a meta-analysis of randomized controlled trials. Can J Anaesth. 2011;58(1):22–37.
53. Lirk P, Berger R, Hollmann MW, Fiegl H. Lidocaine time- and dose-dependently demethylates deoxyribonucleic acid in breast cancer cell lines in vitro. Br J Anaesth. 2012;109(2):200–7.
54. Sridhar P, Sistla SC, Ali SM, Karthikeyan VS, Badhe AS, Ananthanarayanan PH. Effect of intravenous lignocaine on perioperative stress response and post-surgical ileus in elective open abdominal surgeries: a double-blind randomized controlled trial. ANZ J Surg. 2015;85(6):425–9.
55. McCartney CJ, Sinha A, Katz J. A qualitative systematic review of the role of N-methyl-D-aspartate receptor antagonists in preventive analgesia. Anesth Analg. 2004;98(5):1385–400.
56. Bell RF, Dahl JB, Moore RA, Kalso E. Perioperative ketamine for acute postoperative pain. Cochrane Database Syst Rev. 2006;(1):CD004603.
57. Elia N, Tramer MR. Ketamine and postoperative pain: a quantitative systematic review of randomised trials. Pain. 2005;113(1–2):61–70.
58. Carstensen M, Moller AM. Adding ketamine to morphine for intravenous patient-controlled analgesia for acute postoperative pain: a qualitative review of randomized trials. Br J Anaesth. 2010;104(4):401–6.
59. Fu ES, Miguel R, Scharf JE. Preemptive ketamine decreases postoperative narcotic requirements in patients undergoing abdominal surgery. Anesth Analg. 1997;84(5):1086–90.
60. Fawcett WJ, Baldini G. Optimal analgesia during major open and laparoscopic abdominal surgery. Anesthesiol Clin. 2015;33(1):65–78.
61. Tiippana EM, Hamunen K, Kontinen VK, Kalso E. Do surgical patients benefit from perioperative gabapentin/pregabalin? A systematic review of efficacy and safety. Anesth Analg. 2007;104(6):1545–56.
62. Hurley RW, Cohen SP, Williams KA, Rowlingson AJ, Wu CL. The analgesic effects of perioperative gabapentin on postoperative pain: a meta-analysis. Reg Anesth Pain Med. 2006;31(3):237–47.
63. Gilron I. Review article: The role of anticonvulsant drugs in postoperative pain management: a bench-to-bedside perspective. Can J Anaesth. 2006;53:562–71.
64. Zhang J, Ho KY, Wang Y. Efficacy of pregabalin in acute postoperative pain: a meta-analysis. Br J Anaesth. 2011;106(4):454–62.
65. Ramaswamy S, Wilson JA, Colvin L. Non-opioid-based adjuvant analgesia in perioperative care. Contin Educ Anaesth Crit Care Pain. 2013;13:152–7.
66. Blaudszun G, Lysakowski C, Elia N, Tramer MR. Effect of perioperative systemic alpha2 agonists on postoperative morphine consumption and pain intensity: systematic review and meta-analysis of randomized controlled trials. Anesthesiology. 2012;116(6):1312–22.
67. De Oliveira GS Jr, Almeida MD, Benzon HT, McCarthy RJ. Perioperative single dose systemic dexamethasone for postoperative pain: a meta-analysis of randomized controlled trials. Anesthesiology. 2011;115(3):575–88.
68. Waldron NH, Jones CA, Gan TJ, Allen TK, Habib AS. Impact of perioperative dexamethasone on postoperative analgesia and side-effects: systematic review and meta-analysis. Br J Anaesth. 2013;110(2):191–200.

69. Vignali A, Di Palo S, Orsenigo E, Ghirardelli L, Radaelli G, Staudacher C. Effect of prednisolone on local and systemic response in laparoscopic vs. open colon surgery: a randomized, double-blind, placebo-controlled trial. Dis Colon Rectum. 2009;52(6):1080–8.
70. Katz J, Clarke H, Seltzer Z. Review article: Preventive analgesia: quo vadimus? Anesth Analg. 2011;113(5):1242–53.
71. Taylor BK, Brennan TJ. Preemptive analgesia: moving beyond conventional strategies and confusing terminology. J Pain. 2000;1:77–84.
72. Katz J, McCartney CJ. Current status of preemptive analgesia. Curr Opin Anaesthesiol. 2002;15(4):435–41.
73. Moiniche S, Kehlet H, Dahl JB. A qualitative and quantitative systematic review of preemptive analgesia for postoperative pain relief: the role of timing of analgesia. Anesthesiology. 2002;96(3):725–41.
74. Richebe P, Rivat C, Liu SS. Perioperative or postoperative nerve block for preventive analgesia: should we care about the timing of our regional anesthesia? Anesth Analg. 2013;116(5):969–70.
75. Barreveld A, Witte J, Chahal H, Durieux ME, Strichartz G. Preventive analgesia by local anesthetics: the reduction of postoperative pain by peripheral nerve blocks and intravenous drugs. Anesth Analg. 2013;116(5):1141–61.
76. Andreae MH, Andreae DA. Local anaesthetics and regional anaesthesia for preventing chronic pain after surgery. Cochrane Database Syst Rev. 2012;(10):CD007105.
77. Joshi GP, Schug SA, Kehlet H. Procedure-specific pain management and outcome strategies. Best Pract Res Clin Anaesthesiol. 2014;28(2):191–201.
78. Challapalli V, Tremont-Lukats IW, McNicol ED, Lau J, Carr DB. Systemic administration of local anesthetic agents to relieve neuropathic pain. Cochrane Database Syst Rev. 2005;(4):CD003345.
79. Shavit Y, Lewis JW, Terman GW, Gale RP, Liebeskind JC. Opioid peptides mediate the suppressive effect of stress on natural killer cell cytotoxicity. Science. 1984;223(4632):188–90.
80. Singleton PA, Moss J. Effect of perioperative opioids on cancer recurrence: a hypothesis. Future Oncol. 2010;6(8):1237–42.
81. Exadaktylos AK, Buggy DJ, Moriarty DC, Mascha E, Sessler DI. Can anesthetic technique for primary breast cancer surgery affect recurrence or metastasis? Anesthesiology. 2006;105(4):660–4.
82. Gach K, Wyrebska A, Fichna J, Janecka A. The role of morphine in regulation of cancer cell growth. Naunyn Schmiedebergs Arch Pharmacol. 2011;384(3):221–30.
83. Doornebal CW, Vrijland K, Hau CS, Coffelt SB, Ciampricotti M, Jonkers J, et al. Morphine does not facilitate breast cancer progression in two preclinical mouse models for human invasive lobular and HER2(+) breast cancer. Pain. 2015;156(8):1424–32.
84. Cha YI, DuBois RN. NSAIDs and cancer prevention: targets downstream of COX-2. Annu Rev Med. 2007;58:239–52.
85. Forget P, Collet V, Lavand'homme P, De Kock M. Does analgesia and condition influence immunity after surgery? Effects of fentanyl, ketamine and clonidine on natural killer activity at different ages. Eur J Anaesthesiol. 2010;27(3):233–40.
86. Forget P, Vandenhende J, Berliere M, Machiels JP, Nussbaum B, Legrand C, et al. Do intraoperative analgesics influence breast cancer recurrence after mastectomy? A retrospective analysis. Anesth Analg. 2010;110(6):1630–5.
87. Monk TG, Weldon BC, Garvan CW, Dede DE, van der Aa MT, Heilman KM, et al. Predictors of cognitive dysfunction after major noncardiac surgery. Anesthesiology. 2008;108(1):18–30.
88. Deiner S, Silverstein JH. Postoperative delirium and cognitive dysfunction. Br J Anaesth. 2009;103(Suppl 1):i41–6.
89. Bruce AJ, Ritchie CW, Blizard R, Lai R, Raven P. The incidence of delirium associated with orthopedic surgery: a meta-analytic review. Int Psychogeriatr. 2007;19(2):197–214.
90. Steinmetz J, Christensen KB, Lund T, Lohse N, Rasmussen LS, Group I. Long-term consequences of postoperative cognitive dysfunction. Anesthesiology. 2009;110(3):548–55.
91. Aubrun F, Marmion F. The elderly patient and postoperative pain treatment. Best Pract Res Clin Anaesthesiol. 2007;21(1):109–27.

Opiate Medication and Routes of Delivery

3

Oana Predescu and Gabriele Baldini

Key Points

1. Opioids have been a cornerstone in the treatment of surgical pain since the beginnings of medicine.
2. Novel formulations and routes of delivery have been implemented with the aim of reducing the incidence of opioid-side effects and improve patients' long-term outcome.

Historical Perspective

Opioids have been known since 3400 BC, when poppy was cultivated in Mesopotamia, and used for its euphoric effect. Three thousand years later, Hippocrates, the father of medicine, acknowledged the effect of opium as a narcotic. Around 330 BC, Alexander the Great introduced opium to India. During the same era the Romans, Arabs and Greeks used opium as a sedative.

In approximately 250 AD, Hua Tuo, the ancient Chinese physician, was the first to use anaesthesia during surgery: he gave his patients a mixture prepared with opium and cannabis indica to swallow before surgery.

In Europe, during the Inquisition times opium was considered to come from the devil, therefore there are no notes of its use until 1527 when Paracelsus, the German-Swiss alchemist and inventor of toxicology, introduced the opium pill and tincture to be used as analgesic. Paracelsus mixture was called laudanum, from the Latin laudare or "to praise."

In 1680 in England, Thomas Sydenham, known as the "English Hippocrates" introduced the Sydenham laudanum, containing opium, sherry and herbs. He said:

O. Predescu · G. Baldini (✉)
Department of Anesthesiology, McGill University Health Centre,
Montreal General Hospital, Montreal, QC, Canada
e-mail: gabriele.baldini@mcgill.ca

A. Krige, M. J. P. Scott (eds.), *Analgesia in Major Abdominal Surgery*,
https://doi.org/10.1007/978-3-319-94482-1_3

"Of all the remedies it has pleased almighty God to give man to relieve his suffering, none is so universal and so efficacious as opium" [1].

In the 1800s, during the civil war, morphine was used as a painkiller. Morphine is named after Morpheus, the Ancient Greek god of dreams.

In the 1990s, extended release technology has been used for morphine, fentanyl, oxycodone and hydromorphone.

In 2000 the World Health Organisation defined pain treatment as a human right, and pain became "the fifth vital sign". The International Association for the Study of Pain (IASP), "ladder of pain", recognized opioids as the standard of care for treating severe acute and chronic pain.

Pain after abdominal surgery is common, whether surgery is performed laparoscopically, or open. The pathogenesis of surgical pain is multifactorial and therefore a multimodal pain management approach is commonly advised. In fact, although opioids are considered a cornerstone in the treatment of moderate to severe surgical pain, analgesic treatments, which exclusively use opioids to relieve surgical pain, should be discouraged due to the high incidence of opioid side effects.

Classification of Opioids

Opiates are drugs derived from opium. Opioids are compounds that have morphine-like properties and bind to opioid receptors that are widely distributed in the central and peripheral nervous system. The dorsal horn, the periaqueductal grey matter, the raphe nucleus and the thalamus are important zones in the pain pathway, by permitting the suppression of neuronal firing. Figure 3.1 illustrates the ascending pain pathways and the locations of opioid receptors in the nervous system.

Analgesia obtained by opiates binding to opioid receptors is commonly accompanied by various side effects, mediated by peripheral or central mechanisms: constipation, gastroesophageal reflux and nausea due to reduced peristalsis, itchiness, urinary retention, myoclonus, dry mouth, increased sweating, peripheral oedema, arthralgias, cardiac arrhythmias, as well as sedation, confusion, respiratory depression, depression, dysphoria or euphoria, opioid induced hyperalgesia and opioid tolerance [2, 3]. These side effects are dose-dependent, ranging from 2% to 37.1%, and independent from the route of administration [4].

Opioids are classified as naturally occurring, semi-synthetic and synthetic, as well as full agonists, mixed agonist/antagonist, partial agonists and antagonists.

The naturally occurring opioids of clinical significance are morphine and codeine; the semi-synthetic opioids commonly used are the thebaine derivates—oxycodone, buprenorphine, naloxone, naltrexone, nalbuphine, and the morphine derivatives: heroine and hydromorphone. The synthetic opioids include the following:

- Phenylpiperidines: fentanyl, sufentanil, alfentanil, meperidine, remifentanil
- Benzomorphinans: pentazocine

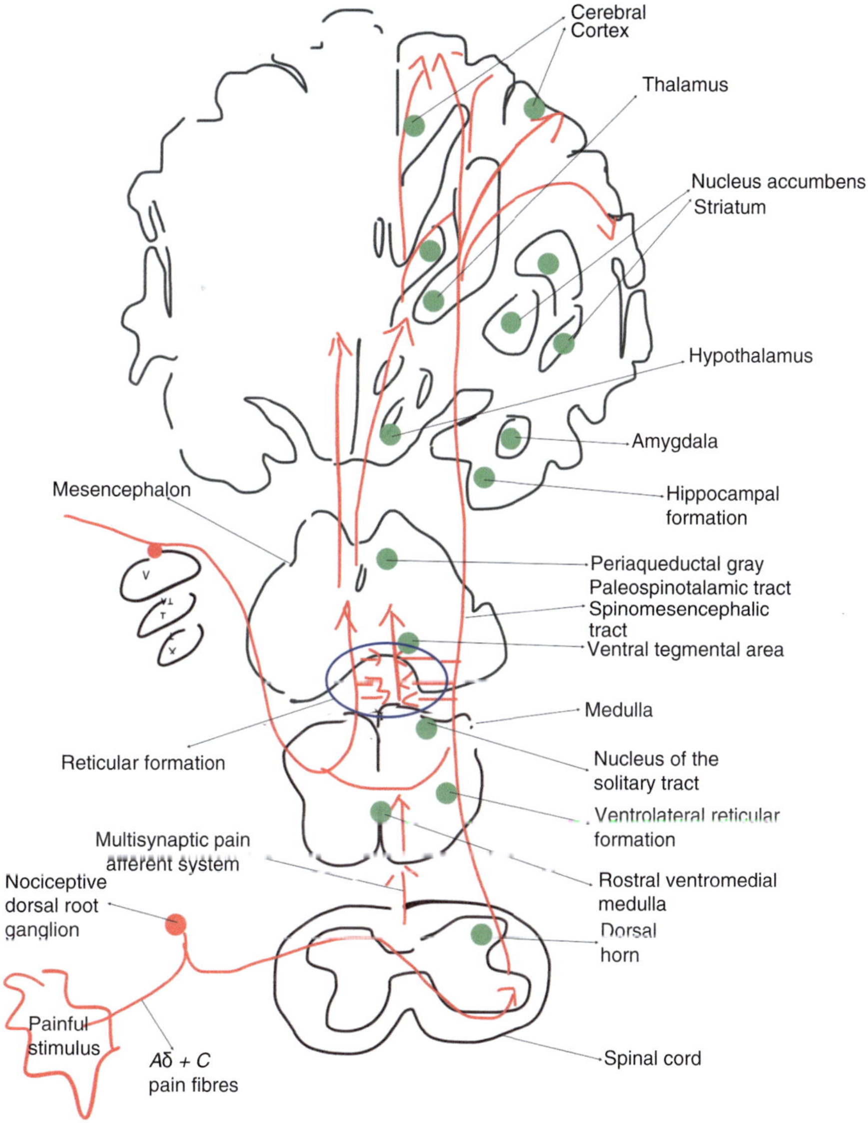

Fig. 3.1 Ascending pain pathways and the locations of opioid receptors in the nervous system

- Diphenylpropylamine: methadone
- Morphinans: levorphanol, butorphanol

The pure opioid agonists most commonly used in clinical practice are morphine, diamorphine (heroin), hydromorphone, fentanyl, meperidine. Pentazocine, butorphanol and nalbuphine are mixed agonist/antagonists and buprenorphine is a partial agonist. Naloxone, naltrexone and alvimopan are opioid antagonists.

Routes of Delivery

Opioids are commonly administered parenterally or orally. Over the years new delivery routes have been used and advanced delivery systems developed to improve patient care. This includes rectal, sublingual, transmucosal, transdermal, subcutaneous, intramuscular, and neuraxial routes of delivery.

Parenteral Route

The intravenous, intramuscular, and subcutaneous administration of opioids are traditional parenteral routes.

Intravenous Administration

The advantage of intravenous administration is that it provides the highest drug bioavailability, a rapid dose titration with more predictable pharmacokinetics, and a fast onset of action.

Intra-operatively and in the early post-operative period, opioids are commonly administered intravenously. These include fentanyl, sufentanil, remifentanil, morphine and hydromorphone. The quality of post-operative analgesia strongly depends on the intra-operative pain management. For an opioid-based anaesthesia, opioid administration can be done intermittently, as continuous infusion, or as target-controlled infusion (TCI). The latter is suggested to provide better intra-operative analgesia and ensure more effective post-operative pain control [5]. Intravenous opioid doses used in clinical practice are reported in Table 3.1.

Oxycodone is a potent opioid that has been recently used intravenously with success to treat post-operative pain [6, 7]. Intravenous morphine, hydromorphone, buprenorphine and fentanyl are widely used in the acute post-operative setting, either as intermittent boluses administered by nurses, or as patient-controlled analgesia (PCA). PCA allows the on-demand, intermittent self-administration of a predetermined dose of analgesic (commonly intravenous opioids or epidural analgesic mixtures of local anaesthetic with opioids) by a patient. PCA with intravenous

Table 3.1 Intra-operative intravenous opioid doses

	Loading dose (μg/kg)[a]	Maintenance infusion rate	Additional boluses	Effect-site concentration (Ce) ng/mL
Alfentanil	25–100	0.5–2 μg/kg/min	5–10 μg/kg	45–75
Fentanyl	4–20	2–10 μg/kg/h	25–100 μg	0.5–1.2
Remifentanil	1–2	0.1–1 μg/kg/min	0.1–1 μg/kg	3–15
Sufentanil	0.25–2	0.5–1.5 μg/kg/h	2.5–10 μg	0.12–0.20

[a]The upper range of the dosage usually refers to patients undergoing cardiac surgery. However, even in this population, high-dose opioids are less often used

Table 3.2 Common doses of intravenous opioids used during patient-controlled analgesia

Drug	Demand dose	Lockout interval (min)	Basal infusion rate
Fentanyl	10–50 μg	5–10	≤50 μg/h
Hydromorphone	0.25–0.5 mg	5–10	≤0.4 mg/h
Morphine	1–2 mg	5–10	≤0.5 mg/h
Remifentanil (labour)	0.5 μg/kg	2	NA
Sufentanil	4–6 μg	5–10	≤5 μg/h
Tramadol	10–20 μg	5–10	≤10 mg/h

opioids maintains the same advantages related to intravenous opioid administration, but with the added benefit of better pain control and increased patient satisfaction [8, 9] than intermittent intramuscular or subcutaneous, nurse-administration. PCA allows efficient titration of opioid requirements and ensures a more stable pain control level, as well as less sedation, respiratory depression and unlimited duration of use [10, 11]. Table 3.2 lists the opioids commonly used in clinical practice and the doses administered during PCA.

Intravenous morphine is considered the "gold standard" opioid used with PCA in the post-operative setting [12]. Hydromorphone is used in morphine intolerant patients, as well as patients with kidney dysfunction due to its liver metabolism. Fentanyl is a very potent opioid, but due to its very short duration of action (approx. 20 min), it is less commonly used. However, it might be a valuable alternative in patients with obstructive sleep apnoea where there is a risk of over-sedation due to opiate sensitivity.

Tramadol PCA offers the same quality of analgesia as morphine, although after lower abdominal surgery it might significantly increase the risk of post-operative nausea and vomiting [13].

When used as continuous infusion, opioid context sensitive half life must be considered. Due to its prolonged context-sensitive half-life analgesia provided by continuous infusion of intravenous morphine is difficult to titrate. In contrast, continuous infusion of remifentanil, which is the opioid with the shortest context-sensitive half-life, quickly achieves therapeutic plasma concentrations. Similarly, its therapeutic effect vanishes 2–5 min after remifentanil is discontinued.

Intramuscular and Subcutaneous Administration

Intramuscular (IM) or subcutaneous (SC) opioid administration is commonly used either as a rescue method when post-operative analgesia is inadequate, or in patients who cannot tolerate oral intake, or in patients with difficult intravenous access. Opioids administered subcutaneously have the same high bioavailability as the intravenous opioids (1:1), and subcutaneous injections are less painful compared to intramuscular injection. However, the pharmacokinetics are less predictable. Continuous subcutaneous administration of opioids is more often used as analgesic treatment for patients with moderate to severe cancer pain than in the acute post-operative setting.

Intramuscular administration of opioids is rarely used in the peri-operative setting and is not supported by current evidence due to its variable bioavailability, pain at the injection site, and the risk of developing sterile abscesses and muscular fibrosis [14].

Enteral Route

Oral (*per os*, PO) administration of opioids offers an easy method to provide analgesia in patients with good oral intake. It has the lowest bioavailability. Slow-release formulations prolong the duration of action, allowing a longer dosing interval [4].

Oral opioids are commonly administered following abdominal surgery, once oral intake is tolerated, by converting daily parenteral opioid consumption to oral opioid equivalent [15, 16]. Several conversions tables are available in the literature. The reader can refer to Table 3.3.

Enteral or systemic opioids are frequently used in the context of a multimodal analgesic regimen to treat breakthrough pain (i.e. used if needed [prn] and not regularly), especially when patients are treated with Enhanced Recovery After Surgery (ERAS) programmes. Common oral opioids used include oxycodone, morphine (PO or SC), hydromorphone (PO or SC), in their immediate release and, or extended release formulations.

Oral opioids can also be administered as oral PCA. This modality follows the same patient-centered care principle as intravenous PCA: opioids tablets are made available at the bedside and they can be taken by patients if analgesia is inadequate during a certain period of time. However, it remains to be determined, especially in patients undergoing abdominal surgery, if oral PCA can be a valuable alternative either to intravenous PCA or to nurse-administered oral analgesia [17].

To decrease opioid side effects analgesic formulations, which include opioid antagonists, have been created: the oxycodone-naloxone combination. The Targiniq

Table 3.3 Oral opioid analgesic conversion table

	Equivalence to oral morphine 30 mg	To convert to oral morphine equivalent, multiply by:	To convert from oral morphine multiply by:
Codeine	200 mg	0.15	6.67
Hydromorphone	6 mg	5	0.667
Meperidine	300 mg	5	0.2
Morphine	30 mg	1	1
Oxycodone	20 mg	1.5	0.667
Transdermal fentanyl	<60 mg = 12 μg/h 61–90 mg = 25 μg/h 90–134 mg = 37 μg/h 180–224 mg = 50 μg/h 225–269 mg = 62 μg/h 270–314 mg = 75 μg/h 315–359 mg = 87 μg/h 360–404 mg = 100 μg/h		

extended release (ER) (Perdue Pharma, Cranbury, NJ) [18], takes advantage of the benefit of a potent extended release opioid and the antagonist effect of naloxone, thus counteracting the opioid induced constipation effect. A starting dose containing 10 mg of oxycodone and 5 mg of naloxone can be administrated PO every 12 h.

Tramadol can also be administered PO as immediate release, or as extended release. It is not only a synthetic opioid, but it also inhibits norepinephrine re-uptake. Similarly, Tapentadol, which is a newer opioid agonist with norepinephrine re-uptake inhibitor activity with better gastric tolerance compared to classical opioids [19]. Alvimopan is a relatively recent FDA-approved peripheral μ-opioid receptor antagonist that does not penetrate the blood-brain barrier, therefore avoiding abolition of the opioid induced analgesic effect while decreasing the opioid-induced constipation [20]. It is indicated to accelerate the time to gastrointestinal recovery following bowel resection surgery leading to a reduction in the duration of post-operative hospital stay by 1 day [20–23].

Neuraxial Route

It has been known for a long time that opioids placed in the epidural or subarachnoid ventricular space provide optimal analgesia in patients with acute and chronic pain, due to their prolonged duration of action. Epidural opioids can be administered as bolus, continuous infusion or patient-controlled epidural analgesia (PCEA) [24, 25]. Commonly, intrathecal opioids are administered as bolus, but in combination with local anaesthetic have also been successfully used as continuous infusion in patients undergoing abdominal surgery [26, 27].

Epidural Opioids

For decades, it has been thought that epidural opioid, particularly lipophilic opioids, diffuse through the wall of radicular arteries as they cross the epidural space and are carried by the radicular blood flow to the spinal cord, where they bind opioid receptors [28]. However, microanalysis studies have shown that radicular blood flow is mainly responsible for washout of opioids from the spinal cord, rather than transporting them to the dorsal horn [29]. Opioid lipid solubility is one of the main determinants of epidural opioid concentration. In fact, highly lipophilic opioids like fentanyl (high octanol: buffer coefficient) are sequestrated into the epidural fat, and reabsorbed into the systemic circulation, and therefore are less available to diffuse into the spinal cord. This explains why several studies have shown that continuous infusion of lipophilic opioids does not produce analgesia by acting on the spinal cord, but rather on the brainstem after they have been reabsorbed into the systemic circulation. Indeed, plasma fentanyl concentrations in patients receiving continuous infusion of epidural fentanyl are similar to those receiving continuous infusion of intravenous fentanyl. In contrast, epidural bolus of opioids, seem to provide analgesia by directly diffusing into the spinal cord and by binding opioid receptors at the level of the dorsal horn [30].

Based on these pharmacokinetic principles, hydrophilic opioids such as epidural morphine are preferred to lipophilic opioids for increasing segmental analgesic spread, and can be particularly useful in patients with long midline incisions [31].

Epidural infusion of a mixture of local anaesthetic and opioid offers better post-operative pain control, and better facilitation of functional recovery compared to epidural infusion of local anaesthetic alone, or systemic opioids [32, 33]. Whilst this has been demonstrated following open abdominal surgery, it remains controversial if epidural analgesia offers any benefits, or if it even delays recovery, in patients undergoing laparoscopic abdominal surgery [34]. Despite its well-proven beneficial physiological effects, the impact of epidural analgesia on morbidity and mortality, as main anaesthesia technique, or in combination with general anaesthesia, remains uncertain [35–38].

The most common epidural opioids administered in clinical practice are fentanyl, morphine and hydromorphone [39], all in a preservative-free formulation. Growing evidence suggests that oxycodone might also be effective after epidural and spinal administration [7, 40, 41].

Extended epidural morphine (EREM) is used for single-dose epidural injection and due to its slow-release properties its analgesic effect lasts for approximately 48 h [19]. However, the evidence for efficacy is lacking for abdominal surgery [42, 43].

Intrathecal Opioids

Intrathecal opioid administration offers adequate post-operative pain control due to good spinal bioavailability. Opioids placed in the intrathecal space exert their action on different targets and compartments [44]: through spinal diffusion, opioids bind opioid receptors located in the white and grey matter; they also bind to the lipophilic structures in the epidural space, after which they are redistributed to the systemic circulation with different kinetics depending on their physicochemical properties [29]. Common opioids used for spinal administration are morphine, hydromorphone, and fentanyl. Diamorphine is frequently used intrathecally, especially in the United Kingdom, due to its rapid onset of action and decreased risk of respiratory depression, as its duration of actions is shorter than that of intrathecal morphine. Intrathecal opioids in combination with general anesthesia have been used in a variety of surgical procedures [45]. Specifically, intrathecal diamorphine or morphine in combination with local anaesthetic has been shown to provide optimal analgesia with minimal side effects in patients undergoing laparoscopic colorectal surgery in the context of an ERAS program [46, 47]. Moreover, it facilitates surgical recovery [48], as it allows early hospital discharge especially when compared to patients receiving epidural analgesia [46]. However, the risk of (early and late) respiratory depression and urinary retention must be considered, especially in elderly patients [45].

Intrathecal doses for morphine, fentanyl, diamorphine and sufentanil are reported in Tables 3.4, 3.5, 3.6, and 3.7.

Table 3.4 Epidural opioid: doses without local anaesthetic

Drug	Solution	Bolus	Basal infusion	Breakthrough dose	Increments in breakthrough
Alfentanil	0.025% (0.25 mg/mL)	10–15 μg/kg	10–18 μg/kg/h	250 μg every 10 min	250 μg
Fentanyl	0.001% (10 μg/mL)	0.5–1.5 μg/kg	0.5–1 μg/kg/h	10–15 μg every 10–15 min	10 μg
Hydromorphone	0.005% (0.05 mg/mL)	0.8–1.5 mg	0.15–0.3 mg/h	0.15–0.3 mg every 10–15 min	0.05 mg
Morphine	0.01% (0.1 mg/mL)	4–6 mg	0.5–0.8 mg/h	0.2–0.3 mg every 10–15 min	0.1 mg
Sufentanil	0.0001% (1 μg/mL)	0.3–0.7 μg/kg	0.1–0.2 μg/kg/h	5–7 μg every 10–15 min	5 μg

Table 3.5 Epidural opioid: doses with local anaesthetic

Drug combination	Solution	Bolus dose of bupivacaine	Basal infusion	Breakthrough
Morphine w. bupivacaine	0.01%		6–8 mL/h	1–2 mL q 10–15 min
Morphine w. bupivacaine	0.05–0.1%	0.5–0.25%	6–8 mL/h	1–2 mL q 10–15 min
Hydromorphone w. bupivacaine	0.0025–0.005%		6–8 mL/h	1–3 mL q 10–15 min
Hydromorphone w. bupivacaine	0.05–0.1%	0.5–0.25%	6–8 mL/h	1–3 mL q 10–15 min
Fentanyl w. bupivacaine	0.001%		0.1–0.15 mL/kg/h	1–1.5 mL q 10–15 min
Fentanyl w. bupivacaine	0.05–0.1%	0.5–0.25%	0.1–0.15 mL/kg/h	1–1.5 mL q 10–15 min
Sufentanil w. bupivacaine	0.0001%		0.1–0.2 mL/kg/h	1–1.5 mL q 10–15 min
Sufentanil w. bupivacaine	0.55–0.25%	0.5–0.25%	0.1–0.2 mL/kg/h	1–1.5 mL q 10–15 min

Table 3.6 Bioavailability of neuraxial opioids

Opioid	Epidural	Intrathecal
Alfentanil	Very low	Very low
Fentanyl	Low as continuous infusion Moderate as a bolus	Moderate
Hydromorphone	High	High
Methadone	Moderate	Moderate
Morphine	High	High
Sufentanil	Low	Moderate

Table 3.7 Intrathecal opioid doses

Diamorphine	0.1–0.5 mg
Fentanyl	12.5–25 μg
Morphine	0.2–0.5 mg (longest duration of action)
Sufentanil	2–10 μg

Transdermal Opioid Patches

Transdermal administration of medication is simple and painless and provides long duration of action. Opioids that are commonly administered transdermally are fentanyl and buprenorphine. The patches are frequently used in chronic and palliative pain patients, although new data support the peri-operative use of fentanyl patches in the context of a multimodal analgesic regimen [49–51]. Transdermal fentanyl patches are easy to administer and less constipating than oral morphine [52, 53]. By using low-dose patches only (12 or 25 μg depending on patient age and weight) the risks of respiratory complications in the post-operative setting are mitigated.

The fentanyl HCl iontophoretic transdermal system (fentanyl ITS), administered as a patient-controlled transdermal fentanyl (PCTS) system, is a PCA system used for treating moderate to severe post-operative pain. It has been shown to have similar analgesic efficacy to intravenous morphine PCA [8, 54–57]. The advantage of inotophoresis systems compared to classical passive diffusion of transdermal fentanyl is the rapid rate of analgesic absorption with no skin depot effect. The device delivers a preprogramed dose of fentanyl over 10 min, for 24 h.

Transmucosal Route

Opioids administered transmucosally, mainly lipophilic opioids, provide a rapid onset of action because of a higher bioavailability compared to oral opioids. Buprenorphine, fentanyl, sufentanil, and butorphanol have been administered intranasally (inhaled) successfully in the recovery room, to treat post-operative pain [58, 59].

Recently, sufentanil sublingual PCA tablets were studied for moderate to severe pain following abdominal surgery and they demonstrated better pain control in the first 72 h compared to intravenous morphine PCA [19, 60].

Analgesic Opioids Commonly Used in Clinical Practice: Available Preparations with Parenteral and Enteral Doses

Alfentanil

- Opioid agonist for parenteral use only, ten times more potent than morphine, used primarily in the operating room.
- Average dose for post-operative analgesia: 10–20 μg/kg/h.

Alvimopan

- Peripherally acting μ-opioid receptor antagonist used to antagonise the constipating effect of systemic opioid to facilitate recovery of bowel function, especially after gastrointestinal surgery.

- 12 mg PO administered 30 min to 5 h pre-operatively, then 12 mg PO every 12 h beginning 1 day after surgery, for a maximum of 7 days; no more than 15 doses.

Buprenorphine

- Partial opioid agonist, highly lipophilic; available for parenteral and sublingual administration.
- 25–50 times more potent than morphine (0.3–0.4 mg of buprenorphine is equivalent to 10 mg morphine).
- It has a slow onset, and duration of action longer than 6 h.
- Analgesic dose: 0.3–0.6 mg IV or IM bolus.

Butorphanol

- Partial agonist, similar to nalbuphine, administered parenterally, epidurally and transnasally.
- It is administered as PCA, and it causes less post-operative ileus compared to other opioid agonists [61].
- Analgesic dose: 0.5–2 mg IV every 3–4 h is indicated for sedation and moderate post-operative pain.

Codeine

- Available for oral and parenteral administration, less potent than morphine.
- Analgesic dose 30–60 mg every 4–6 h.
- Often combined with acetaminophen.
- It is metabolised by the liver to morphine. However, approximately 5–10% of patients do not metabolise codeine and are thus resistant to its analgesic efficacy [62].

Diamorphine

- Available for neuraxial administration: crosses epidural membrane faster and it is cleared from cerebral spinal fluid (CSF) quicker than morphine; it is converted to morphine, and has a long duration of action.
- Analgesic dose: 5–10 mg IV every 4 h.

Fentanyl

- Synthetic opioid agonist, 80 times more potent than morphine.
- Parenteral, transdermal, transmusosal, neuraxial formulations are available.

- Doses for post-operative analgesia: 0.5–1.5 μg/kg every 30–60 min IV prn; 15 μg/kg/h.
- Transdermal iontophoresis system is a novel therapeutic modality to administer fentanyl.

Hydromorphone

- Semi-synthetic opioid, 4–6 times more potent than morphine.
- Available for oral, rectal, parenteral and neuraxial administration.
- Fewer opioid-related side effects compared to morphine.
- Analgesic dose: 0.2–1 mg IV every 2–3 h prn.

Meperidine

- Synthetic opioid agonist with short half-life, available for oral and parenteral administration.
- Due to its neurotoxic metabolite, normeperidine, meperidine can decrease seizure thresholds. It is only indicated for short-term management of acute pain or at low doses to treat shivering during the emergence of anaesthesia.
- Analgesic dose: 50–150 mg PO/IM/SC every 3–4 h. The American Pain Society does not recommend it as first-choice analgesic.

Methadone

- Synthetic broad-spectrum opioid due to its multiple sites of action: μ-receptor agonist, NMDA antagonist, monoamine-oxidase inhibitor.
- Available for oral and parenteral administration.
- More potent than morphine, with a variable, dose-dependent conversion rate.
- Because of its pharmacokinetic properties it provides optimal analgesia with minimal side effects in patients with renal failure or end-stage renal disease.

Morphine

- The "gold standard" opioid which all other analgesics are compared to
- Available for oral, parenteral and rectal administration
- Post-operative analgesia IV doses: 0.03–0.15 mg/kg every 2–4 h prn
- Active metabolites, with analgesic (morphine-6-glucuronide) and hyperalgesic properties (morphine-3-glucuronide morphine).

Nalbuphine

- Agonist/antagonist opioid, equipotent to morphine
- Available for parenteral administration

- 10–20 mg IV reverses respiratory depression induced by opioid agonists, while still maintaining adequate analgesia

Oxycodone

- Opioid agonist, approximately 7.5 times more potent than morphine
- Potent analgesic after oral and parenteral administration, but poor analgesic properties after spinal administration

Pentazocine

- Opioid agonist with weak antagonist action, available for oral and parenteral administration
- Limited use in post-operative pain treatment due to its high incidence of post-operative nausea and vomiting

Remifentanil

- Opioid agonist with very short duration of action, only in parenteral formulation, 100–200 times more potent than morphine.
- Sedative and analgesic doses: 0.05–0.5 μg/kg/min.
- Metabolism does not depend on hepatic and renal function; metabolised by plasma esterases.
- Due to its very short context-sensitive half-life and to its ability to be easily titrated to achieve the desired therapeutic effect, it is frequently used as analgesic and sedative in the intensive care unit, especially in neurosurgical patients.
- Due to its very short duration of action (2–5 min), when remifentanil is used as continuous infusion to provide analgesia during surgery, on emergence of anaesthesia patients require administration of an alternative, longer acting opioid.
- Frequently associated with opioid-induced hyperalgesia. Conflicting evidence suggests that NMDA-antagonists such as ketamine and magnesium can prevent the occurrence of remifentanil induced hyperalgesia [63].

Sufentanil

- Opioid agonist similar to fentanyl, remifentanil, alfentanil, available for parenteral, epidural and oral transmucosal administration
- 1000 times more potent than morphine
- Analgesic doses: 5–50 μg IV every 20–45 min prn

Tramadol

- Synthetic opioid with weak μ-receptor affinity, being 5–10 times less potent than morphine; it also inhibits norepinephrine re-uptake.
- It exists in oral and parenteral formulation.
- It is used to treat moderate post-operative pain, with an analgesic efficacy similar to PCA with intravenous opioids [64].

Conclusions

Opioids still remain the cornerstone of post-operative pain management. However, increasing evidence suggests that multimodal analgesic regimens that include opioid-sparing analgesic strategies aimed at minimising opioid side effects can provide optimal analgesia and hasten recovery. This is particularly important in patients undergoing abdominal surgery and treated within an ERAS programme, in whome opioid side effects significantly delay surgical recovery, prevent early feeding, impede post-operative mobilization and increase the risk of urinary retention [26]. Finally, in vitro and in vivo experimental studies have shown that opioids can suppress cellular immune function, and this might impact on long-term outcomes such as cancer recurrence and metastasis. A completely opioid-free multimodal analgesic regimen is appealing, but further studies are warranted to establish the efficacy and safety in patients undergoing abdominal surgery.

References

1. Waring R, Steventon G, Mitchell S. Molecules of death. 2nd ed. London: Imperial College Press; 2007.
2. Rosenblum A, Marsch LA, Joseph H, Portenoy RK. Opioids and the treatment of chronic pain: controversies, current status, and future directions. Exp Clin Psychopharmacol. 2008;16(5):405–16.
3. Jovey R. Managing pain – the Canadian healthcare professional's reference. 2nd ed. Toronto: Healthcare & Financial Publishing; 2002.
4. Wheeler M, Oderda GM, Ashburn MA, Lipman AG. Adverse events associated with postoperative opioid analgesia: a systematic review. J Pain. 2002;3(3):159–80.
5. Derrode N, Lebrun F, Levron JC, Chauvin M, Debaene B. Influence of peroperative opioid on postoperative pain after major abdominal surgery: sufentanil TCI versus remifentanil TCI. A randomized, controlled study. Br J Anaesth. 2003;91(6):842–9.
6. Pergolizzi JV Jr, Seow-Choen F, Wexner SD, Zampogna G, Raffa RB, Taylor R Jr. Perspectives on intravenous oxycodone for control of postoperative pain. Pain Pract. 2016;16(7):924–34.
7. Sjövall S, Kokki M, Kokki H. Laparoscopic surgery: a narrative review of pharmacotherapy in pain management. Drugs. 2016;16(7):924–34.
8. Power I. Fentanyl HCl iontophoretic transdermal system (ITS): clinical application of iontophoretic technology in the management of acute postoperative pain. Br J Anaesth. 2007;98(1):4–11.
9. Viscusi ER. Emerging techniques in the treatment of postoperative pain. Am J Health Syst Pharm. 2004;61(Suppl 1):S11–4.

10. Momeni M, Crucitti M, De Kock M. Patient-controlled analgesia in the management of post-operative pain. Drugs. 2006;66(18):2321–37.
11. Cashman JN, Dolin SJ. Respiratory and haemodynamic effects of acute postoperative pain management: evidence from published data. Br J Anaesth. 2004;93(2):212–23.
12. Grass JA. Patient-controlled analgesia. Anesth Analg. 2005;101(5 Suppl):S44–61.
13. Ng KF, Tsui SL, Yang JC, Ho ET. Increased nausea and dizziness when using tramadol for post-operative patient-controlled analgesia (PCA) compared with morphine after intraoperative loading with morphine. Eur J Anaesthesiol. 1998;15(5):565–70.
14. Kestenbaum MG, Vilches AO, Messersmith S, Connor SR, Fine PG, Murphy B, Davis M, Muir JC. Alternative routes to oral opioid administration in palliative care: a review and clinical summary. Pain Med. 2014;15(7):1129–53.
15. Baldini G, Fawcett WJ. Anesthesia for colorectal surgery. Anesthesiol Clin. 2015;33(1):93–123.
16. Garimella V, Cellini C. Postoperative pain control. Clin Colon Rectal Surg. 2013;26(3):191–6.
17. Kastanias P, Gowans S, Tumber PS, Snaith K, Robinson S. Patient-controlled oral analgesia for postoperative pain management following total knee replacement. Pain Res Manag. 2010;15(1):11–6.
18. Comelon M, Wisloeff-Aase K, Raeder J, Draegni T, Undersrud H, Qvigstad E, Bjerkelund CE, Lenz H. A comparison of oxycodone prolonged-release vs. oxycodone + naloxone prolonged-release after laparoscopic hysterectomy. Acta Anaesthesiol Scand. 2013;57(4):509–17.
19. Kaye AD, Ali SI, Urman RD. Perioperative analgesia: ever-changing technology and pharmacology. Best Pract Res Clin Anaesthesiol. 2014;28(1):3–14.
20. Absher RK, Gerkin TM, Banares LW. Alvimopan use in laparoscopic and open bowel resections: clinical results in a large community hospital system. Ann Pharmacother. 2010;44(11):1701–8.
21. Curran MP, Robins GW, Scott LJ, Perry CM. Alvimopan. Drugs. 2008;68(14):2011–9.
22. Akça O, Doufas AG, Sessler DI. Use of selective opiate receptor inhibitors to prevent postoperative ileus. Minerva Anestesiol. 2002;68(4):162–5.
23. Vaughan-Shaw PG, Fecher IC, Harris S, Knight JS. A meta-analysis of the effectiveness of the opioid receptor antagonist alvimopan in reducing hospital length of stay and time to GI recovery in patients enrolled in a standardized accelerated recovery program after abdominal surgery. Dis Colon Rectum. 2012;55(5):611–20.
24. Mulroy MF. Epidural opioid delivery methods: bolus, continuous infusion, and patient-controlled epidural analgesia. Reg Anesth. 1996;21(6 Suppl):100–4.
25. Manion SC, Brennan TJ. Thoracic epidural analgesia and acute pain management. Anesthesiology. 2011;115(1):181–8.
26. Fawcett WJ, Baldini G. Optimal analgesia during major open and laparoscopic abdominal surgery. Anesthesiol Clin. 2015;33(1):65–78.
27. Crews JC, Hord AH, Denson DD, Schatzman C. A comparison of the analgesic efficacy of 0.25% levobupivacaine combined with 0.005% morphine, 0.25% levobupivacaine alone, or 0.005% morphine alone for the management of postoperative pain in patients undergoing major abdominal surgery. Anesth Analg. 1999;89(6):1504–9.
28. Cousins M, Bridenbaugh P. Neural blockade. In: Clinical anesthesia and pain medicine. 4th ed. Philadelphia: Lippincott Williams & Wilkins; 2009.
29. Bernards CM, Sorkin LS. Radicular artery blood flow does not redistribute fentanyl from the epidural space to the spinal cord. Anesthesiology. 1994;80(4):872–8.
30. Bernards CM. Sophistry in medicine: lessons from the epidural space. Reg Anesth Pain Med. 2005;30(1):56–66.
31. Rawal N, Allvin R. Epidural and intrathecal opioids for postoperative pain management in Europe—a 17-nation questionnaire study of selected hospitals. Euro Pain Study Group on Acute Pain. Acta Anaesthesiol Scand. 1996;40:1119–26.
32. Finucane BT, Ganapathy S, Carli F, Pridham JN, Ong BY, Shukla RC, Kristoffersson AH, Huizar KM, Nevin K, Ahlén KG, Canadian Ropivacaine Research Group. Prolonged epidural infusions of ropivacaine (2 mg/mL) after colonic surgery: the impact of adding fentanyl. Anesth Analg. 2001;92(5):1276–85.

33. Block BM, Liu SS, Rowlingson AJ, Cowan AR, Cowan JA Jr, Wu CL. Efficacy of postoperative epidural analgesia: a meta-analysis. JAMA. 2003;290(18):2455–63.
34. Hübner M, Blanc C, Roulin D, Winiker M, Gander S, Demartines N. Randomized clinical trial on epidural versus patient-controlled analgesia for laparoscopic colorectal surgery within an enhanced recovery pathway. Ann Surg. 2015;261(4):648–53.
35. Carli F, Kehlet H, Baldini G, Steel A, McRae K, Slinger P, Hemmerling T, Salinas F, Neal JM. Evidence basis for regional anesthesia in multidisciplinary fast-track surgical care pathways. Reg Anesth Pain Med. 2011;36(1):63–72.
36. Guay J, Choi P, Suresh S, Albert N, Kopp S, Pace NL. Neuraxial blockade for the prevention of postoperative mortality and major morbidity: an overview of Cochrane systematic reviews. Cochrane Database Syst Rev. 2014;(1):CD010108.
37. Pöpping DM, Zahn PK, Van Aken HK, Dasch B, Boche R, Pogatzki-Zahn EM. Effectiveness and safety of postoperative pain management: a survey of 18 925 consecutive patients between 1998 and 2006 (2nd revision): a database analysis of prospectively raised data. Br J Anaesth. 2008;101(6):832–40.
38. Pöpping DM, Van Aken HK, Brodner G, Wenk M. It is not the epidural that is dangerous, but the person who gives it. Br J Anaesth. 2014;112(2):392–3.
39. Bujedo BM. Spinal opioid bioavailability in postoperative pain. Pain Pract. 2014;14(4):350–64.
40. Kokki M, Välitalo P, Kuusisto M, Ranta VP, Raatikainen K, Hautajärvi H, Kokki H. Central nervous system penetration of oxycodone after intravenous and epidural administration. Br J Anaesth. 2014;112(1):133–40.
41. de Leon-Casasola OA, Lema MJ. Postoperative epidural opioid analgesia: what are the choices? Anesth Analg. 1996;83(4):867–75.
42. Hartrick CT, Hartrick KA. Extended-release epidural morphine (DepoDurTM): review and safety analysis. Expert Rev Neurother. 2008;8(11):1641–8.
43. Gambling D, Hughes T, Martin G. A comparison of Depodur, a novel, single dose extended-release epidural morphine, with standard epidural morphine for pain relief after lower abdominal surgery. Anesth Analg. 2005;100(4):1065–74.
44. Bujedo BM, Santos SG, Azpiazu AU. A review of epidural and intrathecal opioids used in the management of postoperative pain. J Opioid Manag. 2012;8(3):177–92.
45. Meylan N, Elia N, Lysakowski C, Tramèr MR. Benefit and risk of intrathecal morphine without local anaesthetic in patients undergoing major surgery: meta-analysis of randomized trials. Br J Anaesth. 2009;102(2):156–67.
46. Levy BF, Scott MJ, Fawcett W, Fry C, Rockall TA. Randomized clinical trial of epidural, spinal or patient-controlled analgesia for patients undergoing laparoscopic colorectal surgery. Br J Surg. 2011;98(8):1068–78.
47. Wongyingsinn M, Baldini G, Stein B, Charlebois P, Liberman S, Carli F. Spinal analgesia for laparoscopic colonic resection using an enhanced recovery after surgery programme: better analgesia, but no benefits on postoperative recovery: a randomized controlled trial. Br J Anaesth. 2012;108(5):850–6.
48. Levy BF, Scott MJ, Fawcett WJ, Rockall TA. 23-Hour-stay laparoscopic colectomy. Dis Colon Rectum. 2009;52(7):1239–43.
49. Song JH, Kang C, Hwang DS, Hwang JM, Shin BK. Fentanyl patches to supplement ultrasound-guided nerve blocks for improving pain control after foot and ankle surgery: a prospective study. J Foot Ankle Surg. 2016;55(1):121–4.
50. Lehmann LJ, DeSio JM, Radvany T, Bikhazi GB. Transdermal fentanyl in postoperative pain. Reg Anesth. 1997;22(1):24–8.
51. Reinhart DJ, Goldberg ME, Roth JV, Dua R, Nevo I, Klein KW, Torjman M, Vekeman D. Transdermal fentanyl system plus IM ketorolac for the treatment of postoperative pain. Can J Anaesth. 1997;44(4):377–84.
52. Radbruch L, Sabatowski R, Loick G, Kulbe C, Kasper M, Grond S, Lehmann KA. Constipation and the use of laxatives: a comparison between transdermal fentanyl and oral morphine. Palliat Med. 2000;14(2):111–9.

53. Jeal W, Benfield P. Transdermal fentanyl. A review of its pharmacological properties and therapeutic efficacy in pain control. Drugs. 1997;53(1):109–38.
54. Rawal N, Langford RM. Current practices for postoperative pain management in Europe and the potential role of the fentanyl HCl iontophoretic transdermal system. Eur J Anaesthesiol. 2007;24(4):299–308.
55. Mattia C, Coluzzi F, Sonnino D, Anker-Møller E. Efficacy and safety of fentanyl HCl iontophoretic transdermal system compared with morphine intravenous patient-controlled analgesia for postoperative pain management for patient subgroups. Eur J Anaesthesiol. 2010;27(5):433–40.
56. Sinatra R. The fentanyl HCl patient-controlled transdermal system (PCTS): an alternative to intravenous patient-controlled analgesia in the postoperative setting. Clin Pharmacokinet. 2005;44(Suppl 1):1–6.
57. Viscusi ER, Reynolds L, Chung F, Atkinson LE, Khanna S. Patient-controlled transdermal fentanyl hydrochloride vs intravenous morphine pump for postoperative pain: a randomized controlled trial. JAMA. 2004;291(11):1333–41.
58. Miller R. Miller's anesthesia. Philadelphia: Elsevier Saunders; 2015.
59. Asenjo JF, Brecht KM. Opioids: other routes for use in recovery room. Curr Drug Targets. 2005;6(7):773–9.
60. Melson TI, Boyer DL, Minkowitz HS, Turan A, Chiang YK, Evashenk MA, Palmer PP. Sufentanil sublingual tablet system vs. intravenous patient-controlled analgesia with morphine for postoperative pain control: a randomized, active-comparator trial. Pain Pract. 2014;14(8):679–88.
61. Barash P, Cullen B, Stoelting R. Clinical anesthesia. Philadelphia: Lippincott Williams & Wilkins; 2013.
62. Dean L. Codeine therapy and CYP2D6 genotype. 2012 Sept 20 [updated 2013 Mar 18]. In Medical genetics summaries [Internet]. Bethesda (MD): National Center for Biotechnology Information (US); 2012. Available from: http://www.ncbi.nlm.nih.gov/books/NBK100662/
63. Martinez V, Fletcher D. Prevention of opioid-induced hyperalgesia in surgical patients: does it really matter? Br J Anaesth. 2012;109(3):302–4.
64. Murphy JD, Yan D, Hanna MN, Bravos ED, Isaac GR, Eng CA, Wu CL. Comparison of the postoperative analgesic efficacy of intravenous patient-controlled analgesia with tramadol to intravenous patient-controlled analgesia with opioids. J Opioid Manag. 2010;6(2):141–7.

4 Gabapentinoids

Jeremy Cashman

Key Points

1. Peri-operative gabapentin and pregabalin are associated with a modest reduction in post-operative pain whilst the impact on opioid consumption is more pronounced.
2. In choosing between gabapentinoids there is insufficient evidence to support the use of pregabalin in preference to gabapentin, notwithstanding pregabalin's more favourable pharmacokinetic profile.
3. The appropriate dose and timing of administration of gabapentinoid has yet to be elucidated but it would appear that single dosing whether before or after surgery may be as effective as multiple dosing.
4. Higher doses may be more effective in reducing both acute post-operative pain and persistent post-operative pain, but this advantage is at the expense of a higher incidence of unwanted side effects.
5. Gabapentinoids may shorten hospital stay and are hence useful additions to multimodal analgesia within enhanced recovery after surgery programmes.

Introduction and Historical Perspective

The gabapentinoid gabapentin and its structural analogue pregabalin are second generation anticonvulsants licensed for the treatment of seizures, chronic neuropathic pain arising from diabetes, post herpetic neuralgia and central neuropathic pain. Gabapentin was approved by the United States Food and Drug Administration (FDA) in 1993 initially for use as an anti-epileptic with approval extended in 2004 to include treatment of neuropathic pain. Pregabalin was also

J. Cashman
Department of Anaesthetics, St. George's Hospital, London, UK
e-mail: Jeremy.Cashman@stgeorges.nhs.uk

A. Krige, M. J. P. Scott (eds.), *Analgesia in Major Abdominal Surgery*,
https://doi.org/10.1007/978-3-319-94482-1_4

approved by the FDA in 2004 for the same indications as gabapentin, as well as for generalised anxiety disorders. Since their introduction the gabapentinoids have gained popularity for use in a wide variety of off-label indications, such that gabapentin is now one of the medications with the highest off-label uses (83%) among specific medications [1, 2]. In the United Kingdom there were 8.2 million prescriptions for gabapentin and pregabalin in 2013 (a rise of ~50% over the previous 2 years), and not all for licensed indications [3]. The administration of gabapentinoids for the management of post-operative pain represents one such off-label use.

Mechanism of Action

Gabapentin [1-(aminomethyl)cyclohexaneacetic acid] and pregabalin [(S)-3-(aminomethyl)-5-methylhexananoic acid] are branched chain amino acid analogues of the inhibitory neurotransmitter γ-aminobutyric acid (GABA) (Fig. 4.1).

However, neither drug has any activity in the GABAergic neurotransmitter system. Instead they bind to the α-2δ-1 subunit of presynaptic voltage-gated calcium channels causing decreased calcium entry into nerve endings with decreased release of excitatory neurotransmitters in spinal and supraspinal pathways. In addition to modulation of the N-type calcium channel a variety of other mechanisms of action for analgesia have been suggested including attenuation of stimulus-induced glutamate release from activated pain-transmitting neurones, activation of descending noradrenergic pain-inhibiting pathways, impeding synapse formation and inhibiting neuroinflammation [4]. Thus, it has been postulated that neuropathic pain may involve excessive formation of excitatory synapses and that gabapentin impedes synapse formation between neurones by preventing the synaptogenic protein thrombospondin from binding to the α-2δ-1 subunit [5]. Alternatively, it has been suggested that activation of neuroinflammation contributes to the development of neuropathic pain. Gabapentin and pregabalin have been shown to inhibit substance P mediated activation of nuclear factor-kappa B (NF-κB), one of the transcription factors that regulates levels of cytokines in the central nervous system [6]. This may in turn explain the increased efficacy of gabapentinoids in circumstances of prior inflammation or sensitization where there may be an upregulation of the NFκB-signaling pathway [7].

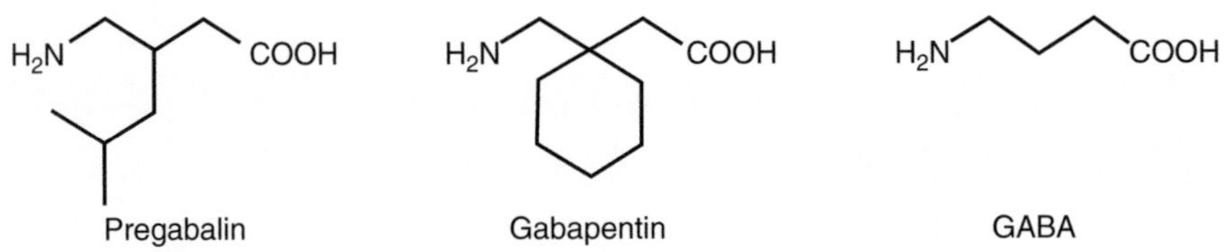

Fig. 4.1 Comparative chemical structures of the gabapentinoids and GABA

Table 4.1 Comparison of the pharmacokinetic parameters of gabapentin and pregabalin

	Gabapentin	Pregabalin
Absorption	Saturable	Non-saturable
Oral bioavailability	60% → 33% (900 mg → 3600 mg)	≥90%
t_{max} (h)	1.7–4	0.7–1.3
VD_{ss} (L/kg)	0.6–0.8	0.5
$t_{½}$ elimination (h)	4.6–8.7	5–7
C_{max} (μg/ml)	2.8–3.8	2.6–3.8

C_{max}: peak plasma concentration; t_{max}: time to reach peak plasma concentration; VD_{ss}: volume of distribution at steady state

Pharmacokinetics

The absorption, distribution, metabolism and elimination properties of gabapentin and pregabalin are outlined below and summarised in Table 4.1.

Absorption

Gabapentin is supplied as an immediate-release oral formulation that is usually administered orally three times a day. Absorption is limited to a relatively small part of the duodenum by a saturable carrier-mediated L-amino acid transporter (LAT) system. Once the active transport system is saturated, progressively higher doses of gabapentin result in progressively smaller increases in blood concentration. Consequently the bioavailability of gabapentin is inversely related to dose, ranging from 60% following 300 mg three times a day, to 33% following 1200 mg three times a day [8]. However, bioavailability can be increased by alterations to the formulation of gabapentin. Gabapentin enacarbil is a transport acycloalkylcarbamate prodrug of gabapentin which undergoes hydrolysis to the parent drug. Absorption is by a proton-linked monocarboxylate transporter (MCT-1) expressed in high levels in the intestinal tract. MCT-1 is not saturated by high doses of drug, consequently the bioavailability of gabapentin approaches 75% with a twice daily oral formulation. Similarly, a modified release formulation of gabapentin using a mucoadhesive gastroretentive delivery system optimizes absorption via a saturable uptake mechanism. The prolonged residence of the gastroretentive tablets in the stomach coupled with the gradual release of gabapentin attenuates saturation of the transporter, thus enhancing absorption and increasing bioavailability with once daily oral administration [9]. Currently, gabapentin enacarbil is marketed in Japan and the United States, whilst modified release gabapentin is only available in the United States. Absorption of pregabalin, by contrast, occurs throughout the small intestine, mediated not just by the LAT system but also by an additional non-saturable pathway. As a result, pregabalin demonstrates linear uptake over its oral dose range of 75–900 mg/day with bioavailability in excess of 90% (Fig. 4.2) [8].

The mean bioavailability of gabapentin is uninfluenced by food but is reduced by about 20% with concomitant use of magnesium and aluminum hydroxide containing antacids. However, the decrease in bioavailability is only 5% when gabapentin is taken 2 or more hours following ingestion of such antacids. Conversely drugs that

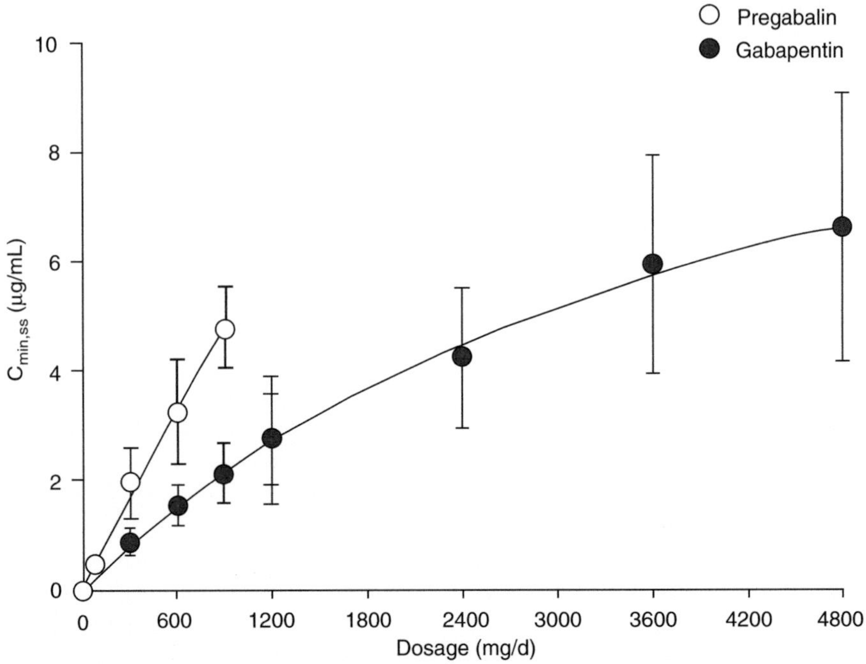

Fig. 4.2 Mean steady-state minimum plasma drug concentration ($C_{min.ss}$) values in healthy subjects given pregabalin or gabapentin every 8 h. Note the nonlinear relationship of gabapentin compared with pregabalin. From [8]; with permission

prolong the transit time in the small intestine such as the opioids, can increase the bioavailability of gabapentin by up to 50% with concomitant increase in side effects, whereas the bioavailability of pregabalin is unaffected by alterations in gastrointestinal transit time [8].

The time to reach peak plasma concentration (C_{max}) following drug administration (t_{max}) is a function of the dose administered for gabapentin but not for pregabalin. Thus t_{max} following single low dose gabapentin occurs at ~1.7 h but increases to 3–4 h following higher doses, whilst t_{max} following single doses of pregabalin up to 300 mg occurs at ~1 h [8].

Less than 3% of gabapentin circulates bound to plasma protein. The apparent volumes of distribution of gabapentin and pregabalin are 0.8 and 0.5 L/kg, respectively, which is similar to that of total body water, reflecting their high aqueous solubility, low lipophilicity and lack of tissue binding. Steady-state predose ($C_{min.ss}$) concentrations of gabapentin in cerebrospinal fluid are approximately 5–35% of the corresponding plasma concentration reflecting gabapentin's CSF-to-plasma partition ratio of 0.1–0.2. The median time to peak CSF concentration of pregabalin occurs at ~8 h following oral administration [8].

Metabolism and Elimination

Neither drug undergoes appreciable hepatic metabolism and approximately 98% of the absorbed dose is excreted unchanged in urine. The elimination half-life of gabapentin is 4.6–8.7 h and is unaltered by the size of dose or multiple dosing. Gabapentin's elimination rate constant, plasma clearance, and renal clearance are directly proportional to creatinine clearance, so dose and frequency should be reduced accordingly in patients suffering from renal dysfunction and in elderly patients. As gabapentin can be removed from the plasma by haemodialysis, a small supplemental dose should be administered posthaemodialysis to provide steady-state plasma levels.

Drug Interactions

No clinically significant drug–drug interactions have been reported with gabapentin or pregabalin because of their low protein binding, lack of hepatic metabolism and low propensity to induce or inhibit hepatic microsomal enzymes.

Indications

Currently the gabapentinoids are only licensed for chronic neuropathic pain, epilepsy and anxiety (pregabalin only). However, they have been widely used as part of a multimodal approach to post-operative pain relief. The rationale for the use of gabapentinoids in the acute setting is that there is a significant neuropathic component to post-operative pain, particularly with operations that damage peripheral nerves (e.g. amputation, thoracotomy and mastectomy). Consequently, gabapentinoids may improve analgesia and reduce opioid consumption by reducing central sensitization.

Acute Post-operative Pain

Analgesic Effect

Although early preclinical models suggested that gabapentinoids possess activity as analgesic agents there does not seem to have been any further interest in this area, possibly because of their low potency as analgesics. A systematic review of four unpublished placebo-controlled studies found that gabapentin, 250 mg, provided some relief in acute dental and orthopaedic post-operative pain but concluded that with NNT 11 it was not clinically useful as a stand-alone analgesic [10]. Similarly, pregabalin, 300 mg, was superior to placebo in a surgical dental pain model [11].

Adjuvant Effect

The use of gabapentinoids as adjuvant drugs to enhance post-operative pain relief has been extensively investigated such that over the last 10 years there have been a succession of systematic reviews [10, 12–22] as well as a several narrative reviews [23–27]. Trials analysed in these meta-analyses have used a range of gabapentin and pregabalin dosing regimens, and there has also been significant clinical and statistical heterogeneity. Therefore, it is possible that some reviews may have overemphasised the benefits of gabapentinoids. Nevertheless, as the number of studies of the efficacy of gabapentinoids has increased it has become clear that peri-operative gabapentin and possibly also pregabalin have significant benefit with regard to acute post-operative pain relief and opioid requirements. The most recent meta-analyses have included more than 130 studies of gabapentin [20] but to date there have been less than half that number of studies of pregabalin available for analysis [21, 22].

Gabapentin and pregabalin are associated with a statistically significant reduction in pain scores. The mean reduction in pain intensity score at 24 h ranges from 5% to 15% for gabapentin [20] but is less consistent with pregabalin, ranging from 0% to 16% [19, 21, 22]. It has been suggested that a reduction in acute pain intensity of 20–33% or ≥2 on a 0–10 numeric rating scale [28, 29] or of 10% in chronic pain [30] constitutes a clinically important response. Consequently, it is debateable whether or not use of gabapentin and pregabalin result in a clinically meaningful reduction in pain score.

Gabapentin and pregabalin are associated with a statistically significant reduction in opioid consumption. The mean reduction in 24-h opioid consumption is of the order 8- to 30-mg morphine equivalent (or about 35–60% reduction), for gabapentin [20, 26] and 8–13 mg morphine equivalent (or about 25% reduction), for pregabalin [21, 26]. This reduction in opioid consumption is associated with a significant reduction in opioid-related side effects such as nausea, vomiting and pruritus. However, despite pregabalin having an opioid-sparing effect that is similar to gabapentin it is associated with a significantly higher incidence of sedation, dizziness and visual disturbances.

Dosing Considerations

Timing of Dose

The beneficial effects of the gabapentinoids on post-operative pain and opioid requirements have been investigated with single and multiple dose regimens, as well as with low- and high-dose regimens. The concept that pre-operative dosing is crucial for reducing post-operative pain and opioid requirement has not been entirely supported by clinical trials. Single-dose crossover trials of pre-operative versus post-operative administration of gabapentin and pregabalin have failed to demonstrate a clear advantage for pre-operative administration [20, 31]. Indeed, one meta-analysis commented that the post-operative effects of gabapentin appeared to be equivalent when given before or after surgery [21]. Furthermore, another study using a surgical dental pain model reported that post-operative administration of pregabalin 75 mg was associated with greater reduction in opioid consumption than pre-operative administration [32]. One might speculate that this could be the result of an analgesic effect of gabapentin as previously discussed [10]. Most single-dose studies have administered the pre-operative dose of gabapentinoid 2 h before surgery, whilst the majority of multiple dose studies have administered the pre-operative dose of gabapentinoid between 1 and 2 h before surgery. However, the time to peak plasma concentration after oral administration is up to 2 h for low-dose gabapentin, up to 4 h for high-dose gabapentin and up to 1 h for pregabalin. Furthermore, the median time to peak pregabalin concentration in cerebrospinal fluid occurs much later, being of the order of 6–8 h after oral administration [8, 33]. Therefore, it is likely that in order to be fully effective, gabapentinoids should be administered several hours pre-operatively.

Single Dose Versus Multiple Dose

Two systematic reviews have stated that the optimal regimen for the peri-operative administration of gabapentin, and in particular single versus multiple dose regimens, needs to be investigated through adequately powered dose-response studies [12, 15]. Ho and colleagues analysed single high dose (1200 mg), single low dose (<1200 mg) and multiple dose gabapentin separately but the number of trials was small and the authors made no comparison between single and multiple dosing [12]. Mishriky and colleagues have investigated whether the frequency of administration of pregabalin impacts on analgesic efficacy. While both single and multiple dosing was associated with a significant opioid-sparing effect the reduction in pain scores was limited to multiple dosing only. Furthermore, the reduction in pain scores was modest and not likely to be clinically relevant [21]. The authors concluded that there appears to be no significant benefit for acute pain outcomes from repeated dosing of pregabalin compared with a single pre-operative dose ≥100 mg. The authors did not specifically address the potential benefit of multiple dosing on CPSP but confined their analysis to the effect of gabapentinoids on acute post-operative pain. In support of their conclusion Mishriky cite a study by Buvanendran and colleagues that reported no difference in acute pain outcomes between groups given pregabalin, either as a single pre-operative 150 mg dose, or three peri-operative 150 mg doses [34]. In contrast, an earlier narrative review suggested that continuing gabapentin or pregabalin post-operatively is likely to be more effective than a single pre-operative dose of either gabapentinoid [31].

Low Dose Versus High Dose

Relatively few studies have attempted to identify the optimal dose of gabapentin or pregabalin for peri-operative use. In a narrative review Schmidt and colleagues identified only five trials; three studied gabapentin and two studied pregabalin. Pain scores were lower in patients who received doses of gabapentin >600 mg and doses of pregabalin >150 mg. Two studies also reported reduction in opioid consumption with higher doses. However, the number of patients studied in each trial group was small. Schmidt and colleagues concluded that higher doses of gabapentin and pregabalin were more effective than lower doses. Interestingly these authors then recommended using even higher doses of gabapentin (1200 mg as opposed to 600 mg) and pregabalin (300 mg as opposed to 150 mg) than were identified as effective in their review [31]. In contrast, Mathiesen and colleagues concluded that the opioid sparing effect of gabapentin was not significantly greater with doses higher than 600 mg [15]. Whilst a more recent review has recommended that future trials should investigate the use of pre-operative gabapentin doses between 600 and 1200 mg [20]. Therefore, it is likely that the optimal dose of gabapentin is between 600 and 1200 mg and the optimal dose of pregabalin is between 150 and 300 mg.

Use of Gabapentinoids in Different Types of Surgery

Whether the type of surgery has a substantial influence on the effectiveness of analgesics is debatable. Thus, it has been suggested that pain level *per se* rather than the extent of the surgical procedure will dictate the effectiveness of analgesics. Indeed, a large observational study has found that the extent of the surgical procedure was not related to post-operative pain intensity [35]. Furthermore, two recent meta-analyses have reported that the analgesic effect of gabapentin and pregabalin were determined by the type of surgery only insofar as the amount of pain caused by the surgery [20, 21]. Thus, the absolute effect of gabapentin is proportionate to the severity of post-operative pain and opioid requirement without gabapentin [22]. Whilst a recent meta-analysis by Eipe and colleagues reported that pregabalin was only effective in surgeries associated with pro-nociceptive pain [22]. Indeed, there is some discussion regarding the types of surgery for which gabapentinoids are indicated. Surgery associated with a high risk of neuropathic pain would seem an appropriate indication. In, addition Mishriky and colleagues undertook a sensitivity analysis according to type of surgery which would seem to suggest that pregabalin is more effective for open abdominal surgery than laparoscopic abdominal surgery [21] although this difference may only reflect the difference in pain.

Side Effects of Gabapentinoids

Between one third and a half of patients experience a side effect associated with gabapentinoid therapy. However, whereas somnolence, ataxia and fatigue are significantly more common in gabapentin and pregabalin treated patients, opioid-related side effects such as nausea, vomiting and pruritus are significantly less common [20, 21]. Pregabalin use is also associated with a significant increase in dizziness and visual disturbances [21]. Furthermore, respiratory depression associated with pregabalin use has been reported in elderly patients and in patients receiving concomitant sedative or hypnotic therapy [22]. In addition, gabapentin is effective in reducing pre-operative anxiety especially in patients with higher anxiety scores. The pre-operative anxiolytic effect of pregabalin has been less clearly demonstrated [21] even at doses that produce significant sedation [36].

Use of Gabapentinoids in Persistent Post-operative Pain

With increasing evidence of a beneficial effect of gabapentinoids on acute post-operative pain their potential for preventing persistent post-operative pain has attracted increasing interest. Clarke and colleagues conducted a systematic review of studies that examined the preventive effects of gabapentinoids on pain that persisted for at least 2 months after surgery (chronic postsurgical pain; CPSP) [37]. There was considerable heterogeneity among the 11 that met the inclusion criteria. Nevertheless, meta-analysis demonstrated a statistically significant reduction in CPSP with gabapentin ($P = 0.04$) and with pregabalin ($P = 0.07$). In addition, both gabapentin and pregabalin improved long-term functional outcome. These authors felt that there was sufficient evidence to suggest that using a high pre-operative dose of gabapentin (1200 mg) was more effective in preventing CPSP and improving functional outcome than using a low pre-operative dose. However, these findings have not been replicated by two subsequent meta-analyses with more rigorous selection criteria. Chaparro and colleagues failed to demonstrate a statistically significant effect of gabapentin on the incidence of CPSP at 3 and 6 months [38], whilst Mishriky and colleagues concluded that there was only limited data to suggest a possible benefit of pregabalin on CPSP at 6 and 12 months [21].

Practical Considerations

Gabapentin or Pregabalin?

Although there have been a greater number of studies of the use of gabapentin than pregabalin, recent meta-analyses have concluded that both peri-operative gabapentin and pregabalin improve post-operative analgesia. A narrative review has suggested that there is more and better evidence for preferring gabapentin over pregabalin to reduce early post-operative pain [31]. However, to date there have been only five comparative studies of gabapentin with pregabalin, and no meta-analyses. Four of these studies compared gabapentin (600–1200 mg) with pregabalin (150–300 mg) as a single pre-operative dose administered prior to institution of spinal anaesthesia for a variety of surgeries [39–42], whilst a fifth study compared gabapentin (600 mg) with pregabalin (150 mg) administered prior to general anaesthesia and continued post-operatively [43]. There was no difference between gabapentin and pregabalin in respect of post-operative pain scores or analgesic requirement with the exception of one study, which found that pregabalin, was superior to gabapentin in reducing post-operative analgesic requirements [42]. Four out of the five studies found that pregabalin was associated with a longer time to request first analgesia. The incidence of side effects was similar.

In summary, whether one agent is more effective or has fewer side effects is unclear and requires further investigation. Despite its more favourable pharmacokinetic profile there is at present insufficient evidence to prefer pregabalin to gabapentin, particularly given the cost advantage in favour of gabapentin.

Guidelines for Rational Prescribing of Gabapentinoids

In 2015 the fourth edition of the Australian and New Zealand College of Anaesthetists (ANZCA) *Acute Pain Management: Scientific Evidence* [44] suggested that, with respect to the gabapentinoids, it was not possible to recommend a particular treatment regimen and was unable to draw any conclusions regarding optimal treatment duration or potential long-term benefits such as reduced CPSP. In 2012, the American Society of Anaesthesiologists published updated practice guidelines for acute pain management in the peri-operative setting [45]. The task force strongly endorsed the use of multimodal pain management therapies whenever possible and suggested that gabapentin and pregabalin should be considered as part of a post-operative multimodal pain management regimen. The task force did not recommend a particular treatment regimen. Indeed there are no official dosing guidelines for the use of gabapentinoids in the management of post-operative pain. Nevertheless, at least two institutions have made available their algorithms for the prescribing of peri-operative gabapentinoids [31, 46]. Combining these with the findings of recent meta-analyses it may be possible to derive rational dosing guidelines.

The Ottawa Hospital (TOH) Acute Pain Service has developed an algorithm for the safe use of pregabalin [46]. According to the algorithm, pregabalin is indicated for:

- Patients with pre-existing opioid dependence or tolerance
- Patients already receiving pregabalin therapy
- Patients with past experience of poorly controlled post-operative pain
- Patients suffering from chronic neuropathic pain
- Anticipated surgery in a site of chronic pain
- Anticipated acute post-operative pain with hyperalgesia

According to the algorithm, pregabalin, 50–75 mg, should be administered 2 h pre-operatively, followed by 50 mg three times a day for 5 days, but with the option to continue for a further 5 days if necessary. The algorithm recommends decreasing the dose by 25 mg for each decade above 50 years of age, so that patients older than 80 years do not receive any pregabalin pre-operatively. In addition, the dose is reduced by 50% for patients with sleep deprivation, neuraxial opioids, renal insufficiency or obstructive sleep apnoea and avoided in any patient found to have more than two of these risk factors. For patients with renal dysfunction, dosing is reduced proportionately based on creatinine clearance to 25 mg once daily for clearance lower than 15 mL/h.

In contrast, Schmidt and colleagues consider that higher dose regimens may be more effective than lower dose regimens in reducing immediate postsurgical pain [32]. Clarke and colleagues have also endorsed using higher doses of gabapentinoids, particularly when the emphasis is on reducing the likelihood of CPSP [37]. Schmidt and colleagues suggest that peri-operative gabapentinoids are particularly indicated for:

Table 4.2 Peri-operative gabapentin and pregabalin dosing regimens[a]

Drug	Pre-operative dose	Post-operative dose
Gabapentin		
Chang et al. [25]	300–600 mg; 1 h preop	1200 mg/day
Clarke et al. [37]	1200 mg; 2 h preop	NA
Doleman et al. [20]	600–1200 mg	NA
Schmidt et al. [31]	1200 mg; 2 h preop	1800 mg a day for 14 days
Weinbroum [24]	600–1200 mg; 1 h preop	1800 mg a day for 3–4 days
Pregabalin		
Eipe et al. [22]	50–75 mg; 2 h preop	150 mg a day for 5 days
Engelman et al. [18]	–	225–300 mg a day
Mishriky et al. [21]	100–300 mg	No benefit
Schmidt et al. [31]	300 mg 2 h preop	300 mg a day for 14 days
Weinbroum [24]	150 mg	300 mg a day for 2 days

[a]Note the regimens presented here represent a synopsis of all the regimens analysed by the authors of each individual review

- Patients who are receiving high doses of opioids pre-operatively
- Patients who are at risk of severe and prolonged post-operative pain where a neuropathic component is likely, such as post-thoracotomy.

These indications are similar to two of the indications in TOH Acute Pain Service's algorithm outlined above. Schmidt and colleagues propose a treatment regimen commencing with either gabapentin 1200 mg or pregabalin 150 mg administered at least 2 h pre-operatively and if possible even the night before surgery, followed by gabapentin 600 mg three times a day for 14 days or pregabalin 150 mg twice a day for 14 days. Schmidt and colleagues conclude that although a pre-operative dose is desirable the failure to administer such a dose should not deter clinicians from post-operative dosing [31].

Apart from the treatment algorithms outlined above it is possible to identify from the various reviews of the gabapentinoids the most common peri-operative gabapentinoid treatment regimens that have been employed in studies. A summary of the doses and treatment regimens of gabapentin and pregabalin is provided in Table 4.2. There is clearly a need for studies investigating the benefits of guidelines on pain outcomes to elucidate the appropriate pre-operative dose, maintenance dose and duration of treatment.

Gabapentinoids as Part of an Enhanced Recovery Programme

A structured approach to peri-operative care, including pain management, is an integral part of an enhanced recovery after surgery (ERAS) programme. Among the many benefits of ERAS are better patient outcomes and reduced length of stay. Consequentially, the opioid-sparing effect of the gabapentinoids may offer potential advantages for ERAS programmes. There is now emerging evidence of an effect of gabapentinoids on hospital length of stay. Thus, one systematic review identified five studies that recorded duration of hospital stay or time to achieve hospital discharge criteria [21]. The authors found that pregabalin-treated patients had a shorter hospital stay or achieved hospital discharge criteria 14 h earlier than controls. More recently, Cheng and colleagues have found that gabapentin reduced opioid use and hospital length of stay in mastectomy patients [47]. In contrast, a randomised, placebo-controlled trial of the effect of a single pre-operative oral dose of gabapentin, 600 mg, in major bowel surgery found no reduction in opioid consumption, opioid-related side effects, time of return of bowel function, or time to hospital discharge [48].

Conclusions

Although not licensed for the management of acute pain, there is now good evidence that peri-operative gabapentin and pregabalin are associated with a modest reduction in post-operative pain whilst the impact on opioid consumption is more pronounced. However, there are fewer studies on which to draw conclusions regarding pregabalin. Conversely it is possible that as a result of clinical and statistical heterogeneity, some reviews may have overemphasised the benefits of gabapentinoids. In choosing between gabapentinoids there is insufficient evidence to support the use of pregabalin in preference to gabapentin, notwithstanding pregabalin's more favourable pharmacokinetic profile. The appropriate dose and timing of administration of gabapentinoid has yet to be elucidated, but it would appear that single dosing whether before or after surgery may be as effective as multiple dosing. In addition, higher doses may be more effective in reducing both acute post-operative pain and persistent post-operative pain, but this advantage is at the expense of a higher incidence of unwanted side effects.

References

1. Radley DC, Finkelstein SN, Stafford RS. Off-label prescribing among office-based physicians. Intern Med. 2006;166:1021–6.
2. Fukuda C, Kohler JC, Boon H, Austin Z, Krahn M. Prescribing gabapentin off label: perspectives from psychiatry, pain and neurology specialists. Can Pharm J. 2012;145:280–4.
3. NHS England. Advice for prescribers on the risk of misuse of pregabalin and gabapentin. www.gov.uk/government/uploads/system/uploads/attachment_data/ file/385791/PHE-NHS_England_pregabalin_and_gabapentin_advice_Dec_2014.pdf.
4. Chincholkar M. Analgesic mechanisms of gabapentinoids and effects in experimental pain models: a narrative review. Br J Anaesth. 2018;120:1315–34.
5. Eroglu C, Allen NJ, Susman MW, et al. The gabapentin receptor α2δ-1 is the neuronal thrombospondin receptor responsible for excitatory CNS synaptogenesis. Cell. 2009;139:380–92.
6. Park S, Ahn ES, Han DW, Lee JH, Min KT, Kim H, Hong Y-W. Pregabalin and gabapentin inhibit substance P-induced NF-κB activation in neuroblastoma and glioma cells. J Cell Biochem. 2008;105:414–23.
7. Gale JD, Houghton LA. Alpha 2 delta (α(2)δ) ligands, gabapentin and pregabalin: what is the evidence for potential use of these ligands in irritable bowel syndrome. Front Pharmacol. 2011;2:28.

8. Bockbrader HN, Wesche D, Miller R, Chapel S, Janiczek N, Burger P. A comparison of the pharmacokinetics and pharmacodynamics of pregabalin and gabapentin. Clin Pharmacokinet. 2010;49:661–9.
9. Chen C, Cowles VE, Sweeney M. The intestinal absorption mechanism of gabapentin makes it appropriate for gastroretentive delivery. Curr Clin Pharmacol. 2013;8:67–72.
10. Straube S, Derry S, Moore RA, Wiffen PJ, Mcquay HJ. Single dose gabapentin for established acute postoperative pain in adults. Cochrane Database Syst Rev. 2010;5:CD008183.
11. Hill CM, Balkenohl M, Thomas DW, Walker R, Mathé H, Murray G. Pregabalin in patients with postoperative dental pain. Eur J Pain. 2001;5:119–24.
12. Ho KY, Gan TJ, Habib AS. Gabapentin and postoperative pain: a systematic review of randomized controlled trials. Pain. 2006;126:91–101.
13. Seib RK, Paul JE. Preoperative gabapentin for postoperative analgesia: a meta-analysis. Can J Anaesth. 2006;53:461–9.
14. Tippana EM, Hamunen K, Kontinen VK, Kalso E. Do surgical patients benefit from perioperative gabapentin/pregabalin? A syteamtic review of safety and efficacy. Anesth Analg. 2007;104:1545–56.
15. Mathiesen O, Møiniche S, Dahl JB. Gabapentin and postoperative pain: a qualitative and quantitative systematic review, with focus on procedure. BMC Anesthesiol. 2007;7:6. Available at: www.biomedcentral.com/1471-2253/7/6.
16. Peng PWH, Wijesundera DN, Li CCF. Use of gabapentin for perioperative pain control – a meta-analysis. Pain Res Manag. 2007;12:85–92.
17. Moore RA, Straube S, Wiffen PJ, Derry S, Mcquay HJ. Pregabalin for acute and chronic pain in adults. Cochrane Database Syst Rev. 2009;3:CD007076.
18. Engelman E, Cateloy F. Efficacy and safety of perioperative pregabalin for postoperative pain: a meta-analysis of randomized-controlled trials. Acta Anaesthesiol Scand. 2011;55:927–43.
19. Zhang J, Ho KY, Wang Y. Efficacy of pregabalin in acute postoperative pain: a meta analysis. Br J Anaesth. 2011;106:454–62.
20. Dolemnan B, Heinink TP, Read DJ, Faleiro J, Lund JN, Williams JP. A systematic review and a meta-regression analysis of prophylactic gabapentin for postoperative pain. Anaesthesia. 2015;70:1186–204.
21. Mishriky BM, Waldron NH, Habib AS. Impact of pregabalin on acute and persistent postoperative pain: a systematic review and a meta-analysis. Br J Anaesth. 2015;114:10–31.
22. Eipe N, Penning J, Yazdi F, Mallick R, Turner L, Ahmadzai N, Ansari MT. Perioperative use of pregabalin for acute pain—a systematic review and meta-analysis. Pain. 2015;156:1284–300.
23. Baidya DK, Agarwal A, Khanna P, Arora MK. Pregabalin in acute and chronic pain. J Anaesthesiol Clin Pharmacol. 2011;27:307–14.
24. Weinbroum AA. Non-opioid IV adjuvants in the perioperative period: pharmacological and clinical aspects of ketamine and gabapentinoids. Pharm Res. 2012;65:411–29.
25. Chang CY, Challa CK, Shah J, Eloy JD. Gabapentin in acute postoperative pain management. Biomed Res Int. 2014;2014:631756. https://doi.org/10.1155/2014/631756.
26. Dahl JB, Nielson RV, Wettersley J, Nikolaisen L, Hamunen K, Kontinen VK, et al. Postoperative analgesic effects of paracetamol, NSAIDs, glucocorticoids, gabapentinoids and their combinations: a topical review. Acta Anaesthesiol Scand. 2014;58:1165–81.
27. Schug S, Goddard C. Recent advances in the pharmacological management of acute and chronic pain. Ann Palliat Med. 2014;3:263–75.
28. Farrar JT, Berlin JA, Strom BL. Clinically important changes in acute pain outcome measures: a validation study. J Pain Symptom Manage. 2003;25:406–11.
29. Cepeda MS, Africano JM, Polo R, Alcal R, Cepeda DB. What decline in pain intensity is meaningful to patients with acute pain? Pain. 2003;105:151–7.
30. Dworkin RH, Turk DC, Wyrwich KW, Beeton D, Cleeland CS, Farrar JT, et al. Interpreting the clinical importance of treatment outcomes in chronic pain clinical trials: IMMPACT recommendations. J Pain. 2008;9:105–21.
31. Schmidt PC, Ruchelli G, Mackey SC, Carroll IR. Perioperative gabapentinoids: choice of agent, dose, timing, and effects on chronic postsurgical pain. Anesthesiology. 2013;119:1215–21.

32. Cheung CW, Choi WS, Leung YY, Lui F, Ng JK, Hei-Ho AM, Irwin MG. A double-blind randomized crossover study to evaluate the timing of pregabalin for third molar surgery under local anesthesia. J Oral Maxillofac Surg. 2012;70:25–30.
33. Buvanendran A, Kroin JS, Kari M, Tuman KJ. Can a single dose of 300 mg of pregabalin reach acute antihyperalgesic levels in the central nervous system? Reg Anesth Pain Med. 2010;35:535–8.
34. Buvanendran A, Kroin JS, Della Valle CJ, Morica M, Turman KJ. Cerebrospinal fluid neurotransmitter changes during the perioperative period in patients undergoing total knee replacement: a randomized trial. Anesth Analg. 2012;114:434–41.
35. Gerbershagen HJ, Aduckathil S, van Wyck AJM, Peelen LM, Kalkman CJ, Meissner W. Pain intensity on the first day after surgery: a prospective cohort study comparing 179 surgical procedures. Anesthesiology. 2013;118:934–44.
36. White PF, Tufanogullari B, Taylor J, Klein K. The effect of pregabalin on preoperative anxiety and sedation levels: a dose-ranging study. Anesth Analg. 2009;108:1140–5.
37. Clarke H, Bonin RP, Orser BA, Englesakis M, Wijesundera DN, Katz J. The prevention of chronic postsurgical pain using gabapentin and pregabalin: a combined systematic review and meta-analysis. Anesth Analg. 2012;115:428–42.
38. Chaparro LE, Smith SA, Moore RA, Wiffen PJ, Gilron I. Pharmacotherapy for the prevention of chronic pain after surgery in adults. Cochrane Database Syst Rev. 2013;7:CD008307.
39. Saraswat V, Arora V. Preemptive gabapentin vs pregabalin for acute postoperative pain after surgery under spinal anaesthesia. Indian J Anaesth. 2008;52:829–34.
40. Ghai A, Gupta M, Hooda S, Singla D, Wadhera R. A randomized controlled trial to compare pregabalin with gabapentin for postoperative pain in abdominal hysterectomy. Saudi J Anaesth. 2011;5:252–7.
41. Bafna U, Rajarajeshwaran K, Khandelwal M, Verma AP. A comparison of effect of preemptive use of oral gabapentin and pregabalin for acute post-operative pain after surgery under spinal anesthesia. J Anaesthesiol Clin Pharmacol. 2014;30:373–7.
42. Rajendran I, Basavareddy A, Meher BR, Srinivasan S. Prospective, randomised, double blinded controlled trial of gabapentin and pregabalin as pre emptive analgesia in patients undergoing lower abdominal and limb surgery under spinal anaesthesia. Indian J Pain. 2014;28:155–9.
43. Ozgencil E, Yalcin S, Tuna H, Yorukoglu D, Kecik Y. Perioperative administration of gabapentin 1,200 mg day^{-1} and pregabalin 300 mg day^{-1} for pain following lumbar laminectomy and discectomy: a randomised, double-blinded, placebo controlled study. Singapore Med J. 2011;52:883–9.
44. Schug SA, Palmer GM, Scott DA, Halliwell R, Trince J, editors. Acute pain management: scientific evidence. 4th ed. Melbourne: Australian and New Zealand College of Anaesthetists and Faculty of Pain Medicine; 2015. www.anzca.edu.au/resources/college-publications.
45. American Society of Anesthesiologists Task Force on Acute Pain Management. Practice guidelines for acute pain management in the perioperative setting: an updated report by the American Society of Anesthesiologists Task Force on Acute Pain Management. Anesthesiology. 2012;116:248–73.
46. Eipe N, Penning J. Postoperative respiratory depression associated with pregabalin: a case series and a preoperative decision algorithm. Pain Res Manag. 2011;16:353–6.
47. Cheng ZH, Frenk V, Bishop JD, Bowling T, Pass HA. Multimodality perioperative analgesia with paravertebral nerve block and gabapentin reduces narcotic use and hospital length of stay in mastectomy patients. Cancer Res. 2015;75(9 Suppl):P2-13-11.
48. Siddiqui NT, Fischer H, Guerina L, Friedman Z. Effect of a preoperative gabapentin on postoperative analgesia in patients with inflammatory bowel disease following major bowel surgery: a randomized, placebo-controlled trial. Pain Pract. 2014;14:132–9.

Peri-operative Ketamine for Acute Pain Management

5

Naveen Eipe

Key Points

1. Ketamine is useful as a co-analgesic and antihyperalgesic, thereby decreasing post-operative pain, opioid analgesic requirements and opioid related side-effects following major abdominal surgery.
2. High-dose ketamine is >1 mg/kg as bolus and >1 mg/kg/h as infusion; low-dose constitutes 0.1–1 mg/kg bolus and 0.1–1 mg/kg/h infusions and ultra-low dose is <0.1 mg/kg and <0.1 mL/kg/h infusion.
3. Post-operatively it may be added to an opioid for PCA use.
4. This will assist the patient in achieving their ERAS goals, i.e., early mobilization, early nutrition and discharge with improved satisfaction.

Introduction

Ketamine was first introduced into clinical practice over 50 years ago as a dissociative anaesthetic [1]. It has since been used for pre-medication, sedation, induction and maintenance of general anaesthesia and for post-operative analgesia. Despite this long standing and wide use both as an anaesthetic and analgesic, its peri-operative role has enjoyed a somewhat waxing and waning popularity. In pain management, ketamine's use has ranged from treating battlefield trauma and burn injuries to acute and chronic, cancer and non-cancer pain. The peri-operative use of ketamine is now backed by extensive experience and good quality evidence [2].

The peri-operative role of multimodal analgesia has been discussed in detail in the preceding chapter on intravenous lidocaine. An acute pain management framework

N. Eipe
Department of Anesthesiology and Pain Medicine, The Ottawa Hospital, University of Ottawa, Ottawa, ON, Canada
e-mail: neipe@toh.on.ca

A. Krige, M. J. P. Scott (eds.), *Analgesia in Major Abdominal Surgery*,
https://doi.org/10.1007/978-3-319-94482-1_5

based on the WHO ladder concept provides us with a step-wise, severity-based, opioid-sparing approach. This has been accepted and implemented widely in simple and standardised peri-operative protocols. The dual appreciation of the role of pronociception in acute pain and the emerging understanding of opioid-induced and opioid-resistant hyperalgesia has led to the recognition for the need for appropriate non-opioid adjuvants with anti-hyperalgesic properties (*see* Chap. 6, Fig. 6.2).

Due to the concurrent introduction of laparoscopic surgery, and the emergence of the principles of Enhanced Recovery after Surgery (ERAS) for abdominal surgery in the past two decades, the entire peri-operative paradigm has shifted from 'bigger and slower' to 'smaller and faster'. In parallel with these surgical changes, there has been a quest for a suitable alternative to epidural analgesia coupled with a renewed interest in *parenteral* non-opioid analgesia. It is in this context that ketamine (and lidocaine) can play a major role by ensuring adequate pain relief coupled with minimal immediate side effects and quantifiable long-term benefits.

Another aspect of multimodal analgesia is that despite recent advances in the pharmacotherapy of acute pain, ketamine remains the *numero uno* non-opioid anti-hyperalgesic adjuvant available for use in peri-operative pain management. Therefore, the role of ketamine in pain management after abdominal surgery cannot be ignored or underestimated [2, 3].

To incorporate ketamine into acute pain management after abdominal surgery it is therefore important to understand the pharmacology of this drug, critically evaluate the evidence for its use and appreciate the practicalities of using ketamine in a rational peri-operative pain management plan.

Pharmacology of N-Methyl-D-Aspartate (NMDA) Receptors (NMDARS)

The NMDARs belong to a class of ionotropic glutamate receptors that also includes the α-amino-3-hydroxy-5-methyl-4-isoxazolepropionic acid (AMPA) receptors (AMPARs) and kainate receptors. Excitatory synaptic transmission in the vertebrate brain relies on the release of L-glutamate from presynaptic terminals that diffuses across the synaptic cleft and binds to postsynaptic AMPARs and NMDARs. Activation of AMPARs is fast and transient, causing brief depolarizations that last no longer than a few milliseconds. NMDARs are not critical for this basal synaptic transmission, but instead they regulate functional and structural plasticity of individual synapses, dendrites, and neurons by allowing activation of specific calcium (Ca^{2+}) dependent signaling cascades [4].

NMDARs are densely expressed at nociceptive synapses in the spinal cord dorsal horn. At resting membrane potentials, external magnesium (Mg^{2+}) ions enter the NMDAR pore, but unlike the permeant calcium (Ca^{2+}) ions, they bind tightly and prevent further ion permeation. A depolarization of sufficient amplitude and duration is required to dislodge and repel the Mg^{2+} ions from the pore, thereby allowing the flow of permeant Ca^{2+}ions. As a result, the NMDAR acts as a molecular coincidence detector: efficient activation and ion permeation through the NMDAR requires both a sufficiently strong depolarization and synaptic release of glutamate. This dual input requirement, together with the slow activation and deactivation allows NMDARs to integrate and decode incoming synaptic activity. The additional high Ca^{2+} permeability of NMDARs enables them to transduce specific synaptic input patterns into long-lasting alterations in synaptic strength. Activation of the NMDAR occurring after an intense or repeated stimulus results in increases in cell excitability because of second messenger effects initiated by the calcium influx [1, 2].

This role of NMDAR in nociceptive transmission has been well established in humans. In acute nociceptive pain, the Mg^{2+} ions get pushed out into the synaptic cleft and the NMDAR opens to Ca^{2+}, which then activates the second messenger system that propagates the signal. When prolonged or repetitive signalling through the synaptic cleft occurs, the NMDAR can get involved in sustained neuronal hyperactivity i.e. simple signal propagation can change into transmission persistence despite cessation of input stimulus. Hyper-excitability of the NMDAR also explains the development and maintenance of what can be called "pathologic pain" or pro-nociception, i.e., increased pain perception as a result of pain sensitization and synaptic plasticity [2]. A NMDAR-mediated increase in dorsal horn synaptic efficacy is therefore thought to be an important contributor to the central sensitization of pain pathways seen in acute hyperalgesia, opioid tolerance, opioid-induced hyperalgesia (OIH) and in chronic pain syndromes [5]. Finally, while ongoing and future work may confirm that NMDAR activation is the sentinel event in the progression of acute pain to chronic pain, its pharmacology will continue to play a pivotal role in managing acute pain and hyperalgesia (Fig. 5.1).

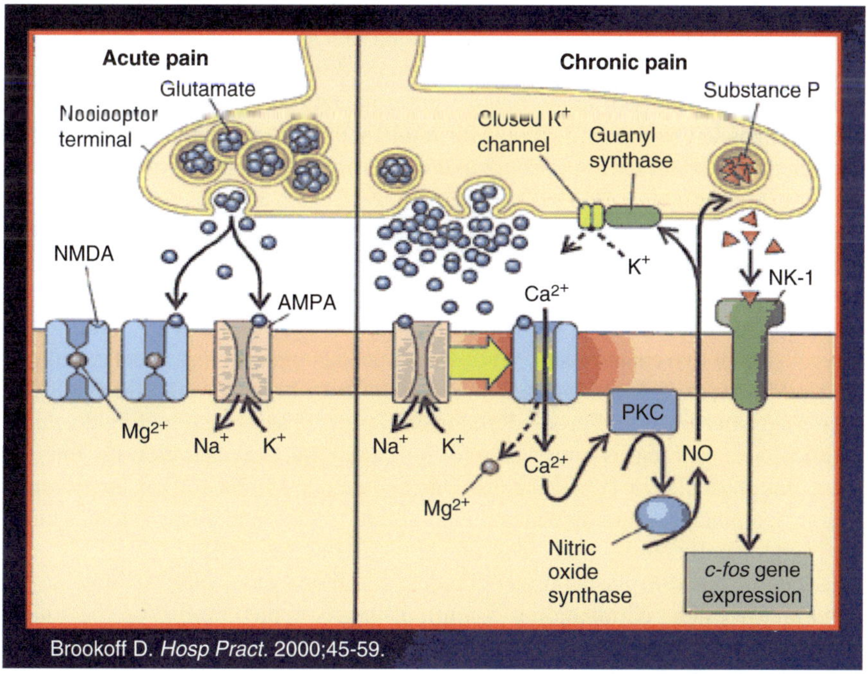

Fig. 5.1 The role of the NMDAR in acute and chronic pain. From [31]; with permission

The clinical relevance of these functions of the NMDARs in pain transmission, amplification and perpetuation is the basis for the use of its antagonists (ketamine, dextromethorphan, nitrous oxide and methadone etc.) in peri-operative pain management [1–3].

Pharmacology of Ketamine

Ketamine is the most widely used, well studied and probably the most potent NMDAR antagonist. It is a phencyclidine (PCP) derivate that was synthesized in 1963 and first used as an intravenous anaesthetic in 1965 [1]. It was approved for clinical use in 1970 and was initially used primarily as an anaesthetic in war-time, natural disasters, other remote and low resource areas. Early experience suggested that wide acceptance would be limited by the side effect profile i.e. the dissociative state during, and the psychomimetic emergence reactions after use. Nevertheless, early users documented the cardio-respiratory stability and the profound analgesia that also lasted well beyond the duration of infusion. Ketamine remains on the WHO's list of Essential Drugs. One of only two intravenous anaesthetics on this list which probably reflects its continued versatility as a relatively safe solo-agent intravenous anaesthetic.

Ketamine has been widely used for decades in veterinary surgery as an anaesthetic and has earned the moniker "horse tranquilizer". This extensive use of ketamine clinically for both human and animal use led to its increased production and subsequent widespread availability. Unfortunately, this use has indirectly also led to a significant increase in the diversion for non-clinical use and abuse of ketamine. The 'street', 'club' and 'party' use of ketamine (dubbed "Special K") is administered through a variety of routes and has unfortunately cast a shadow on its clinical use. This has led to the requirement for implementation of more stringent control measures with restricted prescribing and dispensing. These two issues, the veterinary use and the abuse, are well known to the public and at times perceived as barriers to use by both patients and other healthcare providers. We believe that it is important to discuss and disclose these issues to patients receiving ketamine for post-operative pain.

Ketamine is 2-(2-Chlorophenyl)-2-(methylamino)cyclohexanone hydrochloride and consists of two enantiomers. While racaemic ketamine is more widely available the world over, the S-ketamine variant is more potent with fewer side effects and has been used extensively in Europe. Ketamine is prepared as a water and lipid soluble hydrochloride salt and is approved only for parenteral administration i.e. intravenous, intramuscular or subcutaneous. Other routes of administration for example neuraxial (spinal, epidural or caudal), enteral (oral, rectal) and others (nasal, sublingual and topical) continue to be described in off-label use [1, 2].

Ketamine has low plasma protein binding and high lipid solubility allowing for rapid uptake (alpha elimination 4–5 min), distribution and elimination (beta half-life of 2–3 h). Most (up to 80%) of the intravenously administered drug will be metabolized in the liver by cytochrome P450 system to norketamine whose potency is approximately a third of the parent drug. Ketamine and norketamine are excreted by the kidneys and can both accumulate in renal failure. The clinical relevance of the pharmacokinetics of ketamine in hepatic and renal impairment is the decreased metabolism and delayed elimination respectively, thereby requiring dose or administration frequency reductions [1].

Ketamine primarily binds noncompetitively to the phencyclidine binding site of NMDARs and also modifies them *via* allosteric mechanisms thereby decreasing the glutamate transmission of synaptic impulses. Since these receptors are present in the thalamus and the limbic system in addition to the spinal cord, depending on the dose, the NMDAR mediated actions can have spinal and supraspinal effects. Ketamine may also have effects on dopamine, noradrenergic, serotonergic and opioid receptors. These may not be clinically relevant in the management of peri-operative pain. The cardiovascular, respiratory and gastrointestinal effects of ketamine could have an impact on the pain management of some patients and these have been well described elsewhere [2, 3].

The clinical effectiveness of ketamine in pain management requires the careful determination of the optimal balance that would provide benefit (analgesia) and avoid side effects (psychomimetic and disassociation). In our experience, the patient-to-patient variability with regards to analgesia from ketamine is small. The clinical presentation i.e. the cause of pain, severity, presence of acute hyperalgesia and concurrent opioid administration may be more important for the determination of the appropriate dose for each patient. Patients presenting with acute hyperalgesia, higher pain scores and increasing opioid requirements demonstrate the greatest benefit from the administration of ketamine. If an objective diagnosis of acute neuropathic pain is required to determine the need for ketamine, the DN4 questionnaire may be effectively used.

The clinical effects of ketamine can be described depending on the dose administered. In our experience, irrespective of most patient characteristics, these effects are almost always consistently observed. The dose of ketamine used peri-operatively can be arbitrarily divided into “high”, “low” and “ultra-low”.

It is unusual to use ketamine for pain relief in ‘anaesthetic dose’ or ‘high dose’ range (>1 mg/kg IV or >1 mg/kg/h infusion). At these levels, despite the profound analgesia, the patient will have unpredictable and persistent CNS effects i.e. loss of consciousness and airway reflexes, apnoea, labile cardiovascular effects, disassociation and lasting psychomimetic effects. The most significant latter can include unpleasant dreams, nightmares, abnormal sensations, emergence agitation, delirium, hallucinations and acute psychosis. In fact, at these doses, ketamine can be used to treat ECT-resistant depression and has even been reported to produce a pharmacologically induced model of schizophrenia [1].

When administered in a sub-anaesthetic “low dose” range (0.1–1 mg/kg IV bolus or 0.1–1 mg/kg/h infusion), ketamine’s analgesic efficacy correlates well with analgesia (or anti-nociception). It is induced directly at the spinal level (inhibition of NMDAR mediated pain facilitation) and indirectly at supraspinal level by decreasing the activity of brain structures that respond to noxious stimuli. It has also been shown that ketamine is able to modulate the transmission of pain impulses via interactions with the other receptors and pathways. Depending on the dose of ketamine, this anti-nociception may be due to the facilitated inhibition of the spinal opioid receptors or activation of the descending pain inhibitory monoaminergic pathways expressed at the spinal level by the alpha 2-adrenoceptors. Interestingly, the antinociception of ketamine at 0.3 mg/kg is not reversed by naloxone, suggesting that the opioid receptor agonistic activity was not involved in pain control [6].

"Ultra-low dose" ketamine refers to the use of less than 0.1 mg/kg bolus or less than 0.1 mg/kg/h [7]. This is probably the most useful dose of ketamine for post-operative use, especially in awake patients, as it avoids any CNS side effects. It probably works at the spinal level as a true co-analgesic adjuvant as it improves the analgesic effects of co-administered opioids. The affinity of ketamine for NMDA receptors is several-fold higher than for the non-NMDA receptors (mu and alpha receptors or the monoamine transporter sites). Therefore, at the lowest doses, it is possible that ketamine could interact almost exclusively with NMDA receptors rather than with the alpha receptor. This may explain its effective modulation of pain impulse transmission or anti-pronociception. There is some evidence from animal studies that at low dose ketamine may also directly provoke peripheral nociceptors, inducing analgesia and modulation within the peripheral nervous system. Animal studies have shown that locally administered ketamine effectively prevented withdrawal in formalin and thermal hyperalgesia testing in rats. Although ketamine exhibits promise as a potential topical analgesic in humans, the mechanistic basis of its peripheral actions is not well understood [8].

There may also be a significant synergistic interaction between opioids and NMDA antagonists. It has been postulated that ketamine can prevent central sensitization because while opioids can block the initial response of dorsal horn nociceptive neurons to C-fiber stimulation, NMDA antagonists inhibit the potentiation of abnormal and exaggerated responses on sustained or repeated stimulation [9].

There are two other important clinical situations where ketamine may also be useful. Firstly, it is well known that opioids themselves can worsen pain—*opioid-induced hyperalgesia* (OIH). Secondly, when increasing doses of opioids produce diminishing analgesic effects, clinical *opioid tolerance* is suspected. Both these paradoxical effects of opioid use are not restricted to the long term or long acting formulation use and can be seen in the early post-operative period. They are likely due to the interactions between, and activation of, the NMDARs by the mu-receptor agonists [6]. Ketamine may therefore be the drug of choice to prevent and or treat OIH and prevent the development of opioid tolerance in acute pain management [3].

Evidence for Efficacy

As mentioned earlier, clinical evidence for the use of ketamine dates back more than 4 decades [1]. The intra-operative cardio-respiratory stability was well documented in earlier studies, which also supports the safe use of this drug with minimal monitoring after surgery [10, 11]. The profound analgesia reported was also documented to last beyond the duration of injection or infusion. This was then a poorly understood analgesic effect but nevertheless probably further encouraged its continued and wider use as an anaesthetic in a variety of remote and low-resource settings, e.g., warfare, natural disasters, humanitarian outreach programs etc. Despite the safety profile, the use of ketamine as a sole anaesthetic or analgesic agent was, and is, limited by the potential for psychomimetic side effects and emergence like phenomena. These considerations continue to limit the dose, duration and overall use of ketamine for acute post-operative pain [2, 13].

Ketamine has been shown to be useful in the reduction of acute post-operative pain and analgesic consumption in a variety of surgical interventions with variable routes of administration [12]. Interest in the analgesic properties of low-dose ketamine has prompted clinical trials comparing opioids and ketamine [13]. Others have reported that peri-operative low-dose ketamine may be useful in a variety of clinical settings [14]. They also suggested that ketamine may be given at any point (pre-emptively, intra-operatively, post-operatively) and in any method (bolus, infusion, patient-controlled analgesia co-administration), but would be most useful when the anticipated post-operative visual analog scale (VAS) score is greater than 7/10 and when the site of surgery (and possibly the extent of the incision) has an impact on the efficacy of ketamine as a peri-operative adjuvant drug. However, they postulate that pain severity is more important than surgical site and conclude that abdominal surgery patients should receive ketamine, especially those patients or procedures where significant post-operative pain is expected [14].

Although many studies have suggested that peri-operative ketamine administration could be useful to control post-operative pain, their results are often difficult to compare due to the various ketamine dose regimens used [15]. The distinction of the infusion dose as being 'high', 'low' and 'ultra-low' dose (see preceding section) will probably contribute in the future to an improved understanding and increased confidence leading to wider and safer peri-operative use of this drug.

The importance of an 'adequate' dose of ketamine has been emphasized, in order to prevent the induction of central sensitization caused by stimulation of peripheral nociception together with blocking the wind-up phenomenon [13]. Studies have reported the adequacy of using a ketamine bolus of 0.5 mg/kg IV bolus followed by a 0.12 mg/kg/h infusion [15]. This was calculated to obtain a theoretical plasma ketamine concentration in the range of 100 mcg/mL previously described as being the therapeutic plasma concentration of ketamine for analgesia. At this and lower plasma concentrations, both psychomimetic effects and accumulation are likely to be avoided [15].

The dose of ketamine may also require adjustment according to the procedure. An arbitrary distinction into 'painful' and 'less painful' procedures has also been suggested. For the former a 0.5 mg/kg slow bolus injection of ketamine before or after induction of general anesthesia, was suggested. This may be followed by a continuous infusion of 0.5 mg/kg/h. In procedures expected to be less painful, a 0.25 mg/kg ketamine bolus before incision is recommended followed by infusions of 0.25 mg/kg/h. The continuous intra-operative infusion may also be replaced by appropriate hourly boluses. For procedures lasting longer than 2 h, these authors recommend that the infusion cease at least 60 min before surgery to prevent prolonged recovery [2].

In open abdominal surgery, continuous epidural analgesia is still probably the 'gold standard' for post-operative analgesia. Despite the use of local anaesthetics containing opioids insufficient epidural analgesia after surgery is not infrequent. This inadequacy of epidurals can be caused by epidural blockade failures, unilateral blockade, dose infusion limitations, developing relative or absolute contraindications (sepsis, anticoagulation, localized infection, delirium etc.) and/or patient intolerance to side effects (hypotension, postural symptoms, inability to ambulate etc.).

It has been suggested that combined and pre-emptive administration of ketamine with epidural analgesia may improve the quality of epidural analgesia in the post-operative period [16]. Neuraxial opioids may also result in acute tolerance to opioids and systemic ketamine may be required to prevent the development of acute tolerance to opioids. It has been postulated that viscero-peritoneal nociception is transmitted by multiple spinal nerves and the vagus nerve [17]. This nociception induces central sensitization not only segmentally, but also multi- and supra-segmentally. One of the analgesic action sites of ketamine is known to be supraspinal i.e. ketamine might block brainstem sensitization via the vagus or phrenic nerve during upper abdominal surgery. This may explain the frequently observed effect of ketamine in potentiating the epidural analgesic effects of the neuraxial opioid and local anaesthetic, which otherwise would only act segmentally [16, 17].

Level I evidence from systematic reviews confirm that low dose ketamine when combined with morphine not only reduced pain intensity but also improved wakefulness and PONV when compared with the higher dose of morphine alone [3, 14]. This is despite a significant number of clinical trials (17 of 38, 45%) demonstrating no benefit of adding ketamine to the existing standard practice opioid analgesia. The intensity of pain, type of surgery, other co-analgesics used and the ketamine administration protocol may have influenced the results of those clinical trials. Ketamine should be considered when post-operative pain requires large doses of opioids, such as major abdominal and thoracic surgery [13].

Ketamine and Opioids

Opioid escalation in acute pain can sometimes be futile, with inadequate pain control despite very high doses. In addition, some types of pain, particularly central neuropathic and vascular ischaemic pain, can be refractory to opioid therapy. Ketamine is well described in a number of clinical trials for pain refractory to high-dose opioids. Such use is based on preclinical data demonstrating an important role for the NMDA receptor in opioid-induced hyperalgesia and in persistent pain from inflammation, nerve injury and cancer [5, 8].

Ketamine is also useful to reduce the area of punctuate mechanical hyperalgesia surrounding the surgical incision for several days after surgery. While the significance of acute hyperalgesia may be related to progression to chronic pain, the pre-emptive administration of ketamine also consistently decreases the post-operative morphine consumption. Whether the mechanical hyperalgesia is related to the opioid administration (OIH) or occurs *de novo* remains unknown. Irrespective of the cause of this pro-nociception ketamine is probably the most potent anti-hyperalgesic available for clinical use. This has been clearly demonstrated after abdominal surgery and lasts for 48 h after ketamine anaesthesia. This anti-hyperalgesic mechanism is not fully appreciated but supports the pre-emptive and persistent analgesic effect of ketamine [16, 17].

There has been considerable interest in the combination of ketamine with the peri-operative opioids administered. Opioids are traditionally used as a part of general anaesthesia and for the treatment of acute post-operative pain. Recent research indicates that opioids produce not only analgesia, but also hyperalgesia. Consequently, peri-operative (pre, per, and post-operative) opioids may paradoxically increase post-operative pain and opioid requirements. Central sensitization includes an altered processing of innocuous, tactile impulses from myelinated afferents so that activation of these fibres produces painful sensations. The neurophysiological and biochemical mechanisms of these alterations include a decrease in inhibitory input or an increase in synaptic efficacy or membrane excitability, mediated by wind-up and neurokinin and N-methyl-D-aspartic acid receptor mechanisms (NMDA receptors) [18].

In the post-operative period, opioid containing intravenous patient-controlled analgesia (PCA) are frequently used for analgesia [19, 20]. The addition of ketamine to the morphine PCA has been described in a number of clinical trials. The concerns for the stability of these drugs have also been addressed [20]. Intravenous patient-controlled analgesia (PCA) with subanaesthetic ketamine and morphine dosaging following transthoracic lung and heart surgery has been shown to result in lower pain scores, reduced morphine consumption, shorter post-operative IV-PCA dependence, associated cardiovascular stability and better respiratory parameters. The potentiation of opioid-induced analgesia and the opioid-sparing effect of ketamine were observed in paediatric patients [21]. The parameters of the PCA settings: opioid bolus size, lockout intervals and hourly limits remain unchanged. In some situations, continuous infusion of the combination of morphine and ketamine delivered by the PCA will be better than either the opioid alone or a PCA approach alone, because of a stable NMDA receptor block [19]. We emphasize that the magnitude of the PCA bolus may need to be adapted to the individual patient, according to analgesic efficacy and side effects. The ratios described in these studies vary, but the most frequently described one is of morphine: ketamine in 1:1 ratio [19, 21]. (See further details in section Practical Application below.)

Benefits of Post-operative Ketamine

It has been a challenge to consistently demonstrate an effect of ketamine on pain scores. This again may be due to the type of surgery, ketamine dosing protocol, other multimodal analgesia drugs and/or clinical measurements. Some studies have shown a larger improvement in dynamic pain scores, while others show both rest and dynamic pain improvements [16]. The other major benefit of ketamine observed is a reduction in opioid analgesic consumption [2, 5, 21].

This interaction of ketamine with opioids may become clinically relevant especially when pain is poorly controlled or increasing opioids are required to provide adequate analgesia.

Preclinical studies have reported that opioid mu receptor activation leads to a sustained increase in glutamate synaptic effectiveness at the level of NMDA receptors. Opioids when used alone in large doses for a prolonged period induce tolerance, which may also lead to increased post-operative pain. Ketamine, by blocking these NMDA receptors, can reduce pain, opioid requirements and prevent the development of tolerance. This has been studied extensively in animals and consistently produced positive results.

This is one of the fundamental concepts that has led to the use of ketamine as an adjuvant to opioids in multiple clinical trials and consolidated the position of ketamine in the multimodal analgesia paradigm [13]. In the study by Choe et al. administration of morphine and ketamine prior to surgery reduced the need for supplemental analgesics [9].

There are other benefits of the concomitant administration of low-dose morphine and ketamine. Studies have shown that in combination these drugs improve the adequacy of respiration measured by the oxygen saturation (SpO_2) level. This may be secondary to pain reduction thus enabling patients to breathe more deeply, cough better, and maintain adequate minute ventilation with only negligible upper-airway obstruction compared with heavily (opioid) sedated post-operative patients. In the same study, because morphine did not control pain as well as the combination of morphine and ketamine did, SpO_2 in the morphine-alone group also remained lower. In addition, ketamine characteristically increases respiratory muscle tone, which could have also contributed to airway patency and better SpO_2, even though a subanaesthetic dose of ketamine was applied. All the above-mentioned reasons could also have contributed to the maintenance of a normal respiratory rate and depth in the patients receiving a combination of morphine and ketamine [6].

This is an important clinical caveat—the metaphoric 'double-edged sword' of pain management in abdominal surgery—incisional pain prevents adequate respiration; its treatment with opioids can also lead to sedation and respiratory depression. Low dose or ultra-low dose ketamine can reduce pain without sedation or respiratory depression and should therefore be a standard part of the multimodal analgesia for abdominal surgery.

Even in patients with high risk of respiratory depression, secondary to obesity and sleep apnoea, ketamine in combination with other intravenous agents is being used to provide opioid-free anaesthesia (OFA). Another significant benefit of this OFA technique is the reduction in PONV which again indirectly implies the contribution of opioids to this gastrointestinal side-effect [22]. A trend toward less PONV is seen in patients receiving ketamine and these reductions in PONV parallel the decreased opioid consumption and improved analgesia seen with ketamine [6, 13, 14].

Hyperalgesia and Progression to Chronic Pain

The prompt and sustained abolition of pain resistance to morphine by a single bolus injection of morphine and ketamine in up to 65% of the treated patients has been well documented [6]. At the same time they observed when comparing the total dose of morphine in both groups that the effect of ketamine was greater than additive. This supports the contention of an interaction of ketamine with NMDA receptors that could have been activated by either or both of the peri-operative nociceptive inputs and by the administration of morphine.

The smallest ketamine plasma concentration to counteract hyperalgesia while producing minimal side effects was shown to be 60 μg/mL. This concentration has been achieved by giving an initial bolus dose of ketamine 0.5 mg/kg, followed by a continuous infusion of 0.12 mg/kg/h. The average ketamine consumption in many studies is significantly lower which might explain some of the negative clinical trial results in terms of pain scores and/or analgesic consumption.

When given in the sub-anaesthetic or 'low' dose, intra-operative ketamine is known to reduce mechanical hyperalgesia and improve post-operative analgesia. Even a small dose of ketamine given before skin incision decreases post-operative pain and reduces morphine consumption after open renal surgery [16]. A small intravenous dose of ketamine before the first incision followed by a 24-h infusion had a morphine-sparing effect after total hip arthroplasty and decreased post-operative chronic pain up to 6 months after surgery [21].

The effect of adding ketamine to opioids or multimodal analgesic regimens on wound hyperalgesia has been reported in clinical trials. Wound hyperalgesia was evaluated by punctuate mapping with Von Frey hair filaments and pressure pain detection thresholds. The area of hyperalgesia tested by Von Frey hair filament was significantly less in ketamine groups in a majority of trials. Though the clinical implication of hyperalgesia remains poorly understood and not well studied, it is an indicator of central sensitization. It has been hypothesized that a reduction in the area of hyperalgesia could be a measure of the prevention of central sensitization by ketamine. The reduction in the area of hyperalgesia may not be associated with improvement in acute post-operative pain outcome measures, but may decrease the persistence of wind-up pain at 7 days [23]. When followed up at 2 weeks, 1 and 6 months and 1 year after surgery, patients who received IV ketamine had significantly reduced long-term pain [24]. It may also be worthwhile to note that all patients studied by these investigators had undergone surgery for rectal adenocarcinoma, a typically difficult pain model to treat. Thus, even without any effect on acute nociceptive pain, low-dose ketamine may have a role in reducing pathological pain, which in these patients was chronic, neuropathic and malignancy related.

Apart from patients with malignancy related surgery, patients undergoing surgical procedures which are associated with the risk of development of chronic post-operative neuropathic pain such as thoracotomy and amputation, will benefit from peri-operative ketamine [13].

Another group of patients who may benefit from peri-operative ketamine are those who have already developed chronic pain and/or those who are opioid tolerant. Loftus et al. demonstrated that intra-operative preventative ketamine reduces opiate consumption in the acute post-operative period by 37% in opiate-dependent patients with chronic pain who are undergoing painful back surgery. In addition, it seems to reduce pain intensity post-operatively in the PACU and at 6 weeks as well as reduced morphine consumption at the first post-operative visit. The results of these trials have shown that intermediate and long-term outcomes produced by the addition of ketamine was far superior to that produced by opioid analgesics [12]. Other than the reduction in pain intensity at 6 weeks, research has also found significantly less antidepressant use at the first post-operative visit compared with placebo, despite no significant difference between groups pre-operatively [12].

Understanding the utility of preventative NMDA receptor antagonism in patients with a history of chronic pain has also led to its use in patients on chronic opiate medication. This has been suggested as a primary target for future research. It is well known that patients with chronic pain and chronic opioid use are at increased risk of suboptimal post-operative pain management and consequently at increased risk of cardiopulmonary complications and further exacerbation of existing chronic postsurgical pain [12].

Influence on Carcinogenesis

In addition to their analgesic effects, opioids have well established immune-modulatory effects. Despite experimental and animal studies implicating peri-operative opioids in cancer metastasis and recurrence the evidence from clinical trials are conflicting. It is theorized that various agents (anaesthetics, analgesics, blood transfusions etc.) activate specific genes during the peri-operative period, which may contribute to cancer recurrence and metastasis [25].

Ketamine is known to exhibit immuno-modulatory effects on macrophages, lymphocytes, and mast cells in experimental studies. Despite its inhibition of the dendritic cell-mediated maturation of T cells in a mouse model, it must be noted that the ketamine concentration used was two to three times higher than that used in human clinical setting. One study reports the effect of low-dose ketamine (0.15 mg/kg) on immune function in patients undergoing elective abdominal surgery [26]. It indicated that ketamine attenuated production of the proinflammatory cytokines, IL-6 and TNFα, and suppressed NK cell cytotoxicity after operation. The clinical relevance of these findings is not fully understood [25, 26].

The contribution of other factors (especially opioids) on immune-modulation, neuro-endocrine and inflammatory response influencing tumor metastasis and/or recurrence cannot be ruled out. Nevertheless, ketamine offers a promising non-opioid option in abdominal surgery and until further evidence in this area becomes available, is probably safe (and safer than opioids alone) to administer to patients with abdominal surgery, especially those with malignancies [25].

Other Benefits of Ketamine

Another reported benefit of ketamine is in the treatment of post-operative shivering with a faster onset than meperidine at ultra-low dose (<0.1 mg/kg) [27]. Low-dose ketamine is commonly used to treat distressing states such as anxiety and depression [28]. It is unclear whether changes in stress hormone concentrations are beneficial or harmful in pain and depression. This study found that even at low doses, ketamine doubles cortisol production [29].

Side Effects

Widespread use of ketamine has been limited by clinicians' concerns about adverse effects such as dysphoria, hallucinations, and dissociative symptoms. Furthermore, the dosing of ketamine is inconvenient in chronic pain patients as it is relatively short acting and is unavailable in an oral formulation [5].

The side effects of ketamine have been described in the preceding sections. Whilst these are dose dependant, some patients demonstrate intolerance to the central nervous system side effects i.e. sedation, nausea and vomiting, catalepsy and locomotor depression, dependence and tolerance [8]. Side effects from ketamine were more commonly observed at higher doses and sedation is commonly described at these doses [30].

It has been observed in healthy human volunteers that high dose ketamine can significantly alter mood states and produce dose-related impairment of sensory perception or even impact the process of sensory integration [6]. It has been reported that more than one third of the patients may experience unpleasant dreams or acute psychosis-like symptoms that may or may not be associated with hallucinations on emergence when anaesthetic doses (1–3 mg/kg) of ketamine are administered. Sub-anaesthetic doses (0.1–1 mg/kg) of ketamine in healthy human volunteers can produce subtle cognitive dysfunction, e.g., attention-free recall and recognition memory. Clinical studies in patients with acute pain receiving such sub-anaesthetic doses showed no changes in cognition, perception, or mood swings in any patients even 24 h after ketamine administration [6]. This difference can be explained by the fact that the healthy volunteers are different from the patients experiencing acute pain. Consequently, patients who do not have poorly controlled pain or acute hyperalgesia should not be prescribed ketamine—they may experience adverse side-effects without any clinical benefit.

It is probably important to note that many of the central nervous system side effects (dizziness, diplopia, dysphoria, dreams, hallucinations disorientation, strange sensations, light headedness, sleep difficulties, and confusion) described in ketamine-treated patients is also seen with opioids.

Making a clear distinction between the etiologies of these presentations, especially in patients receiving both opioids and ketamine, may be clinically challenging, if not impossible.

Practical Considerations

Intra-operative Ketamine

A novel method of ketamine administration during surgery was developed at our center. We combine ketamine with fentanyl and lidocaine and infuse this 'cocktail' (called fentaketacaine or FLK) during surgery under general anaesthesia.

At or after induction, patients identified as appropriate for ketamine (and lidocaine) receive 0.2–0.5 mg/kg (max 20 mg IV) followed by lidocaine (1–2 mg/kg, max 100 mg IV). We then initiate an infusion of FLK (syringe containing Fentanyl 10 μg/mL + Lidocaine 10 mg/mL + Ketamine 1 mg/mL). This is prepared by taking a 20 mL syringe and adding 200 μg Fentanyl (4 mL of 50 μg/mL), 200 mg Lidocaine (10 mL of 2%), 20 mg ketamine (2 mL of 10 mg/mL) and saline (4 mL) to make it a total of 20 mL. We program the pump as though there is only lidocaine 10 mg/mL in the syringe at 1–2 mg/kg/h. Because of the ratios in the mixture, the pump will also deliver Fentanyl 1–2 μg/kg/h. and Ketamine 0.1–0.2 mg/kg/h. The infusion rate can be reduced or increased depending on the haemodynamics. For obese and morbidly obese patients, it is important to use their ideal body weight (IBW). Additional boluses of ketamine, lidocaine or longer acting opioids are rarely required, unless the patient is opioid tolerant or is demonstrating other signs of inadequate analgesia. There may be an anaesthetic (MAC) sparing effect and it may be advisable to monitor the depth of anaesthesia, especially in long procedures and/or vulnerable patients (younger, older, past history etc.).

This infusion of FLK can be continued for 4–6 h without accumulation and usually stopped at or before wound closure. Patients usually wake up comfortably, especially after laparoscopic procedures and some will require early post-operative resumption of their multimodal analgesia, including titration of longer acting opioids. The two main indications for the use of FLK are (1) alternative to epidurals and (2) difficult-to-treat pain patients. These indications have been elaborated in Table 5.1.

Post-operative Ketamine

It is often challenging to achieve good quality analgesia following abdominal surgery. While epidural analgesia and other regional anaesthesia techniques described

Table 5.1 Indications for intra-operative ketamine as fentaketacaine (FLK) infusion

1. Alternatives to epidurals
• Epidural contraindicated, refused or failed
• Epidural attempted, inadequate or not tolerated
• Epidural not done—minimally invasive (laparoscopic) surgery
2. Difficult-to-treat pain
• Surgery at a site of chronic pain
• Chronic pain elsewhere, e.g., fibromyalgia
• Opioid-use, abuse, dependence or tolerance
• Poorly controlled pain: acute hyperalgesia
• Experience in past of poorly controlled pain

elsewhere in this book are very useful, they are not always possible, may fail or become inadequate. Two of the frequently encountered side effects with opioid based analgesia are respiratory depression and post-operative nausea and vomiting (PONV). These may have a significant impact on the recovery of patients after abdominal surgery. After any surgery, especially abdominal surgery, the patient may remain in a fasting state (NPO) and have enteral drainage or feeding tubes that would preclude the use of the gut for oral/enteral multimodal analgesia. As described in the chapter on lidocaine, parenteral multimodal analgesia based on the WHO step ladder (step-wise, severity-based and opioid-sparing) with adequate anti-pronociception is vital to ensure high quality analgesia with low side effects.

It is in this context that ketamine (and lidocaine) are essential parts of the acute pain management armamentarium for abdominal surgery. While the use of lidocaine is described in detail elsewhere, the use of the DN4 questionnaire will be useful to determine the need to add ketamine to the post-operative plan. As discussed previously, ketamine is a very potent anti-hyperalgesic and is clearly indicated to treat both mechanical and opioid-induced hyperalgesia. The other patients who would benefit from post-operative ketamine include those with poorly controlled pain, failed or inadequate epidural or other regional anesthesia techniques, opioid escalation or side-effects especially ileus, nausea/vomiting, sedation and respiratory depression, opioid tolerant or dependant, chronic neuropathic/non-cancer pain or malignancy related pain.

One of the most effective and safe ways of administering ketamine in the post operative period is via a PCA system. With ketamine delivered in a fixed ratio with the parenteral opioid. Ketamine administered via the PCA allows the patient to self-titrate their requirements within a safe hourly limit. This in turn decreases opioid use and associated side-effects, decreases the need for health care provider intervention and empowers the patient with a sense of autonomy. Moreover, as discussed above, the indications for ketamine in the post-operative period includes patient and procedural indications that are otherwise poorly controlled with opioids alone (Table 5.2). Adding ketamine to the opioid PCA therefore provides excellent analgesia with improved patient safety and satisfaction.

At our center, two morphine-ketamine ratio choices were made available as a premixed solution for use in the PCA. These ratios served to accommodate a wide range of opioid requirements, without exceeding a fixed amount of ketamine

Table 5.2 The Ottawa Hospital (TOH) Acute Pain Service (APS) indications for adding ketamine to IV PCA

1. **T**rauma: multiple and/or major injuries; burns, degloving and crush injuries, rib fractures
2. **A**cute Pain: poorly controlled, acute on chronic pain, prevention of Chronic Post-Surgical Pain (CPSP), opioid tolerance and/or dependence, substance abuse
3. **N**europathic pain: acute hyperalgesia opioid induced or opioid resistant, malignancy related, vascular insufficiency and ischemia, sickle cell crises etc.
4. **G**astro-Intestinal Surgery: with or without epidural analgesia, laparoscopic procedures and laparoscopic converted to open, ERAS
5. **O**bese, OSA and elderly: sensitive to opioids or having opioid side effects

available for use on demand. The general principle is to keep the hourly dose of intravenous ketamine to less than 10 mg/h. At this ultra-low dose the patient would benefit from the NMDA antagonist anti-hyperalgesic effects while avoiding the psychomimetic side-effects. In our extensive experience of over 15 years, the patients whose PCA contains the morphine and ketamine combination continue to be monitored as per the opioid PCA modality and do not require any extra or special monitoring *per se*.

Morphine, 1 mg/mL, with Ketamine, 1 mg/mL, is prescribed for patients expected to use less than 10 mg/h of morphine. These would include almost all abdominal surgery in most of the opioid naïve patients. Morphine, 5 mg/mL, with ketamine, 1 mg/mL, is suggested for patients expected to require between 25 and 50 mg/h of morphine on an ongoing basis (i.e., >12 h). This would be used in opioid-tolerant patients, polytrauma patients, those with vascular ischemia and those with malignancy related pain. Even when using the ketamine PCA mixtures, the orders and the pump program remains unchanged with *bolus*, *lockout*, *basal* and *hourly limit* set according to the morphine requirement.

For opioid-tolerant patients or others with poorly controlled pain, it is preferable to increase the bolus size and hourly limit, rather than change the lockout or add a basal infusion [20]. The variable magnitude of the bolus dose was probably the result of the well-known interindividual variability in drug requirement to achieve satisfactory analgesia.

The use of ketamine requires careful consideration in patients at particular risk for respiratory depression from conventional opioid-only, e.g., morbidly obese patients, those with suspected OSA and or untreated OSA, elderly and renal insufficiency. Extended or increased cardiorespiratory monitoring may be required for these patients, especially until their pain is well controlled.

Also of importance to note is that when ketamine is added to the post-operative pain management, pain scores and consequently opioid requirements can fall dramatically. It is therefore pertinent to monitor these patients and reduce any fixed dose or long-acting opioids that they may be receiving. If sedation, respiratory depression or any other signs or symptoms of opioid overdose occur after the ketamine is started, they should be treated as per standard opioid overdose guidelines.

In some situations, especially in intensive care and other monitored areas, ketamine can also be administered as a continuous intravenous infusion. This is most likely to provide stable antihyperalgesia, but less likely to provide situational analgesia as required by the patient. In our experience this has been useful in sedated, intubated and ventilated patients in the critical care areas. Again, the aim would be to keep the hourly limit of ketamine to less than 10 mg/h.

Conclusions

The combination of our understanding of the pharmacology, vast clinical experience and the available evidence support a wide role for the use of ketamine in the peri-operative period. Ketamine is useful as a co-analgesic and anti-hyperalgesic thereby decreasing post-operative pain, opioid analgesic requirements and opioid related side-effects following major abdominal surgery. Low and ultra-low dose ketamine can be used as an infusion during surgery. Post-operatively it may be added to an opioid for PCA use. This will assist the patient in achieving their ERAS goals, i.e., early mobilization, early nutrition and discharge with improved satisfaction.

References

1. Tawfic QA. A review of the use of ketamine in pain management. J Opioid Manag. 2013;9:379–88.
2. Himmelseher S, Durieux ME. Ketamine for perioperative pain management. Anesthesiology. 2005;102:211–20.
3. Ding X, Jin S, Niu X, Wang T, Zhao X, Ren H, Tong Y, Li Q. Morphine with adjuvant ketamine versus higher dose of morphine alone for acute pain: a meta-analysis. Int J Clin Exp Med. 2014;7:2504–10.
4. Blanke ML, Vandongen AMJ. Activation mechanisms of the NMDA receptor. In: Van Dongen AM, editor. Biology of the NMDA receptor. Boca Raton, FL: CRC Press; 2009. Chapter 13.
5. Grande LA, O'Donnell BR, Fitzgibbon DR, Terman GW. Ultra-low dose ketamine and memantine treatment for pain in an opioid-tolerant oncology patient. Anesth Analg. 2008;107:1380–3.
6. Weinbroum AA. A single small dose of postoperative ketamine provides rapid and sustained improvement in morphine analgesia in the presence of morphine-resistant pain. Anesth Analg. 2003;96:789–95.
7. Tawfic QA, Eipe N, Penning J. Ultra-low-dose ketamine infusion for ischemic limb pain. Can J Anaesth. 2014;61:86–7.
8. Romero TR, Galdino GS, Silva GC, Resende LC, Perez AC, Côrtes SF, Duarte ID. Ketamine activates the L-arginine/nitric oxide/cyclic guanosine monophosphate pathway to induce peripheral antinociception in rats. Anesth Analg. 2011;113:1254–9.
9. Choe H, Choi YS, Kim YH, Ko SH, Choi HG, Han YJ, Song HS. Epidural morphine plus ketamine for upper abdominal surgery: improved analgesia from preincisional versus postincisional administration. Anesth Analg. 1997;84:560–3.
10. Slogoff S, Allen GW, Wessels JV, Cheney DH. Clinical experience with subanesthetic ketamine. Anesth Analg. 1974;53:354–8.
11. Waxman K, Shoemaker WC, Lippmann M. Cardiovascular effects of anesthetic induction with ketamine. Anesth Analg. 1980;59:355–8.
12. Loftus RW, Yeager MP, Clark JA, Brown JR, Abdu WA, Sengupta DK, Beach ML. Intraoperative ketamine reduces perioperative opiate consumption in opiate-dependent patients with chronic back pain undergoing back surgery. Anesthesiology. 2010;113:639–46.
13. Subramaniam K, Subramaniam B, Steinbrook RA. Ketamine as adjuvant analgesic to opioids: a quantitative and qualitative systematic review. Anesth Analg. 2004;99:482–95.
14. Laskowski K, Stirling A, Mckay WP, Lim HJ. A systematic review of intravenous ketamine for postoperative analgesia. Can J Anaesth. 2011;58:911–23.
15. Zakine J, Samarcq D, Lorne E, Moubarak M, Montravers P, Beloucif S, Dupont H. Postoperative ketamine administration decreases morphine consumption in major abdominal surgery: a prospective, randomized, double-blind, controlled study. Anesth Analg. 2008;106:1856–61.
16. Kararmaz A, Kaya S, Karaman H, Turhanoglu S, Ozyilmaz MA. Intraoperative intravenous ketamine in combination with epidural analgesia: postoperative analgesia after renal surgery. Anesth Analg. 2003;97:1092–6.
17. Aida S, Yamakura T, Baba H, Taga K, Fukuda S, Shimoji K. Preemptive analgesia by intravenous low-dose ketamine and epidural morphine in gastrectomy: a randomized double-blind study. Anesthesiology. 2000;92:1624–30.

18. Bell RF, Dahl JB, Moore RA, Kalso E. Peri-operative ketamine for acute post-operative pain: a quantitative and qualitative systematic review (Cochrane review). Acta Anaesthesiol Scand. 2005;49:1405–28.
19. Sveticic G, Farzanegan F, Zmoos P, Zmoos S, Eichenberger U, Curatolo M. Is the combination of morphine with ketamine better than morphine alone for postoperative intravenous patient-controlled analgesia? Anesth Analg. 2008;106:287–93.
20. Schmid R, Koren G, Klein J, Katz J. The stability of a ketamine-morphine solution. Anesth Analg. 2002;94:898–900.
21. Lee SK. The use of ketamine for perioperative pain management. Korean J Anesthesiol. 2012;63:1–2.
22. Ziemann-Gimmel P, Goldfarb AA, Koppman J, Marema RT. Opioid-free total intravenous anaesthesia reduces postoperative nausea and vomiting in bariatric surgery beyond triple prophylaxis. Br J Anaesth. 2014;112:906–11.
23. Stubhaug A, Breivik H, Eide PK, Kreunen M, Foss A. Mapping of punctuate hyperalgesia around a surgical incision demonstrates that ketamine is a powerful suppressor of central sensitization to pain following surgery. Acta Anaesthesiol Scand. 1997;41:1124–32.
24. De Kock M, Lavand'Homme P, Waterloos H. 'Balanced analgesia' in the perioperative period: is there a place for ketamine? Pain. 2001;92:373–80.
25. Lee BM, Cata JP. Impact of anesthesia on cancer recurrence. Rev Esp Anestesiol Reanim. 2015;62:570–5.
26. Heaney A, Buggy DJ. Can anaesthetic and analgesic techniques affect cancer recurrence or metastasis? Br J Anaesth. 2012;109(Suppl. 1):i17–28.
27. Dal D, Kose A, Honca M, Akinci SB, Basgul E, Aypar U. Efficacy of prophylactic ketamine in preventing postoperative shivering. Br J Anaesth. 2005;95:189–92.
28. Parsaik AK, Singh B, Khosh-Chashm D, Mascarenhas SS. Efficacy of ketamine in bipolar depression: systematic review and meta-analysis. J Psychiatr Pract. 2015;21:427–35.
29. Khalili-Mahani N, Martini CH, Olofsen E, Dahan A, Niesters M. Effect of subanaesthetic ketamine on plasma and saliva cortisol secretion. Br J Anaesth. 2015;115:68–75.
30. Kose EA, Dal D, Akinci SB, Saricaoglu F, Aypar U. The efficacy of ketamine for the treatment of postoperative shivering. Anesth Analg. 2008;106:120–2.
31. Brookoff D. Chronic pain: a new disease? Hosp Pract (Off Ed). 2000;35:45–52. 59

Intravenous Lidocaine

6

Naveen Eipe

Key Points

1. Peri-operative IV lidocaine infusions lead to significant decreases in pain scores and reduced opioid analgesic consumption and opioid related side effects, notably nausea, vomiting and ileus.
2. Identification of acute hyperalgesia is an important concept that is being increasingly recognised and for which IV lidocaine has a role.
3. IV lidocaine is a useful non-opioid analgesic, anti-inflammatory and antihyperalgesic, which can contribute to significant improvements in patient outcomes, especially after abdominal surgery.
4. Dosing is a bolus of 1–2 mg/kg followed by an infusion of 1–2 mg/kg/h (use ideal body weight [IBW] if the body mass index [BMI] >30 and do not exceed a maximum dose of 100 mg bolus or 100 mg/h)
5. Safety is maintained by adhering to the correct dose, adjusting the dose for high risk patients (renal or liver dysfunction, on interacting medication or those with certain cardiac disease or seizure disorders) and appropriate monitoring for toxicity.

Introduction

Acute pain management has witnessed numerous innovations and advances in the past three decades. Evolution of these strategies has had to keep pace with the changes and advancements in surgical technique. Notable amongst these was the introduction of minimally invasive and laparoscopic surgery in the

N. Eipe
Department of Anesthesiology and Pain Medicine, The Ottawa Hospital, University of Ottawa, Ottawa, ON, Canada
e-mail: neipe@toh.on.ca

A. Krige, M. J. P. Scott (eds.), *Analgesia in Major Abdominal Surgery*,
https://doi.org/10.1007/978-3-319-94482-1_6

1990s. The paradigm of improving patient safety and outcomes has become better measured using clearly defined goals derived from the work done in Enhanced Recovery after Surgery (ERAS).

An optimally working thoracic epidural has been the 'gold standard' for open abdominal surgery, but its role in laparoscopic surgery and ERAS is being questioned [1]. When abdominal surgery is conducted without continuous epidural analgesia, conventional acute pain management has to rely on other methods of analgesia such as truncal blocks and opioids as the main stay of analgesia. Side effects of 'conventional' opioid-based acute pain management regimes are well known to contravene many of the ERAS principles. Most prominent amongst these opioid side-effects in the peri-operative period are nausea, vomiting and ileus. These side-effects prevent early oral nutrition, delay patient ambulation and hospital discharge thus having a major impact.

The search continues for a non-opioid analgesic adjuvant (preferably parenteral) that would provide peri-operative analgesia without interfering with gut function recovery and/or healing integrity. Intravenous (IV) lidocaine is a unique therapeutic component of peri-operative multimodal analgesia that may provide these and other additional benefits in abdominal surgery. In so doing it may help patients realize many of the ERAS goals and outcomes, while minimizing the need for conventional opioid-based analgesia [2].

Multimodal Analgesia: The Foundation for Successful IV Lidocaine

A structural and functional framework for acute pain management is the first requirement prior to the introduction and application of any innovative treatment modality like IV lidocaine. We also need to standardize our pain management protocols and therefore it is useful to revisit (and adhere to) some acute pain management principles. A useful place to start is the well established and widely respected WHO step ladder (Fig. 6.1). The World Health Organization (WHO) step ladder provides us with four basic principles which remain applicable to modern acute pain management. It describes a (1) severity based, (2) stepwise approach that further aims to (3) minimize the use and/or need for opioids. This also (4) introduces and encourages the use of non-opioid adjuvants for acute pain at any level (or every step) of pain (or the ladder).

At this stage we need to clearly define the role of the above-mentioned adjuvants. We believe that acute hyperalgesia or 'pronociception' occurs more frequently than previously recognized in acute pain, especially in certain procedures and patients. Adjuvants directed towards this pronociception (notably ketamine, lidocaine and gabapentinoids, etc.) will ensure adequate treatment of this presentation of acute neuropathic pain [3]. It is also now well-established that opioids are not only ineffective in treating acute hyperalgesia and neuropathic pain; they can paradoxically worsen pain, by producing opioid-induced hyperalgesia (Fig. 6.2).

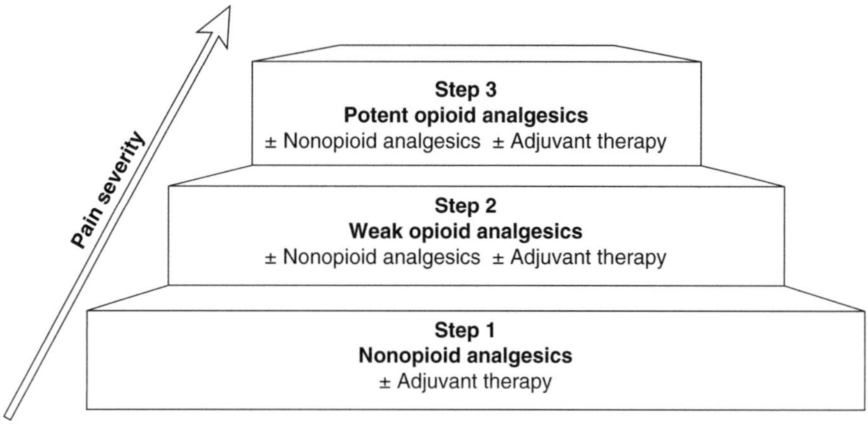

Fig. 6.1 World Health Organization pain step ladder. Image created by Perry Ng

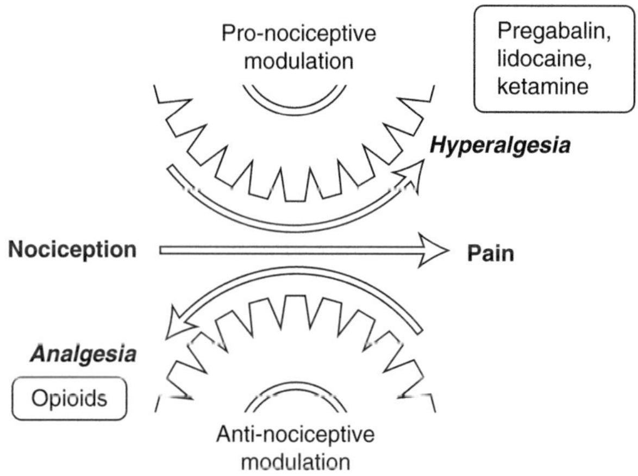

Fig. 6.2 Opioids are not only ineffective in treating acute hyperalgesia and neuropathic pain; they can paradoxically worsen pain, by producing opioid-induced hyperalgesia. Image created by Perry Ng

While clinical research in the past two decades has supported the use of these adjuvant drugs in the management of post-operative pain, their exact positioning within the original WHO Step Ladder paradigm continues to evolve.

In our opinion, the use of these adjuvants should be based on the identification of pronociception or acute neuropathic pain presenting as hyperalgesia [2]. The diagnosis of acute neuropathic pain can be made objectively using the well-validated DN4 questionnaire first described by Bouhassira [4].

This appreciation of the role of acute neuropathic pain, often coexisting and independent of severity with nociceptive pain, is in our opinion, a very important addition to the concept of the original WHO Step Ladder (Fig. 6.3). We also believe

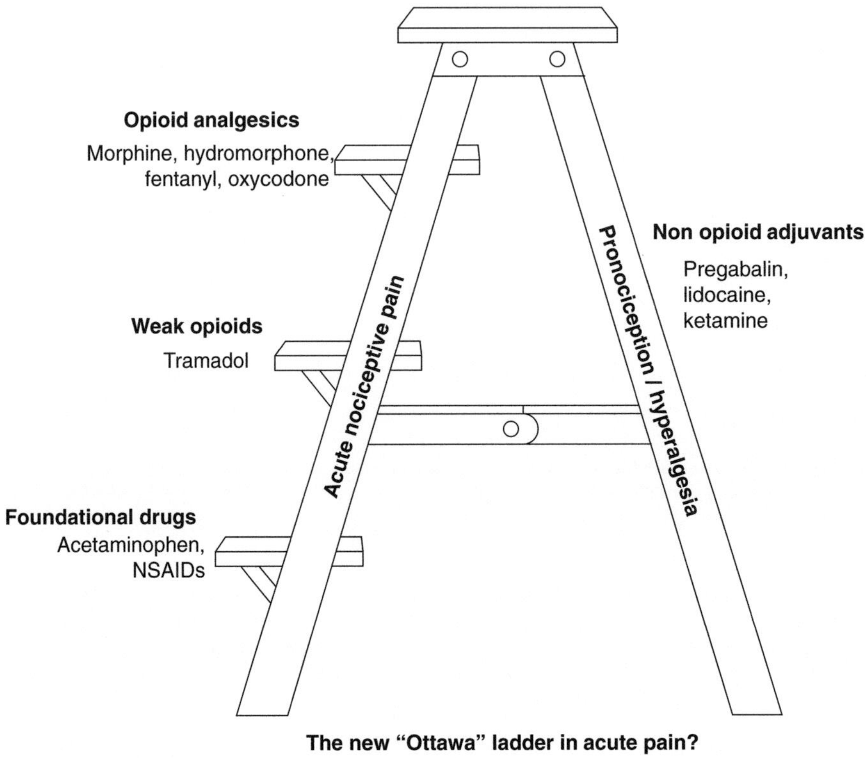

Fig. 6.3 Updated concept of the original WHO Step Ladder

that this will simplify the understanding and explanation of the role of drugs like ketamine and IV lidocaine for acute pain.

Management of acute pain after abdominal surgery is well described through the work done in ERAS with the emphasis on multimodal opioid-sparing analgesia. Another important aspect of using multimodal analgesia in abdominal surgery is the controversial association of NSAIDs with poor wound healing, particularly their implication in causing GI anastomotic leaks [1]. IV lidocaine may not only avoid the need for NSAIDs, but also provide pharmacological effects that provide added protection to GI healing with early feeding and return of gut function. It is in this context that IV lidocaine can play a key role in the management of acute pain after abdominal surgery—as an analgesic, anti-inflammatory and antihyperalgesic with direct prokinetic effects on the gastrointestinal (GI) tract [5].

Pharmacology

While the 'local' anaesthetic lidocaine is best known when applied on or in tissues to be anaesthetised, the intravenous use for pain is neither novel nor new [6]. Lidocaine was first used via this route as an antiarrhythmic and the cardiology literature provides a wealth of information on its systemic use and safety profile. In anaesthesia, its intravenous use was introduced to blunt airway reflexes and sympathetic responses to laryngoscopy and tracheal intubation. Later, with the introduction of the otherwise painful propofol on injection its availability, acceptance and familiarity of use at anaesthetic induction became widespread. Regarding pain management, it was first used in chronic pain, where it continues to be used as a short-term infusion in ambulatory and outpatient clinic settings. All this clinical experience and familiarity with IV lidocaine is also supported by its wide availability, relative ease of administration and cost effectiveness in pain management.

Mechanism of Action

Lidocaine is an amide type local anaesthetic that blocks sodium ion channels on the cell membranes and stabilizes the membrane. In neural tissues, lidocaine inhibits the generation, transmission and propagation of neural impulses. There may also be a relevant role in the inhibition of spontaneous neuronal firing in damaged and dysfunctional nerves. While this effect is best described when the drug is applied directly to nerves; it probably and at least in part, explains the mechanistic basis for systemic analgesic effects of IV lidocaine.

While the exact mechanisms of systemic lidocaine continue to be described, when given intravenously, the systemic effects of intravenous (IV) lidocaine result in direct and indirect effects on the GI tract. At the primary afferent pathway, apart from the described sodium channel blockade, IV lidocaine may effect changes in the NMDA receptors, potassium channels, calcium channels and G-coupled receptors, though the significance of these latter effects are less clear or clinically relevant. At the neuronal level, it is hypothesized that lidocaine has a dual effect. It may directly stimulate the intestinal smooth muscle while inhibiting the intrinsic sympathetic nervous innervation. At the level of the spinal reflex, it blocks the afferent and/or efferent parts of the reflex arc. It may also have inhibitory effects on colonic distention via the mechano-insensitive nociceptors, which themselves are known to trigger tissue injury-induced and/or inflammatory hyperalgesia.

Beyond the above-mentioned effects on the GI tract and its innervation, IV lidocaine's most prominent effects are probably anti-inflammatory in nature. Lidocaine reduces the release of cytokines by reducing neutrophil activation. Systemic lidocaine attenuates the production of IL-8, which is identified as the first endogenous mediator for evoking hyperalgesia involving the sympathetic nervous system. In GI surgery, these may have a beneficial impact on the peritoneal inflammatory response secondary to incision (in open surgery) or even distention (in laparoscopic surgery). A more generalized attenuation of the peri-operative stress hormone response in non-GI surgery has also been attributed to IV lidocaine, but clinical trials studying this effect have either not demonstrated it at all or been able to do so consistently [7–10].

Overall, the pharmacological effect of IV lidocaine involves multiple pathways (peripheral and central) and mechanisms (direct and indirect), which in turn may explain the frequently observed clinical benefits that last beyond the duration of the lidocaine infusion [7–10].

In clinical trials for GI surgery, the indirect effect of opioid sparing of IV lidocaine also translates into lower pain scores, analgesic consumption and side-effects. The most clinically relevant outcome after abdominal surgery from the opioid-sparing effect of IV lidocaine is in the reduction of nausea-vomiting and ileus.

Integrated within a severity-based, step-wise opioid-sparing multimodal analgesia protocol, IV lidocaine provides well-managed pain. This allows for the patient to deep breathe and cough, mobilise, resume feeding and achieve early discharge, all with few side effects, better satisfaction and measurable quality of recovery scores. These are the key ERAS outcomes dependent on acute pain management and IV lidocaine consistently produces this effect.

Pharmacokinetics

Dosage: The most widely described and implemented dose of IV lidocaine for acute pain is 1–2 mg/kg as a bolus. Because of its relatively short plasma half-life of 6 min, to maintain the therapeutic plasma levels, this bolus needs to be followed with a continuous infusion of 1–2 mg/kg/h. The target plasma concentration for therapeutic effect is between 2.5 and 3.5 μg/ml, which is achieved with the above-mentioned dosing schedule.

Safety: To study the safety of these prolonged infusions we have used a 3-compartment model with age, height and weight as covariates to simulate the pharmacokinetics of a prolonged infusion [2]. This was done for two doses of infusions: 1 and 2 mg/kg/h. We have found that without an initial bolus the levels of lidocaine rise gradually over 4 h and then stabilize at about 8 h (Fig. 6.4). They remain stable over the next few days in the models and then rapidly decline upon discontinuation of the infusion (Fig. 6.5).

Toxicity [2]: Despite the well-described safety in numerous clinical trials, it must be reiterated that systemic lidocaine has a very narrow therapeutic index i.e. central nervous system (CNS) toxicity occurs (>5 μg/ml) slightly above the therapeutic plasma level (2.5–3.5 μg/ml) (Table 6.1). The factors that influence the plasma concentration of free lidocaine include the dose and/or speed of injection, acid-base status, hypercapnia and hypoxia, low plasma protein level and diminished hepatic or renal function. Very rarely do patients actually have a hypersensitivity, idiosyncrasy or diminished tolerance to systemic lidocaine that is independent of the above-mentioned factors. As the plasma concentrations rise above 5 μg/ml, the patient will exhibit central nervous system symptoms that follow an almost predictable progression. It is only when the plasma concentrations exceed 10 μg/ml that cardiovascular signs manifest. Appreciation of this aspect of the pharmacology of IV lidocaine supports the requirement for continuous cardiac monitoring and physician presence for the first 40 min after the bolus dose. In our experience, this infusion can probably be safely continued for 2–3 days without continuous electrocardiogram (ECG) monitoring, as long as routine clinical monitoring of the patient includes carefully seeking the symptoms and signs of lidocaine toxicity.

The progression of the clinical presentation in lidocaine toxicity closely mirrors the increasing plasma concentration. When the plasma concentration of lidocaine exceeds 5 μg/ml, patients will first exhibit central nervous system (CNS) symptoms

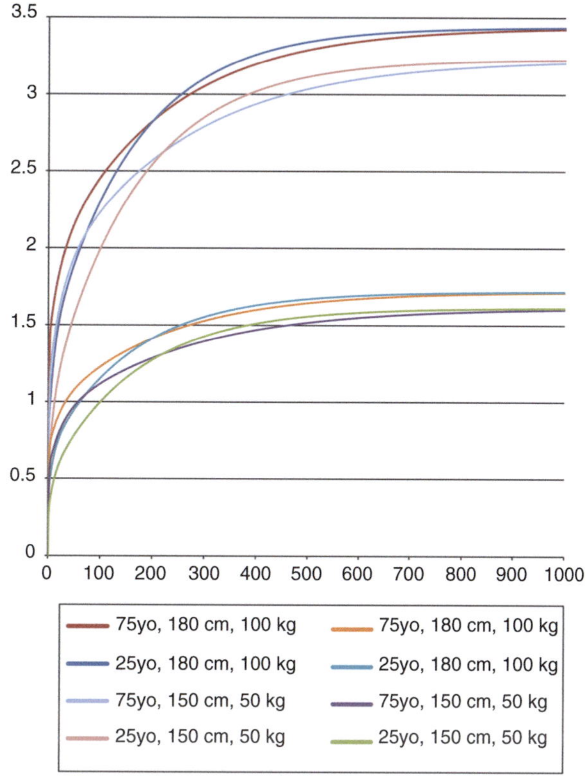

Fig. 6.4 Pharmacokinetic simulation for IV lidocaine infusion (without bolus) with plasma concentration in µg/ml represented on the *Y*-axis and time in minutes on the *X*-axis

of toxicity. This begins around 6 µg/ml and is quite definite at 10 µg/ml. In awake patients, these CNS symptoms follow an almost predictable progression. It begins with numbness of the tongue, a metallic taste, a feeling of light-headedness followed by tinnitus. Visual disturbances progress to muscle twitching, unconsciousness followed by seizures. If undetected or untreated these will proceed into a coma, and the patient will probably suffer a respiratory arrest and/or cardiovascular collapse. In clinical practice, the more common complaints as systemic lidocaine approaches toxic levels are 'ketamine-like' effects i.e. sedation, sleepiness, lightheadedness, relaxation, euphoria, unreality and "flying and drunkenness." Toxicity with lidocaine results in cardiovascular system (CVS) signs in awake patients far less frequently than CNS symptoms for two reasons. Firstly, lidocaine itself is less cardiotoxic than the better known and more lipophilic bupivacaine. Secondly, and probably more importantly, these CVS events occur when the serum levels exceed 10 µg/ml, which is well after the exhibition of CNS toxicity levels (5–10 µg/ml). These CVS signs include negative inotropy (greater in patients with conduction problems or after myocardial infarctions), effects on conduction (widened PR interval and QRS duration, sinus tachycardia, sinus arrest and partial or complete atrioventricular dissociation) and effects on vascular tone (where hypertension often precedes hypotension). Once again, these are potentiated by acidosis, hypercapnia

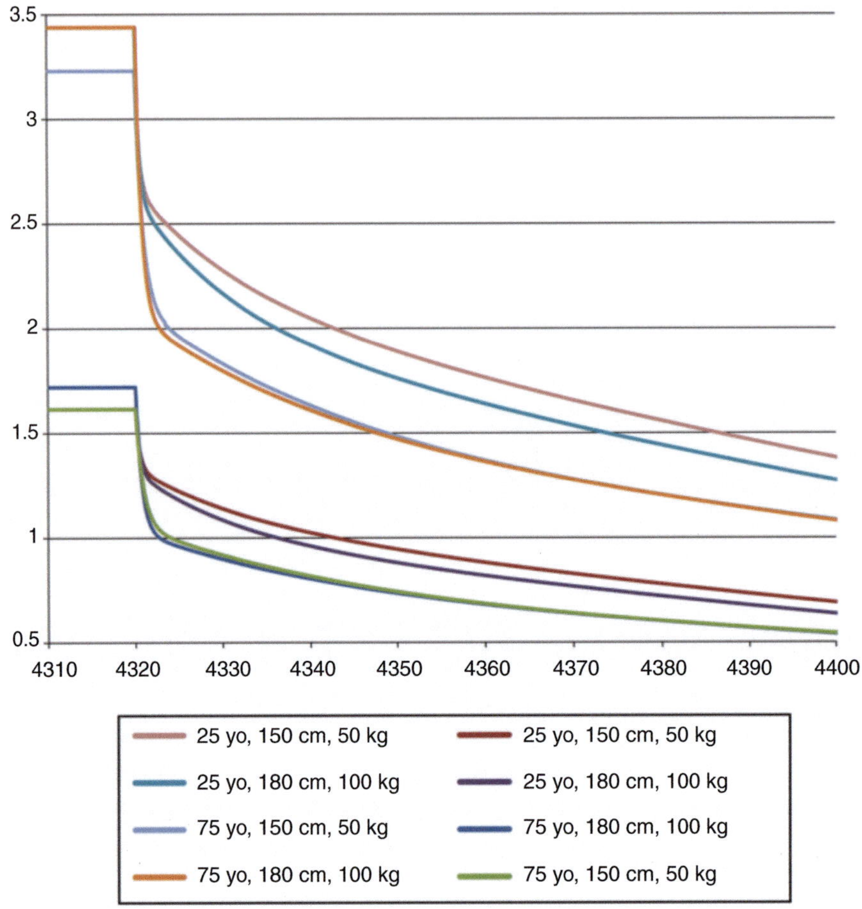

Fig. 6.5 Pharmacokinetic simulation for IV lidocaine on discontinuation of infusion-plasma concentration in μg/ml is represented on the *Y*-axis and time (since initiation) in minutes on the *X*-axis

and hypoxia, which in turn also worsen cardiac suppression, increase arrhythmias and may prove to be fatal.

An important clinical *correlate* of understanding the IV lidocaine toxicology is that as long as the patients are awake (or are easily aroused from sleep), and remain communicative, the CNS symptoms will occur first and therefore should be carefully sought after by the nursing staff (see Table 6.1). A *corollary* to this concept is that the cardiac signs will be the primary presentation if the CNS symptoms have been missed. And a *caveat* to the safety of IV lidocaine is that dosing must be reduced and continuous cardiac monitoring must be instituted in patients with cardiac, hepatic or renal dysfunction, and in those who are deeply sedated or anaesthetized (usually in the operating rooms, recovery units or in the ICU) [2].

Table 6.1 Summary of The Ottawa Hospital Policy for IV lidocaine [2]

Stage	Treatment	Monitoring	Comments
Preparation	The initial dose is administered in a **clinical area** where continuous cardiac monitoring, non-invasive blood pressure, pulse oximetry and resuscitative equipment/cardiac arrest cart is available	• Assess clinical status, vital signs and pain scores at rest and with activity • The patient or health care professional may also complete a Brief Pain Inventory (**BPI**) and/or **DN4** questionnaire • Weight—If patient's BMI is more than 30, use Ideal Body Weight (**IBW**)	The physician must be available to remain in attendance with the patient for at least 15 min **after** administration of the lidocaine bolus
Initiation	**Bolus** Dose IV lidocaine = 1.5 mg/kg by slow IV push over 2–4 min followed by infusion (see below)	• Assess pain q15 min until pain is stable, or as determined by the physician • Continuous visual patient monitoring during first 20 min after initiation of infusion, and then as per Physician's orders • Oxygen saturation, blood pressure and heart rate: q5 min for first 20 min, then q30 min for 1 h, then as per Physician's orders • **Side effects**—Sedation score: *None*—Fully awake, alert. *Mild*—Occasionally drowsy, easily aroused. *Moderate*—Frequently drowsy; easily roused, drifts off to sleep during conversation. *Severe*—Somnolent; difficult to arouse, minimal or no response to stimuli Sleep-Normal sleep; easily aroused, RR > 10 and even, not shallow • ECG monitoring may be carried out at the discretion of the attending physician • Administer Midazolam 1–2 mg IV PRN if patient develops twitching, or tremors	• In patients with co-morbidities or at the discretion of the physician, the bolus dose can be reduced or infusion duration may be increased (given over 1 h) • If the patient develops symptoms or signs of toxicity further treatment can be adjusted or avoided

(continued)

Table 6.1 (continued)

Stage	Treatment	Monitoring	Comments
Infusion	• Usual range for a lidocaine infusion is 0.5–2 mg/kg/h • The usual starting dose is 1 mg/kg/h • This infusion can be increased or decreased by 0.25–0.5 mg/kg/h based on clinical response (pain scores) or signs of toxicity • Allow 8 h for steady-state serum levels to be achieved before making dosage adjustments	• Observe for **signs of toxicity** including twitching, tremors or seizures. Hypertension may be an early warning sign of toxicity • The most common symptoms of toxicity include sedation, tinnitus, metallic taste and perioral numbness • These symptoms usually disappear with cessation of the infusion for 1–2 h and resumption of the infusion at a decreased rate • Other signs of toxicity include respiratory depression, dizziness, confusion, blurred vision, double vision, visual hallucinations, bradycardia, hypotension, and agitation • Page/Call APS **stat** if patient develops any signs or symptoms of toxicity and/or if there is no change in pain scores and analgesic consumption	• Routine serum lidocaine level testing is not necessary • However, in the event of life-threatening symptoms that may be attributed to lidocaine toxicity, serum lidocaine levels should be obtained and sent for analysis • These symptoms may include: hypotension, abrupt/severe change in the level of consciousness and bradycardia • In all these cases, the lidocaine infusion must be stopped immediately • **Note**: serum lidocaine levels take several days or weeks to be reported and are therefore of limited usefulness for APS patients • Mild sedation or other mild symptoms of lidocaine toxicity (peri-oral numbness, heavy tongue, tinnitus) should not require lidocaine blood level testing
Infusion-titration and termination	• Lidocaine infusion for APS patients may be **discontinued** at the discretion of attending anesthesiologist once bowel recovery is underway and oral analgesics are both tolerated and sufficient for pain control	• Patients may experience a sudden reduction in their pain scores and opioid analgesic requirements in the first 24 h after starting lidocaine • Continue to optimize multimodal analgesia • Anti-hyperalgesic medications (e.g. pregabalin) may be required to replace or supplement IV lidocaine	• Mild to moderate sedation can be secondary to lidocaine or opioids • Typical duration of infusion is 12–72 h, but may be extended at the discretion of APS physician to achieve bowel recovery and opioid-sparing pain control

Lidocaine is metabolized in the liver and excreted by the kidneys, and therefore depends on adequate functioning of these organ systems for clinical effectiveness and safety. Lidocaine has a high hepatic extraction and its metabolism depends not only on hepatic metabolic capacity, but also on hepatic blood flow. Monoethylglycinexylidide (MEGX) and glycinexylidide (GX) are the two major metabolites of lidocaine. MEGX has similar convulsant and anti-arrhythmic potency as lidocaine. However, MEGX is rapidly metabolized by the liver to GX. MEGX has also been shown to decrease the clearance of lidocaine. GX has significantly less activity than lidocaine and is both metabolized and excreted by the kidney. MEGX has been known to cause toxicity in patients with cardiac failure and GX is known to accumulate in patients with renal failure. There is no specific pharmacological antidote for systemic lidocaine toxicity. As such, early detection and standard supportive treatment are required to prevent and treat lidocaine toxicity, respectively [2].

Evidence for Efficacy

Peri-operatively, when IV lidocaine is administered as a continuous infusion at clinically relevant doses (1–2 mg/kg/h) it usually results in plasma concentrations that remain below 5 μg/ml. At this plasma level, it is adequate to attenuate sympathetic responses, decrease pain and demonstrate a significant volatile anaesthetic and opioid sparing effect. This use of lidocaine for up to 24 h has been widely reported to show a significant decrease in pain, reduced analgesic requirements, a faster return of gastrointestinal function and an overall reduction in side effects.

One of the first clinically relevant studies was published by Gunnar Rimback and colleagues in 1990 [7]. They had previously observed that intraperitoneal lidocaine reduced the incidence of post-operative ileus. They enrolled 30 patients undergoing open cholecystectomy who were given radio-opaque markers to swallow prior to their surgery. They observed that the patients randomized to IV lidocaine treatment (100 mg bolus followed by 3 mg/min for 24 h) showed significant recovery in bowel motility that was confirmed by serial radiographs. These patients also had less pain, less opioid requirements and recovered faster. Rimback suggested that the IV lidocaine reduced the ileus and/or enhanced gut function recovery through one or more of five mechanisms—excitatory effect on gut smooth muscle (direct), reducing pain and opioid requirements (indirect), blockade of sympathetic reflexes, reducing catecholamines and/or an anti-inflammatory effect.

Scott Groudine and coworkers reported the next study that provided additional useful information regarding our understanding of peri-operative IV lidocaine in 1998 [8]. They randomized 40 patients undergoing open radical prostatectomy to receive placebo or lidocaine (bolus 1.5 mg/kg followed by 3 mg/min continued until 60 min after skin closure). They serially estimated the plasma concentrations and found them to remain within the therapeutic range (between 1.3–3.7 μg/ml). They reported a significant reduction in opioid analgesic requirements, decreased pain scores with greater satisfaction and earlier return of bowel activity in the patients receiving lidocaine. They also noted that on the third post-operative day, when the surgical drains were being removed, most patients receiving lidocaine had either passed flatus or had a bowel movement, were ambulant and had progressed to a full diet.

These patient outcomes are precisely those sought by enhanced recovery after surgery (ERAS) protocols and this study highlighted the important role played by IV lidocaine in achieving clinically relevant ERAS outcomes.

Wolfgang Koppert and co-workers demonstrated another ERAS outcome in 2004 [9]. They confirmed that patients receiving lidocaine after undergoing major abdominal surgery had no side effects and maintained safe plasma concentrations. Additionally, they observed that the lidocaine benefits (decreased analgesic requirements and pain scores) became more prominent 36 h after the lidocaine infusion had been terminated. This effect of intra-operative lidocaine administration—a positive impact that is not only sustained but also increases with time—has been seen elsewhere but not well understood or explained. Rimback first described this effect in their landmark study mentioned previously [7].

In a group of patients undergoing open colorectal surgery without epidural analgesia (either refused or contraindicated), Herroeder and co-workers demonstrated that those randomized to treatment with IV lidocaine had an earlier recovery of bowel function and shorter length of stay. They also measured a group of inflammatory markers, all of which were significantly blocked by IV lidocaine as demonstrated by a marked reduction in their rise. They concluded that "systemic lidocaine may provide a convenient and inexpensive approach to improve outcome for patients not suitable for epidural anesthesia" [10].

As ERAS protocols became more widely adopted and meticulously implemented, the impact of single modalities or interventions became more difficult to define, demonstrate or prove. Nevertheless, Abdourahamane Kaba's study, published in 2007, showed that IV lidocaine could play an important role even in a standardized colorectal ERAS protocol [11]. They randomized 45 patients undergoing laparoscopic colonic resections to receive placebo or IV lidocaine (bolus of 1.5 mg/kg followed by 2 mg/kg/h for 24 h). Other than decreasing pain scores, analgesic consumption and side-effects well beyond the duration of the lidocaine infusion; they observed two other important findings. When titrated with a depth of anesthesia monitor, patients receiving lidocaine required a significantly lower amount of volatile anaesthetics. More importantly, these patients had a significant improvement in their dynamic pain scores. In other words, although the rest pain scores were similar, the patients receiving lidocaine were able to mobilize, deep breathe and cough better than those receiving a standard opioid based analgesic protocol.

At least three studies have compared IV lidocaine to epidural analgesia. In 2006, Kuo studied patients undergoing open colonic resections and randomized them into three groups—epidural, intravenous lidocaine and placebo [12]. While patients with epidurals had better pain relief, lower opioid consumption, earlier return of bowel function and reduced cytokine production compared to IV lidocaine during the 72 h after colonic surgery; compared to the control group, these outcomes were significantly improved in the group receiving IV lidocaine compared with the placebo group. This study, demonstrated that thoracic epidurals had the best outcomes for open surgery but that IV lidocaine may offer a good alternative, especially when epidurals are contraindicated, refused or fail. In 2010, Brian Swenson and colleagues randomized 45 patients undergoing open colorectal surgery to receive either an epidural with bupivacaine or IV lidocaine. Post-operatively, they continued the epidural or lidocaine until the return of bowel function or 5 days (whichever was earlier). They found no differences between the groups for any of the outcomes—pain scores, analgesic consumption, side effects, return of bowel function or hospital length of stay; suggesting these modalities were comparable in their impact [13]. In 2011, Wongyingsinn and co-workers compared IV lidocaine to epidural analgesia for laparoscopic colonic resections in a standardized ERAS protocol [14]. They reported no difference in post-operative pain intensity, time out of bed, dietary intake, duration of hospital stay, and post-operative complications. This study confirms that even in well-established protocols for laparoscopic colorectal surgery, lidocaine can ensure the same ERAS outcomes as epidural analgesia.

To have a balanced view of the use of IV lidocaine, it is important to highlight that in other models of acute pain less consistent benefits have been reported. These include patients undergoing hip arthroplasty (Martin, Anesthesiology 2008), hysterectomy (Bryson, CJA 2009) and others where the investigators failed to demonstrate a clinical and/or statistically significant analgesic benefit from IV lidocaine [15, 16]. Despite these results, trials with IV lidocaine in ambulatory surgery, experimental ischemic pain in volunteers, post amputation stump pain and in preventing persistent pain after breast surgery continue to provide encouraging results [17–19]. We expect more trials in a wide variety of surgical models to be conducted and reported.

To date there have been four published systematic reviews with meta-analyses (Level 1 evidence) for the peri-operative use of IV lidocaine [5, 20–23]. Sun and co-investigators published the most recent systematic review, which only included clinical trials on abdominal surgery [5]. They included 21 placebo controlled double blind randomized controlled trials, of which 15 were for open surgery, and 6 for laparoscopic procedures. In their sub-group analysis, they found that compared to placebo, those patients who received IV lidocaine while undergoing open procedures showed significant benefit in terms of decreased pain scores, analgesic consumption and side effects. In the laparoscopic sub-group, despite the clear trend towards benefit, these differences did not achieve statistical significance. Across all procedures, and again more so for open procedures, IV lidocaine improved recovery of bowel function and shortened hospital length of stay.

Practical Considerations

Intra-operative

There are a significant number of indications for the use of intravenous lidocaine based on the pharmacology, evidence and experience. These are listed in Table 6.2. In abdominal surgery, the use of IV lidocaine is considered an alternative to epidural or other regional anaesthesia techniques.

Table 6.2 Summary of indications for IV lidocaine

	Alternative to regional anaesthesia	Acute pain with pronociception (hyperalgesia)
Intra-Operative	1. Epidural—contraindicated or failed 2. Laparoscopic surgery 3. Enhanced recovery protocols 4. Trauma—multiple, significant injuries	1. Opioid dependence or tolerance 2. Surgery at a site of chronic pain 3. Previous experience of poorly controlled pain 4. Substance abuse
Post-Operative	1. Epidural—inadequate or failed 2. Laparoscopic converted to open 3. Trauma—burns, degloving, crush injury 4. Rib, clavicle or sternal fractures 5. Prevention or treatment of ileus	1. Acute neuropathic pain—DN4+ 2. Opioid sparing technique—Obese, OSA, elderly and those with opioid side effects 3. Difficult to treat patients—chronic pain/opioid tolerance/substance abuse 4. Neuropathic pain models—Spine surgery and limb amputations

As mentioned before, intra-operative epidural analgesia with continuous administration of local anaesthetics is still the "gold standard" after open abdominal surgery. However, these can be associated with a very high failure rate—up to one in three fail to provide adequate analgesia because the catheter is either removed prematurely or malpositioned [20]. In addition, the continuous epidural technique requires standardization and individualization so that with careful adjustment of the infusion (drug, dose and delivery) adequate analgesia is achieved without three major side-effects: hypotension, urinary retention and motor blockade.

Intravenous lidocaine is, on the other hand, devoid of these three issues and Level 1 evidence has established that intravenous lidocaine significantly decreases the intensity of post-operative pain and reduces opioid consumption [5]. Consequently, lidocaine appears to be an appropriate alternative option for pain relief when epidural analgesia is not possible or when it is inappropriate due to patient, surgical procedure or provider factors. These contraindications for continuous epidural analgesia may include patient refusal, localized or systemic infections, anatomical and/or post-surgical abnormalities of the spine that make the epidural placement difficult and those with failed, patchy or unilateral epidural blockade.

The concomitant use of IV lidocaine with another regional anaesthesia technique (e.g., epidural, TAP block) requires careful consideration and is probably best avoided because of possible local anaesthetic toxicity. If both techniques are required, the bolus of only one should be administered and simultaneous continuous infusions of both are probably contraindicated.

One exception to this would be the use of spinal opiate analgesia, typically as a primary analgesic technique for laparoscopic abdominal surgery, where the systemic dose of intrathecal bupivacaine is low enough too safely allow the addition of IV lidocaine intra-operatively. This approach was implemented in 2016 at national level in Scotland as part of their ERAS protocol for laparoscopic colorectal surgery (Personal Communication from Dr. Anton Krige).

The widespread implementation of minimally invasive and laparoscopic surgery has resulted in the move away from epidural techniques. We believe IV lidocaine should be a component of every laparoscopic procedure, irrespective of its duration, invasiveness and desired outcomes. There is considerable experience and good quality evidence to support this. The infusion can be terminated at the end of the surgery or continued for a few hours into the post-operative period.

A very important use of intra-operative IV lidocaine therapy is in situations where laparoscopic procedures are 'converted' to open, especially when there was no epidural placed. As evident from several clinical trials with open abdominal surgery, these patients with 'conversions' will benefit from the continuation of lidocaine into the post-operative period [8–10, 12, 13]. We would recommend continuing the IV lidocaine for 3–5 days or until the bowel function returns, pain is well-controlled and/or the patient can tolerate oral medications.

Outside of GI surgery, evidence supports the benefits for the use of lidocaine for patients with chronic pain undergoing other major surgery [17, 18]. In our experience, patients with 'difficult to manage' acute pain, either in the past or currently, benefit from IV lidocaine. Some of these are patients with chronic pain, opioid tolerance and/or opioid dependence, substance abuse and complex neuropsychiatric disorders. Table 6.2 summarizes the indications for the use of IV lidocaine as an infusion during surgery.

It should be noted that the intra-operative use of lidocaine can reduce the requirements of volatile agents, especially when titrated with depth of anesthesia monitoring (BIS). In fact an accidental intra-operative lidocaine overdose was detected with a drop in BIS value [11, 12, 24–27].

Post-operative Lidocaine

When a patient is identified as being at risk of developing acute hyperalgesia, we recommend the use of anti-hyperalgesic medications such as IV lidocaine, ketamine or gabapentinoids. The objective diagnosis of acute neuropathic pain can be made using Bouhassira's widely accepted DN4 questionnaire [28]. The initiation of IV lidocaine in the post-operative period has similar indications as mentioned in Table 6.2. The difference in initiation and duration of this therapy is that it has to take into consideration the clinical presentation of the patient.

One of the most important uses of IV lidocaine after abdominal surgery may be in the prevention and/or treatment of post-operative ileus. Truly, irrespective of the type of surgery the patient has undergone, lidocaine may be useful for this. The effect of IV lidocaine on GI function has been demonstrated clearly in a number of trials and also confirmed in the systematic reviews [5]. Though the mechanism by which lidocaine prevents and treats post-operative ileus is unclear, as mentioned in preceding sections, it is probably a combination of direct and indirect effects [12–18]. Of these factors, the spinal reflex arc and sympathetic hyperactivity, activated by abdominal pain, is widely accepted as the predominant cause for inhibited intestinal motility and propulsive activity. Lidocaine accelerates post-operative intestinal motility by blocking the afferent or efferent link of the sympathetic inhibitory spinal and prevertebral reflexes, by reducing the inflammatory response and by providing an opioid-sparing effect.

It is worthwhile reviewing a remarkable case series published by Baumann where they describe the management of ileus secondary to spinal cord injury

[28]. These authors report that in patients with ileus (duration 4–10 days) after a serious spinal cord injury (refractory to medical management), five of seven of these patients experienced resolution of their ileus with a lidocaine infusion of 10–20 h duration. This finding suggests that lidocaine may have a more direct effect on the gut than what was previously considered. We have observed this effect in patients who have undergone spinal surgery and present with an ileus. It is our opinion that IV lidocaine may be the drug of choice in the management of post-operative ileus.

Depending on local acute pain management strategies, patients who have received continuous epidural analgesia post-operatively may develop an ileus after the epidural is discontinued. We routinely use and recommend IV lidocaine as a 'rescue' for these patients. In others who are NPO or have a naso-gastric tube still draining, we 'prophylactically' start lidocaine infusions for such patients on the day their epidural is turned off. Again, this practice is based on evidence from trials that have shown IV lidocaine to be non-inferior to epidurals in this respect [12–14].

Developing a Local Policy

In 2009, we proposed a formal protocol to guide the administration of IV lidocaine for acute pain management on the standard surgical wards (see Table 6.1) [2]. Proper and continued training of the nursing staff is of vital importance for the safe and successful implementation of this protocol. On the surgical floor IV lidocaine may be used, but trained personnel and standard resuscitative equipment should be available for immediate use. In our center, immediate in-house availability of the Acute Pain Service (APS) team during the daytime and on-call anaesthesia team after hours ensures round the clock support to the nursing staff.

An important caveat is that the initiation of this therapy is clearly defined as requiring the anesthesiologist in attendance and takes place in a monitored setting. Most of our patients receiving IV lidocaine post-operatively will have received a bolus (1–2 mg/kg to maximum of 100 mg in less than 1 min) as part of their anaesthetic induction. The remainder, for whom this is initiated while they are awake in the post-operative period (in the post-anaesthetic care unit or PACU), receive the bolus (similar dose) over 2–4 min. The infusion is started immediately after the bolus, both during the anaesthetic and in PACU at a rate of 1 mg/kg/h. In the awake patient, this rate can be adjusted upwards to 1.5 or 2 mg/kg/h. The lidocaine infusions are run for 2–3 days and can be reduced back to 1.5 or 1 mg/kg/h depending on the benefit. All patients will also receive our standardized multimodal analgesia APS protocols. When the patient leaves the PACU to the surgical floor, a protocol is printed and attached to the patient chart. For patients on IV lidocaine, we ensure careful bedside monitoring (see Table 6.1) by the nursing staff, meticulous and regular follow up by the APS team, along with proper handover and communication between them and surgical teams.

We summarize our experience with IV lidocaine and focus on patient safety factors:

1. *Patient Selection*:
   Patients who may benefit from IV Lidocaine are summarized in Table 6.2. IV lidocaine may have adverse effects on cardiac conductivity, myocardial contractility and precipitate partial or grand mal seizures. Hence caution is warranted in patients with history of any degree of heart block, heart failure or seizure disorder. Impaired liver and renal function or drug interactions may also impair lidocaine clearance; hence this needs to be carefully considered. A thorough list of potential drug interactions and medical conditions that place patient at increased risk was listed in the formal policy.
2. *Regional Anaesthesia Techniques*:
   IV lidocaine is contraindicated when other regional anaesthesia techniques are concurrently used (with the exception of intrathecal local anaesthetic), especially where bolus or large doses of any local anaesthetic are administered. Examples include epidural, plexus blocks and TAP blocks. IV lidocaine infusion can be initiated 4–8 h after the discontinuation of these regional techniques, and a bolus dose is best avoided. In the case of a failed epidural, as long as the epidural infusion was stopped without an epidural bolus (test dose), IV lidocaine can be initiated immediately-again without a bolus dose. Individual patient factors may also need consideration in all these situations and extended monitoring may be justified.
3. *Physician and Nursing factors*:
   IV lidocaine may only be ordered by anaesthesiologists—all nurses on the wards where this treatment modality is to be implemented should be educated regarding the policy and procedures associated with IV lidocaine for acute pain management.
4. *Maintenance of IV lidocaine on the standard ward*:
   When intravenous lidocaine therapy is started in the OR, a critical care area such as PACU or ICU, therapeutic levels (2.5–3.5 μg/ml) may be maintained on the standard ward with no need for continuous ECG monitoring. Assessments of level of sedation, etc. are done as per IV PCA standards. However, ECG monitoring, pulse oximetry and BP measurement devices should all be immediately available.
5. *Dose*:
   The usual rate of IV lidocaine therapy is 1 mg/kg/h. Acceptable range is 0.5–2 mg/kg/h. Need for continuation of therapy to be assessed on a daily basis.
6. *Initiation of IV lidocaine therapy*:
   Patients with ASA status 1 or 2 with no concern for adverse effect or drug interactions with IV lidocaine may be considered for initiating therapy on the standard wards. Consider portable continuous ECG, pulse oximetry and BP monitors during loading dose and for 15 min after. The anaesthesiologist may administer 1.5 mg/kg (total max. of 100 mg) IV by intermittent bolus over 4 min. The anaesthesiologist should stay in attendance for 15 min after completing the loading dose.
7. *High-Risk Patients*:
   Less healthy patients (especially the elderly, obese and those with hepatic and renal dysfunction) are at risk for respiratory depression in the first few hours

after initiation of lidocaine treatment, secondary to the opioids administered prior to initiation of lidocaine therapy. It may be reasonable to initiate and continue the IV lidocaine therapy in a higher dependency monitored area like PACU, step-down unit or ICU. Once the dose of lidocaine has been titrated, they should remain closely monitored for 4–8 h while the plasma concentrations stabilize. The titration of therapy and level of care needs to be individualized to the patient needs.

8. *Equipment and Administration*:
    (a) Use 250 ml commercially supplied bags of a standard 0.4% lidocaine solution. Ensure the bags are well labelled in their stock area and avoid confusion with 500 ml IV bags. It is preferable to use IV administration pumps with preprogrammed settings (0.4% and 250 ml) from a drug library for IV lidocaine. Once IV lidocaine is chosen only the patients weight and dose (in mg/kg/h) need to be programmed. Programming of the pump is performed by the primary bedside nurse and cross-checked by another nurse before initiation. There must be protection against the possibility for gravity free-flow of the IV lidocaine. This is easily achieved by only administering the IV lidocaine via the side-port of a PCA Y-connector that has an anti-free-flow valve (often referred to as an anti-siphon valve) built into the Y-connector (Fig. 6.6).
    (b) Clinically, and in our extensive experience with this drug, the most common cause of toxicity is dose, programming and/or unintentional rapid infusion due to equipment failure or personnel error. Careful and meticulous dose calculation and pump programing, two-person crosscheck, along with vigilant patient monitoring, is the cornerstone of safety in peri-operative IV lidocaine therapy.
    (c) It is very important to stock only preservative and epinephrine free lidocaine for intravenous use on the anaesthetic drug carts. If bags of IV lidocaine are used, they should be labelled or packaged clearly and kept well separated from the intravenous fluids.
    (d) It should be emphasized that the dose of IV lidocaine should be calculated based on ideal body weight (IBW) and reduced for age, cardio-respiratory insufficiency and hepato-renal dysfunction, all of which predispose the patients to toxicity.
    (e) The safe duration of continuous infusion is not widely reported or well established. The context sensitive half time after a 3-day infusion of lidocaine is approximately 20–40 min and there is no accumulation over time in healthy individuals. These remain stable for days and decrease rapidly when discontinued. We have used this drug for 2–3 days in over 75% of our patients requiring this drug. Our pharmacokinetic modelling is also reassuring and in keeping with our current clinical practice. Other investigators have reported up to 14 days of continuous infusion without toxicity [29].

Conclusions

The benefits of peri-operative IV lidocaine infusions have been confirmed with good quality evidence and growing clinical experience. These include significant decreases in pain scores and reduced opioid analgesic consumption with resul-

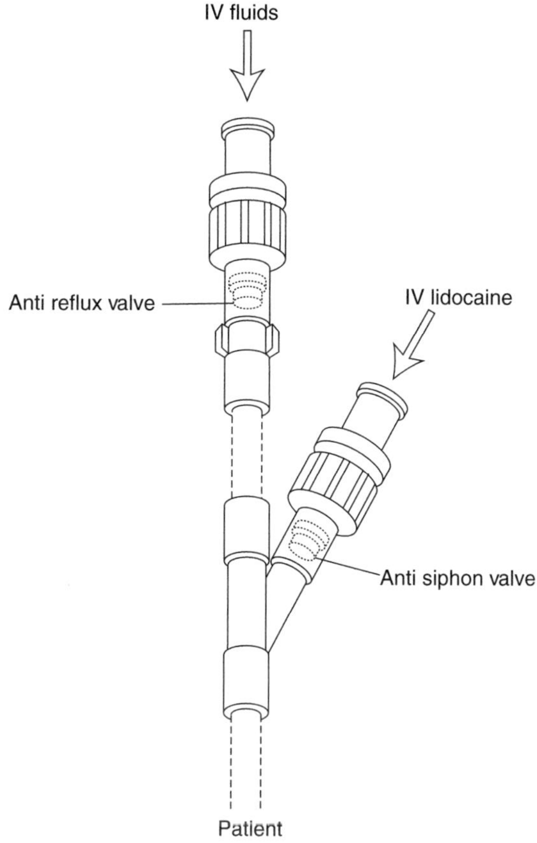

Fig. 6.6 Anti-siphon valve built into the Y-connector. Image created by Perry Ng

tant reduction in opioid related side effects, notably nausea, vomiting and ileus. The concepts of multimodal analgesia and therapeutic use of non-opioid adjuncts in the management of acute post-operative pain are still evolving. Identification of acute hyperalgesia is an important concept that is being increasingly recognized; IV lidocaine has an important role in this aspect of acute pain management. IV lidocaine is a useful non-opioid analgesic, anti-inflammatory and anti-hyperalgesic, which can contribute to significant improvements in patient outcomes, especially after abdominal surgery.

References

1. Eipe N, Penning J. Bowel surgery and multimodal analgesia: same game, new team? Anesth Analg. 2009;109:1703–4.
2. Eipe N, Gupta S, Penning J. Intravenous lidocaine for acute pain—an evidence based clinical update. BJA Educ. 2016;16:292–8.
3. Eipe N, Penning J, Yazdi F, et al. Perioperative use of pregabalin for acute pain—a systematic review and meta-analysis. Pain. 2015;156:1284–300.
4. Bouhassira D, Attal N, Alchaar H, et al. Comparison of pain syndromes associated with nervous or somatic lesions and development of a new neuropathic pain diagnostic questionnaire (DN4). Pain. 2005;114:29–36.

5. Sun Y, Li T, Wang N, et al. Perioperative systemic lidocaine for postoperative analgesia and recovery after abdominal surgery: a meta-analysis of randomized controlled trials. Dis Colon Rectum. 2012;55:1183–94.
6. de Oliveira CM, Issy AM, Sakata RK. Intraoperative intravenous lidocaine. Rev Bras Anestesiol. 2010;60:325–33.
7. Rimbäck G, Cassuto J, Tollesson PO. Treatment of postoperative paralytic ileus by intravenous lidocaine infusion. Anesth Analg. 1990;70:414–9.
8. Groudine SB, Fisher HA, Kaufman RP Jr, et al. Intravenous lidocaine speeds the return of bowel function, decreases postoperative pain, and shortens hospital stay in patients undergoing radical retropubic prostatectomy. Anesth Analg. 1998;86:235–9.
9. Koppert W, Weigand M, Neumann F, et al. Perioperative intravenous lidocaine has preventive effects on postoperative pain and morphine consumption after major abdominal surgery. Anesth Analg. 2004;98:1050–5.
10. Herroeder S, Pecher S, Schönherr ME, et al. Systemic lidocaine shortens length of hospital stay after colorectal surgery: a double-blinded, randomized, placebo-controlled trial. Ann Surg. 2007;246:192–200.
11. Kaba A, Laurent SR, Detroz BJ, et al. Intravenous lidocaine infusion facilitates acute rehabilitation after laparoscopic colectomy. Anesthesiology. 2007;106:11–8.
12. Kuo CP, Jao SW, Chen KM, et al. Comparison of the effects of thoracic epidural analgesia and i.v. infusion with lidocaine on cytokine response, postoperative pain and bowel function in patients undergoing colonic surgery. Br J Anaesth. 2006;97:640–6.
13. Swenson BR, Gottschalk A, Wells LT, et al. Intravenous lidocaine is as effective as epidural bupivacaine in reducing ileus duration, hospital stay, and pain after open colon resection: a randomized clinical trial. Reg Anesth Pain Med. 2010;35:370–6.
14. Wongyingsinn M, Baldini G, Charlebois P, et al. Intravenous lidocaine versus thoracic epidural analgesia: a randomized controlled trial in patients undergoing laparoscopic colorectal surgery using an enhanced recovery program. Reg Anesth Pain Med. 2011;36:241–8.
15. Martin F, Cherif K, Gentili ME, et al. Lack of impact of intravenous lidocaine on analgesia, functional recovery, and nociceptive pain threshold after total hip arthroplasty. Anesthesiology. 2008;109:118–23.
16. Bryson GL, Charapov I, Krolczyk G, et al. Intravenous lidocaine does not reduce length of hospital stay following abdominal hysterectomy. Can J Anaesth. 2010;57:759–66.
17. De Oliveira GS Jr, Fitzgerald P, et al. Systemic lidocaine to improve postoperative quality of recovery after ambulatory laparoscopic surgery. Anesth Analg. 2012;115:262–7.
18. Frölich MA, Mckeown JL, Worrell MJ, Ness TJ. Intravenous lidocaine reduces ischemic pain in healthy volunteers. Reg Anesth Pain Med. 2010;35:249–54.
19. Wu CL, Tella P, Staats PS, et al. Analgesic effects of intravenous lidocaine and morphine on post amputation pain: a randomized double-blind, active placebo-controlled, crossover trial. Anesthesiology. 2002;96:841–8.
20. Marret E, Rolin M, Beaussier M, Bonnet F. Meta-analysis of intravenous lidocaine and postoperative recovery after abdominal surgery. Br J Surg. 2008;95:1331–8.
21. Mccarthy GC, Megalla SA, Habib AS. Impact of intravenous lidocaine infusion on postoperative analgesia and recovery from surgery: a systematic review of randomized controlled trials. Drugs. 2010;70:1149–63.
22. Vigneault L, Turgeon AF, Côté D, et al. Perioperative intravenous lidocaine infusion for postoperative pain control: a meta-analysis of randomized controlled trials. Can J Anaesth. 2011;58:22–37.
23. Kranke P, Jokinen J, Pace NL, et al. Continuous intravenous perioperative lidocaine infusion for postoperative pain and recovery. Cochrane Database Syst Rev. 2015;7:CD009642.
24. Wu CT, Borel CO, Lee MS, et al. The interaction effect of perioperative co-treatment with dextromethorphan and intravenous lidocaine on pain relief and recovery of bowel function after laparoscopic cholecystectomy. Anesth Analg. 2005;100:448–53.
25. Saadawy IM, Kaki AM, Abd El Latif AA, et al. Lidocaine vs. magnesium: effect on analgesia after a laparoscopic cholecystectomy. Acta Anaesthesiol Scand. 2010;54:549–56.

26. Kuipers JA, Boer F, de Roode A, et al. Modeling population pharmacokinetics of lidocaine: should cardiac output be included as a patient factor? Anesthesiology. 2001;94:566–73.
27. Gaughen CM, Durieux M. The effect of too much intravenous lidocaine on bispectral index. Anesth Analg. 2006;103:1464–5.
28. Baumann A, Audibert G, Klein O, Mertes PM. Continuous intravenous lidocaine in the treatment of paralytic ileus due to severe spinal cord injury. Acta Anaesthesiol Scand. 2009;53:128–30.
29. Williams DR, Stark RJ. Intravenous lignocaine (lidocaine) infusion for the treatment of chronic daily headache with substantial medication overuse. Cephalalgia. 2003;23:963–71.

Spinal Analgesia as an Adjunct to General Anaesthesia for Laparoscopic Major Abdominal Surgery

7

Sabrina Dhillon and Michael J. P. Scott

Key Points

1. Spinal anaesthesia (using local anaesthetics and an opioid additive) combined with general anaesthesia has several benefits for laparoscopic and robotic assisted surgery. These include improved initial pain control in the post-anaesthetic care unit (PACU) and an opioid-sparing effect during the post-operative period.
2. Spinal anaesthesia has a good safety profile and low failure rate when compared to epidural anaesthesia.
3. The dosing of local anaesthetic using smaller total volumes of around 2.0 mL reduces the risk of high block in the steep head down position. The dosing of intrathecal opioids should be calculated on a weight and age basis with dosing at the lower therapeutic range. Dosages of 150–200 μg of morphine or 300–600 μg of diamorphine are typically used.
4. Spinal anaesthesia is short acting, with the motor effect wearing off within a few hours allowing for early mobility in keeping with the principle aims of enhanced recovery programs. Given the short duration of a spinal, as compared with an epidural, the need for using post-operative vasopressors and prolonged post-operative intravenous fluids is not necessary. Early mobilization free of intravenous lines or a PCA is achievable.

Introduction

Minimally invasive surgery using laparoscopic or robotic assisted techniques has proven to have several advantages over open surgery in the short term, including a smaller incision with less wound pain, less analgesic use, lower wound morbidity,

S. Dhillon · M. J. P. Scott (✉)
Department of Anesthesiology, Virginia Commonwealth University Health System, Richmond, VA, USA
e-mail: Michael.J.Scott@vcuhealth.org

A. Krige, M. J. P. Scott (eds.), *Analgesia in Major Abdominal Surgery*,
https://doi.org/10.1007/978-3-319-94482-1_7

and potentially a quicker return of gastrointestinal function. Despite these advances any major surgery is still associated with pain, physiological and haemodynamic effects, complications such as infection or thromboembolic events, and a surgical stress response.

Enhanced recovery after surgery (ERAS) protocols involve a set of evidence based elements that aim to decrease the physiologic stress of surgery, improve the metabolic response to surgery, reduce complications, and decrease the hospital length of stay. Surgical stress can be defined in terms of the body's response to surgical injury that affects not only haemodynamics, but also the neuroendocrine, metabolic, and immune systems. Generally speaking, there are two parts to the surgical stress response. The first part involves activation of the sympathetic nervous system with pituitary response. This can result in issues such as muscle catabolism, hyperglycemia, and insulin resistance. The other component of the stress response involves inflammation and immunological changes.

The combination of minimally invasive surgery together with an ERAS protocol has led to shorter length of hospital stays and low morbidity. With rapid recovery of gut function and the ability to give patients oral multimodal analgesia the need for addressing analgesia in these patients with complex catheter based techniques (such as thoracic epidural anaesthesia) or large doses of opioids has been challenged. The more rapid clinical recovery and the reduction in inflammatory mediators in some studies indicate that the stress response is maintained for a shorter duration of time post-operatively in minimally invasive surgery [1]. This has challenged traditional concepts of the role of the stress response in recovery after surgery and whether obtunding the stress response should be a major goal in peri-operative care. However, it is clear that pain and the ascending pathway activation should be viewed not only as a key driver of the stress response but that they impair the return of function, especially mobility and respiratory function, which are key factors in ensuring good outcomes after surgery.

It is within this context that this chapter explores the evidence behind the increasing use of spinal anaesthesia as an adjunct to general anaesthesia in major laparoscopic abdominal surgery. Spinal anaesthesia is being widely used in both laparoscopic and robotic assisted surgery. It is also being used to provide early relief from the visceral component of pain in open surgery where the abdominal wall component of pain relief is being blocked using local anaesthetic techniques such as wound infusion catheters, transversus abdominus plane (TAP) blocks or rectus sheath catheters.

Evidence for Efficacy: Regional Anaesthesia (Spinal or Epidural) with General Anaesthesia

General anaesthesia in combination with thoracic epidural anaesthesia or single shot spinal for major surgery has several advantages. Patients who get a combined anaesthetic tend to have lower requirements for inhaled anaesthetics, as well as intra-operative and post-operative narcotics. Reduction in inhalational anaesthetic is thought to reduce the risks of post-operative cognitive dysfunction. The benefit of opioid reduction is discussed later in this chapter. There is also the benefit of reducing the stress response. Neuraxial anaesthesia can diminish the neuroendocrine stress response, however the duration of reduction is proportional to how long the neuraxial block lasts [2]. Therefore this benefit for spinal anaesthesia is less compared with epidural infusion.

The effects of thoracic epidural analgesia (TEA) in open abdominal surgery have been studied extensively over the past two decades and are discussed in more detail in this book. For open abdominal surgery, TEA provides significantly better analgesia than parenteral opioids for both pain at rest and pain with movement. TEA has been associated with not only superior pain control, but also decreased cardiac and pulmonary morbidity, decreased risk of venous thrombosis, and earlier return of bowel function as compared to intravenous opioid analgesia [3, 4]. However, there are several downsides to epidural analgesia. First, there is a risk of hypotension that is caused by the sympathectomy-induced vasodilation of the blood vessels. Treatment of hypotension with intravenous fluids may lead to fluid overload if vasopressors are not used appropriately to maintain blood pressure once intravascular volume is normal. The resulting intravenous fluid excess can increase downstream complications and ileus. Secondly, there is a failure rate of insertion of epidurals due to anatomical issues or an inadequate analgesia block in the post-operative period, which is relatively common, and will need expert input to troubleshoot. Thirdly, there may be issues with motor blockade, which may be at odds with ERAS pathway goals of early mobility particularly if the epidural is inserted too low for the incision. Lumbar epidurals, with an increased frequency of leg weakness, are less desirable than a thoracic epidural for open abdominal surgery. The concentration of local anaesthetic used may also be a contributing factor with higher concentrations (particularly above 0.2%) having a higher incidence of motor block. Fourthly, there are potential serious neuroaxial complications (spinal cord injury, vertebral canal haematoma or epidural abscess) from epidural catheter insertion although the National Audit Project (NAP)3 study in the UK has shown these to be relatively rare (albeit devastating) for patients [5]. Therefore, certain patients, such as those on anticoagulants or those with coagulation disorders, may not be candidates for TEA given the risk of an epidural hematoma. The lesser complication of accidental dural puncture may result in a post dural puncture headache in 0.5% of patients.

The overall benefits of thoracic epidural (analgesia) in improving recovery or decreasing length of stay in patients undergoing laparoscopic surgery are uncertain. The current evidence base indicates there may be an analgesic benefit in the use of TEA in laparoscopic colorectal surgery. However, this analgesic benefit may not be clinically significant, and when coupled with the negative impact on a number of post-operative outcomes, this makes it difficult to recommend the routine use of TEA for laparoscopic colorectal surgery [6]. TEA may still be beneficial for patients at high risk of cardiorespiratory disease or who have chronic pain issues such as inflammatory bowel disease and should therefore still be considered. Thoracic epidural analgesia is discussed in far greater detail in the chapter that follows. Given the reasons outlined above concerning epidural anaesthesia, a single shot spinal technique may be better suited to combine with a general anaesthetic for patients undergoing laparoscopic abdominal surgery within an ERAS pathway.

The Advantages of Spinal Anaesthesia Over Thoracic Epidural Analgesia in Laparoscopic Surgery

TEA was originally thought to be mandatory for ERAS protocols to be successful. In 2009 this view was challenged when spinal anaesthesia was combined with general anaesthesia for laparoscopic colorectal in the United Kingdom resulting in ultra low length of stays of 23 h along with reduced opioid consumption [7]. However, consistently short hospital stays of around 4 days have been achieved in the USA without the use of any regional anaesthesia as an adjunct [8]. Therefore it is right to question whether adding spinal anaesthesia to general anaesthesia is worth the extra effort and risk compared with performing straight forward general anaesthesia with less invasive truncal local anaesthetic blocks such as TAP blocks and opioids or using newer modalities such as intravenous lidocaine infusions described in other chapters of this book.

Spinal Anaesthesia has similarities to TEA in terms of the benefits of neuraxial blockade such as optimal pain control at rest and with movement and also the opioid-sparing effects. Given its limited duration of action, it is more practical for laparoscopic surgery, which theoretically may have less wound pain than major open abdominal surgery. Spinal anaesthesia is reliable in comparison with the relatively high rate of epidural failure. It is safe with a lower rate of serious complications than epidural anaesthesia, despite having similar contraindications in terms of anticoagulation use and patient specific factors [5]. Spinal anaesthesia tends to be predictable, in terms of anaesthetic level provided assuming that local anaesthetic is dosed per standard guidelines. Spinal anaesthesia has also been associated with a rapid return of gastrointestinal function, a shorter length of hospital stay, lower use of vasopressors and improved early mobility in comparison to TEA [6, 9].

Spinal anaesthesia may cause immediate hypotension due to sympathetic block, which may have serious implications for those patients with cardiac issues such as aortic stenosis, and be quite profound in the elderly or those who are volume depleted. The risk of hypotension should be expected and clinicians should consider vasopressor use as well as invasive blood pressure monitoring to ensure prompt treatment. Delayed respiratory depression due to the opioid in the injectate mixture is the other main complication which readers need to be aware of.

A mixture of local anaesthetic and an opioid such as diamorphine or hydromorphone is commonly used and is correlated with lower pain scores and reduced opioid requirements post-operatively, especially in patients who have undergone abdominal surgery. Diamorphine has been used in one study for a 23-h hospital stay and was safe [7]. One large retrospective study found that the addition of hydromorphone had a significant effect on the total duration of analgesia, and that it is was efficacious and safe. Some studies have found that there may be increased incidence of respiratory depression with spinal morphine in an elderly patient population. The potential risk of respiratory depression and excessive sedation must be taken into account with dosing intrathecal opiates. Higher doses of intrathecal morphine are associated with greater degrees of respiratory depression; so typical dose range is less than 0.1–0.3 mg. Other studies had mixed results regarding time to return of bowel function and length of hospital stay.

A randomised controlled study by Levy et al. in 2011 showed no benefit of TEA over spinal analgesia or intravenous opioids [6]. Although pain scores were lower in the epidural group there was increased nausea. Lengths of stay were similar in the spinal and PCA morphine groups. Importantly, the epidural group had the longest length of stay due to a combination of reduced mobility and fluid gain despite receiving minimal opioids other than the fentanyl in the epidural. However, lengths of stay of 3–4 days were still achieved in the epidural group demonstrating that good outcomes are still possible while using them. A study by Hubner in 2015 in 128 patients also showed a 1-day increase in median recovery in patients having thoracic epidurals compared with PCA in laparoscopic surgery. PCA patients had significantly less overall complications (19 [33%] vs 35 [54%]; $P = 0.029$) [10]. A randomised controlled trial in colorectal resection within an enhanced recovery protocol by Wongyingsinn et al. compared patients receiving general anaesthesia and PCA morphine compared with general and spinal anaesthesia (bupivacaine and 200 mcg of morphine) for analgesia [9]. Mean opioid consumption in the first 24 h was reduced in the spinal group (8 mg vs 37 mg). Quality of analgesia was better but this did not translate into a reduction in length of stay. The nonrandomized study by Virlos et al. of TEA versus intrathecal analgesia with 2.0 mL of 0.5% bupivacaine and 1–1.5 mg of diamorphine for laparoscopic colorectal surgery patients reported a reduced median post-operative pain score (0 vs 3·5; $P < 0{\cdot}001$) There was also an earlier return to mobility (1 vs 4 days; $P < 0{\cdot}001$) and a shorter hospital stay (4 vs 5 days; $P < 0.001$) in favor of the intrathecal analgesia group. Return to normal gut function and post-operative nausea and vomiting were similar in the two groups [11]. A study in open liver resection surgery on 100 consecutive patients comparing epidural analgesia and 300 μg of intrathecal morphine showed a more rapid return to diet and function in the intrathecal morphine group [12].

Evidence for Spinal Anaesthesia and Its Effects on the Stress Response

The surgical stress response, which was alluded to earlier in the chapter, may be blunted transiently under spinal anaesthesia. One study by Day et al. compared the effects on neuroendocrine response in patients who had received spinal anaesthesia with those that had intravenous patient controlled analgesia (PCA) for pain control [2]. Both groups had similar interleukin (IL)-6 levels suggesting that the groups were comparable for the amount of primary tissue injury driving the stress response. The authors found that at the 3-h mark, the spinal anaesthesia group of patients had a statistically significant decrease in glucose and cortisol levels compared to the PCA group. This difference was gone at the 6-h mark, which showed that the stress response was only obtunded for the duration of the local anaesthetic block of the spinal injection. Additional useful data from the study was the reversion of IL6 levels back to normal by 36–48 h after laparoscopic surgery thereby showing the stress response in turn was reverting back to normal at this time point. Therefore, it does not make scientific sense to continue an epidural beyond this point simply for the control of the stress response alone. However, some surgeons will keep an epidural running to block the sympathetic outflow to the bowel to encourage early return of gut function.

Practical Aspects of Performing Spinal Anaesthesia with General Anaesthesia for Laparoscopic Surgery

The key issues of performing a spinal block in patients undergoing laparoscopic colorectal surgery is to perform the block safely and to avoid the danger of a high block because the patient is put into the steep head down position soon after performing the injection. With the practicalities of getting a patient ready for starting surgery after induction with intravenous access, catheters and skin preparation, and so on, 20 min usually elapses before insufflation of the pneumoperitoneum takes place. During initial use of spinal anaesthesia in laparoscopic surgery there was concern that with insufflation of the abdomen and high intra-abdominal pressures that CSF leakage through the dural puncture would lead to either increased headache or CSF pressure changes. There have been no published reports of this and in the author's previous unit there was only one case of post dural puncture headache in over 600 patient episodes. The standard needle used for the spinal injection was a 25 g Whitacre spinal needle.

Performing the Spinal Awake or Asleep?

Medicolegal considerations have led to most anaesthetists performing regional anaesthetic procedures with the patient awake prior to induction of anaesthesia. The problem with this is that the timing can lead to development of a sympathetic block with resultant vasodilatation and hypotension, either whilst the patient is waiting in the presurgical unit, or at the time of induction of anaesthesia. It is important therefore to ensure that a patients' haemodynamic parameters are controlled throughout this period with appropriate use of intravenous fluids and vasopressors. The advantage of performing the block with the patient asleep is that the hemodynamic consequences of induction of anaesthesia and positive pressure ventilation can be addressed prior to the onset of the sympathetic block from the spinal injection. In some countries performing spinal anaesthesia in anaesthetized patients is acceptable practice but the reader must make their own clinical judgement, regarding which is better for the patient, and what is acceptable medico-legal practice.

Patient Position for Performing the Spinal—Sitting or Lateral?

If injectate volumes are low ($\leq$ 2.0 mL) our group has found it makes minimal difference whether the spinals were performed in the sitting or lateral position. If larger volumes are used and the solution is hyperbaric then we would recommend the sitting awake technique with a time period of around 20 min before the patient is put in the steep head down position to allow the local anaesthetic to 'fix' around the lumbosacral region.

Local Anaesthetics Used as the Injectate Mixture

Traditionally spinal anaesthesia has been performed by local anaesthetic injection into the CSF to give a dense sensory and motor block at the spinal cord level at which the injectate comes into contact with. This depends on the position of the patient, level of the injection, speed and volume of injectate and baricity and concentration of local anaesthetic agent used. There are a range of agents and concentrations in a sterile formulation to allow use as a spinal anaesthetic. It is important to avoid high concentration local anaesthetics due to neural toxicity. The most common agents used for spinal anaesthesia are 0.5% plain bupivacaine, 0.5% levo bupivacaine or 0.5% hyperbaric bupivacaine. The duration of block can vary but is commonly 2–4 h depending on the volume used. A 2% hyperbaric prilocaine mixture has recently come onto the market but this is more suitable for ambulatory surgery where the duration of block is under 1 h.

Use of Opioids in the Injectate Mixture

Opioids added to the injectate mixture improve both quality and duration of analgesia. Fentanyl, diamorphine or morphine are drugs commonly added to the injectate mixture.

One on the most feared consequences of adding opiate to the injectate mixture is the risk of delayed respiratory depression, particularly if opiates are re-dosed in the post-operative period. For that reason, fentanyl has the advantage in improving analgesia in shorter procedures such as caesarean section without the downstream risk.

However, despite the risk of delayed respiratory depression being present it appears to be no greater than using opiates in a patient-controlled analgesia (PCA) pump post-operatively. The important thing is to ensure the patient is monitored in the same way as if they had a PCA as this will then pick up any severe consequences of respiratory depression. One single centre retrospective analysis in 5969 patients confirmed the efficacy and patient satisfaction of spinal opiates used for major urologic, orthopedic, general, vascular, thoracic, and gynecologic surgery. Pruritus was the most common complaint from patients. Whilst 3% of patients developed respiratory depression it was easily detectable and always reversed with standard administration of naloxone.

Even if longer acting opiates are used in the injectate mixture a proportion of patients will still need intravenous opiates for breakthrough pain in the PACU. In our own experience this can be up to 40%; however minimal opiates are required after this point provided the patient receives oral multimodal analgesia consisting of a combination of paracetamol 1 g QID and ibuprofen 400 mg TID regularly. The addition of the other non-opioid adjuvants discussed in chapters 4–6 will also reduce this rescue opiate requirement.

The most important effect of adding intrathecal opiates appears to be the downstream reduction in opioid consumption. In three studies by Levy, Day and Wongyingsinn there was up to a sixfold sparing effect in the use of post-operative morphine in those patients receiving spinal opiates in addition to local anaesthetic [2, 6, 9]. A study by Virlos confirmed the opioid-sparing effect of intrathecal opiates but the doses of diamorphine were higher—1–1.5 mg. Despite these higher doses there were no adverse events reported in their intrathecal group of 99 patients [11].

As early adopters of spinal opioids in laparoscopic colorectal surgery the author's unit found success with volumes of around 2.5 mL of 0.5% hyperbaric bupivacaine following trials of various volumes of isobaric and hyperbaric formulations of 0.5% bupivacaine. The spinal was performed sitting before surgery and allowed to fix for at least 20 min before the abdomen was insufflated and the patient put in the steep head down position. More recently by reducing the volume of 0.5% bupivacaine to 2.0 mL we use plain bupivacaine successfully.

Our unit used a spinal injectate mixture with 0.3 mg diamorphine added to it. Diamorphine comes as a sterile white powder and can be diluted as needed and added to the injectate solution. This work was in part based on Saravanan's work in obstetric anaesthesia for dosing of intrathecal diamorphine in caesarean section, which showed the ED_{95} value for intrathecal diamorphine to prevent intra-operative supplementation was 0.39 mg. There was an approximate linear dose relationship between the dose of opioid, the duration of action of analgesia and the incidence of side effects such as pruritus or nausea and vomiting [13]. As the main aim of enhanced recovery protocols is to enable patients to eat soon after surgery any perceived benefit of increasing doses of opioids to negate the need of opiates in the post-operative period can lead to protracted nausea and vomiting and a patient that cannot take their multimodal oral analgesics or mobilize. Our unit therefore uses opioid dosing at the lower end of the range so that there is efficacy and an opiate sparing effect, but patients are at less rick of nausea, vomiting or respiratory depression. As stated previously we find around 40% of patients need breakthrough pain relief in the PACU with intravenous opiates but once they are comfortable they do not require a PCA morphine drip on the ward/floor. Our current dosing is around 0.005 mg/kg of diamorphine, reduced by up to 50% if the patient is over 70 years old. However, Virlos' group used higher doses of diamorphine from 1.0 to 1.5 mg without untoward side effects [11]. In countries where diamorphine is not available other opiates are used such as duramorph. This is preservative-free morphine available as a pre-mixed 1 mg/mL preparation. If we were using this, we would ensure the total injectate volume is less than 2.5 mL but usually in the 2.0–2.2 mL dose range. The dosing range of intrathecal morphine in clinical practice is usually 0.1–0.3 mg. A meta-analysis found that increasing the dose increased the risk of pruritus but not nausea and vomiting. Doses less than 0.3 mg lead to no more respiratory depression than systemic opiates [14].

A meta-analysis of spinal opiate use in abdominal, spine and cardiothoracic surgery included 645 patients. Pain intensity at rest was reduced as was pain on movement. Opioid requirement was decreased intra-operatively and up to 48 h after surgery. There was an increased risk of respiratory depression in the morphine group (odds ratio [OR] 7.86 [95% CI 1.54–40.3], as was the incidence of pruritus [OR 3.85 [95% CI 2.40–6.15]). Interestingly in this paper, the side effects did not appear to be dose related [14].

Use of Other Adjuncts in the CSF

There have been studies on the use of clonidine to try and potentiate and prolong the analgesic effects of spinal anaesthesia. One study in caesarean sections showed no reduction in post-operative morphine with the addition of 75 μg of clonidine, however no opiate was used in the injectate [15]. There have been no studies on adding clonidine to opiates and local anaesthetic spinal mixtures in major abdominal surgery.

Conclusions

ERAS protocols are designed to decrease hospital length of stay, improve outcomes, and reduce surgical stress. Even though the stress response in laparoscopic surgery is reduced it is still important to provide optimal analgesia to restore post-operative function. It is clear that there are many successful ways of providing analgesia for laparoscopic surgery within ERAS with the adoption of multimodal analgesia and opiate sparing techniques at their heart.

Spinal anaesthesia is a simple, safe and proven technique that introduces both local anaesthetic and an opiate into the cerebrospinal fluid. The local anaesthetic effect causes both motor and sensory block. The most commonly used drug is bupivacaine and motor and sensory block ceases by approximately 4 h. The stress response according to one study is only reduced for the duration of this local anaesthetic effect so the benefit to the patient in the immediate post-operative period is limited [2]. However, correctly dosed long acting opiates can have a dramatic opioid sparing effect with the result that patients suffer less opioid side effects, particularly, lethargy, nausea, vomiting and ileus that are linked with traditional PCA morphine. The other benefit of using intrathecal opiates is that patients do not need a PCA/intravenous carrier which requires a drip stand. Finally, the skill set required for insertion is limited compared to many of the other regional techniques allowing easy implementation at large scale and the long duration of a single injection avoids any lack of compliance from ward staff often seen with other techniques requiring continued administration. Therefore, in the setting of an ERAS Protocol when intravenous fluids are stopped the morning after surgery patients are more likely to be able to mobilize independently.

References

1. Scott MJ, Baldini G, Fearon KCH, Feldheiser A, Feldman LS, Gan TJ, et al. Enhanced Recovery After Surgery (ERAS) for gastrointestinal surgery: Part 1. Pathophysiological considerations. Acta Anaesthesiol Scand. 2015;59(10):1212–31.
2. Day AR, Smith RVP, Scott MJP, Fawcett WJ, Rockall TA. Randomized clinical trial investigating the stress response from two different methods of analgesia after laparoscopic colorectal surgery. Br J Surg. 2015;102(12):1473–9.
3. Rigg JRA, Jamrozik K, Myles PS, Silbert BS, Peyton PJ, Parsons RW, et al. Epidural anaesthesia and analgesia and outcome of major surgery: a randomised trial. Lancet. 2002;359(9314):1276–82.
4. Myles PS, Peyton P, Silbert B, Hunt J, Rigg JRA, Sessler DI, et al. Perioperative epidural analgesia for major abdominal surgery for cancer and recurrence-free survival: randomised trial. BMJ. 2011;342(mar29 2):d1491.
5. Cook TM, Counsell D. Major complications of central neuraxial block: report on the Third National Audit Project of the Royal College of Anaesthetists. Br J Anaesth. 2009;102(2):179–90.
6. Levy BF, Scott MJ, Fawcett W, Fry C, Rockall TA. Randomized clinical trial of epidural, spinal or patient-controlled analgesia for patients undergoing laparoscopic colorectal surgery. Br J Surg. 2011;98(8):1068–78.
7. Levy BF, Scott MJP, Fawcett WJ, Rockall TA. 23-Hour-stay laparoscopic colectomy. Dis Colon Rectum. 2009;52(7):1239–43.
8. Delaney CP, Brady K, Woconish D, Parmar SP, Champagne BJ. Towards optimizing perioperative colorectal care: outcomes for 1,000 consecutive laparoscopic colon procedures using enhanced recovery pathways. Am J Surg. 2012;203(3):353–5. discussion 355–6
9. Wongyingsinn M, Baldini G, Stein B, Charlebois P, Liberman S, Carli F. Spinal analgesia for laparoscopic colonic resection using an enhanced recovery after surgery programme: better analgesia, but no benefits on postoperative recovery: a randomized controlled trial. Br J Anaesth. 2012;108(5):850–6.
10. Hübner M, Blanc C, Roulin D, Winiker M, Gander S, Demartines N. Randomized clinical trial on epidural versus patient-controlled analgesia for laparoscopic colorectal surgery within an enhanced recovery pathway. Ann Surg. 2015;261(4):648–53.
11. Virlos I, Clements D, Beynon J, Ratnalikar V, Khot U. Short-term outcomes with intrathecal versus epidural analgesia in laparoscopic colorectal surgery. Br J Surg. 2010;97(9):1401–6.
12. Koea JB, Young Y, Gunn K. Fast track liver resection: the effect of a comprehensive care package and analgesia with single dose intrathecal morphine with gabapentin or continuous epidural analgesia. HPB Surg. 2009;2009(5):1–8.
13. Saravanan S, Robinson APC, Qayoum Dar A, Columb MO, Lyons GR. Minimum dose of intrathecal diamorphine required to prevent intraoperative supplementation of spinal anaesthesia for Caesarean section. Br J Anaesth. 2003;91(3):368–72.
14. Meylan N, Elia N, Lysakowski C. Benefit and risk of intrathecal morphine without local anaesthetic in patients undergoing major surgery: meta-analysis of randomized trials. Br J Anaesth. 2009;102(2):156–67.
15. Tuijl IV, Klei WAV, van der Werff DBM, Kalkman CJ. The effect of addition of intrathecal clonidine to hyperbaric bupivacaine on postoperative pain and morphine requirements after Caesarean section: a randomized controlled trial. Br J Anaesth. 2006;97(3):365–70.

Thoracic Epidural Analgesia

8

Jonathan Antrobus

Introduction

Despite the first description of epidural blockade at the beginning of the twentieth century, it wasn't until the 1970s that clinicians began to use epidural analgesia for major surgery. Finding widespread use in the 1980s through the 1990s, clinicians began to realize that epidural local anaesthetic (LA) infusions not only provided excellent analgesia but also modulated the surgical stress response leading to improvements in recovery, and this heralded a period of research interest into the outcome benefits of epidurals. Much of what we know about epidurals comes from these studies, and meta-analyses of these trials in the 1970s–1990s showed impressive effects on post-operative outcomes claiming improvements in mortality, bowel recovery, cardiac ischaemia, respiratory failure and venous thrombosis. Then, around the turn of this century, Enhanced Recovery Pathways started to become popular as a means of improving recovery and reducing complications, and, recognising the associated outcome benefits, thoracic epidural analgesia (TEA) was seen to be one of the critical elements of an ERAS pathway [1, 2].

However much of this evidence came from small studies published decades ago. Few large, well-conducted RCTs have been performed. There have since been huge strides made in peri-operative medicine with many advances in fluid management and analgesic techniques; minimally invasive surgery is now routinely used for surgery, all leading to better recovery and reduced complications. The patients in these early studies were often managed in a way that would not be considered standard practice today.

Thus, the results of many of these older studies may not be directly applicable to our patients today, and the purported benefits of epidural analgesia are likely to be overstated in today's context. Researchers have recently re-examined

J. Antrobus
Department of Anaesthesia, Borders General Hospital, Melrose, Roxburghshire, UK
e-mail: antrobus@doctors.org.uk

A. Krige, M. J. P. Scott (eds.), *Analgesia in Major Abdominal Surgery*,
https://doi.org/10.1007/978-3-319-94482-1_8

outcomes associated with epidurals in light of changes in peri-operative medicine. Commentators have suggested that TEA is no longer the analgesic panacea that it was once purported to be [3, 4] and clinicians have noted the high failure rate associated with TEA. Consequently, TEA is undeniably less popular now than previously. In a recent US survey of laparoscopic colorectal surgery, only 1.5% of patients were managed with TEA [5], and survey of Australian anaesthetists found that epidural use for abdominal surgery fell from 53% in 1998 to 27% in 2003; respondents citing lack of evidence and fear of litigation [6]. Nevertheless, when efficacious, TEA remains the single most effective technique for managing pain for open abdominal surgery and despite questions raised about the outcome data, some patients are still likely to receive benefit in terms of reduced peri-operative morbidity. TEA may no longer be a panacea but it remains worthy of consideration. As other authors have noted, it is not the act of inserting an epidural but the way in which it is managed that is the key to success [7].

Evidence for Efficacy

Adequate pain management is an essential element of post-operative care. Aside from being deeply unpleasant for the patient, poorly controlled pain may lead to post-operative morbidity and is known to be a risk factor for persistent post-surgical pain [8]. Well-controlled pain therefore may lead to faster recovery and reduce the risk of cardiac and pulmonary complications as well as improving patient satisfaction. An ideal analgesic would completely remove pain with no side effects, either absent or beneficial effects on patient physiology, and leave the patient free to eat, mobilize, and engage with rehabilitation after their surgery. We know that the ideal analgesic does not exist: whatever the surgery and whatever the modality of analgesia, there is a balance between increasing analgesic efficacy and increasing burden to the patient—either in terms of invasiveness, side effects such as nausea and sedation, or organ dysfunction such as hypotension. Therefore, total absence of pain is unrealistic, and will lead to a significant burden to the patient in other terms. Pragmatically, we want our patient to be able to cough effectively, participate actively in physiotherapy, walk around and micturate without need for bladder catheterisation, so a balance should be struck of a level of pain that is tolerable for the patient but with minimized side effects and physiological disequilibrium. Impact on dynamic pain is perhaps more important than impact on pain at rest: it is relief of pain on mobilization that will allow the patient to cough and mobilise, and pain control at rest appears to be a poor marker for pain control on movement [9].

Open Abdominal Surgery

Following abdominal surgery, pain is transmitted along the ventral branches of the spinal segmental nerves from T5 to T12, which innervate the abdominal wall, muscle layers, skin and fascia. A segmental epidural block will lead to reduced transmission of pain along these nerves. The pelvic and abdominal organs receive variable sensory innervation from the autonomic nervous system, arising from both craniosacral parasympathetic outflow and the thoracolumbar sympathetic chain, which can also be blocked by epidural local anaesthetic.

For abdominal surgery through a laparotomy incision, TEA provides significantly better analgesia than systemic opioids for both dynamic and rest pain, and tends to do so for the duration of the epidural infusion. The evidence for this is fairly unequivocal at present and is widely supported by the literature. A meta-analysis for TEA in mixed surgical procedures in 3000 patients [10] found that dynamic pain was significantly reduced in the epidural group at every time point until post-operative day 3. Another meta-analysis specifically assessing colorectal surgery studies [11] found that dynamic pain was significantly reduced on the day of surgery and post-operative day 1 and a Cochrane review for aortic surgery [12] found a significant improvement in dynamic pain for 3 days post-operatively in patients receiving epidurals. A large observational study examined the effect on pain scores of over 10,000 patients undergoing abdominal surgery and found that pain on movement was significantly less in patients with epidurals than those treated with IV morphine PCA, and remained so for 4 days post-operatively. When comparing epidural analgesia to other analgesic modalities there are other end-points to consider other than the pain score. Epidural analgesia may reduce fatigue and attenuate the loss of post-operative functional capacity, and one RCT found that both quality of life scores (SF36) and functional exercise capacity were improved at 3 weeks, but not at 6 weeks, post-operatively [13].

However, some studies suggest the improvement in pain scores with TEA over opioid infusions is not always particularly large, and here, interpretation of the data becomes interesting. Clearly an improvement that is *statistically* significant may not always equate to an improvement that is *clinically* significant. Clearly then this effect would be of questionable benefit. There is still some debate regarding what exactly constitutes a minimal clinically important difference (MCID) in terms of pain scores—a reduction in VAS from 8 to 40 mm depending on aetiology of pain [14, 15]—and anything less than this may not be perceived as a reduction in pain by the patient. One of the largest epidural RCTs to date, the MASTER trial [16], found the separation in pain scores between the epidural and IV morphine PCA groups was at its greatest for pain on coughing on the morning of post-operative day 1, where the mean 0–10 cm VAS in the epidural group was 3.9 and in the IV morphine PCA group was 5.5 thus giving a difference of 1.6 cm. Although pain on coughing remained statistically superior in the epidural group for the duration of the 3-day infusion, from post-operative day 2 onwards the benefit in pain score was less than 1 cm, and pain at rest was only statistically better on the morning of post-operative day 1. This was partly related to an intention to treat analysis in the trial design and a 40% failure rate in the epidural group. An RCT examining the efficacy of TEA in elderly patients found the reduction in pain on coughing was only >2 cm VAS on extubation, and the difference was less than 2 cm from every time point onwards [17].

Post-operative analgesia has changed considerably in recent decades, and clinicians are using many other interventions in their multimodal analgesic armamentarium. Intravenous lidocaine (Chap. 6) can reduce pain and nausea after abdominal surgery and may reduce hospital stay, and peri-operative magnesium [18] has been shown to reduce opioid consumption and pain. Regional analgesic techniques such as transversus abdominus plane (TAP) blocks (Chap. 11) and continuous wound infiltration (CWI) of local anaesthetic (Chap. 13) have been shown to reduce post-operative pain when compared to PCA alone. Moreover, these techniques may also negate many of the problems associated with epidural analgesia such as motor block, hypotension, and the need for a urinary catheter, whilst removing concerns regarding neuraxial complications associated with an epidural catheter.

The majority of published epidural studies use an opioid PCA (or even intramuscular opioids) as the control group. It could be argued that systemic opioids alone are no longer the 'standard' post-operative analgesic against which TEA should be compared. We do not know, therefore, if the TEA outcome benefits still exist when it is compared with the aforementioned novel, opioid sparing analgesic regimens. In fact, CWI has been shown to provide as effective analgesia as TEA for abdominal surgery for both dynamic and rest pain [19] and, when compared to CWI for hepatic surgery, TEA only reduced pain on the first post-operative day while opioid consumption, bowel recovery or hospital stay were unchanged [20]. Indeed, other studies have confirmed this finding in patients undergoing hepatic surgery, with CWI providing analgesia equivalent to TEA [21, 22] and CWI being associated with a shorter hospital stay. Another study, which compared four-quadrant TAP blocks to TEA for abdominal surgery found that post-operative pain scores, bowel recovery, time out of bed and hospital stay were equivalent, with earlier removal of the urinary catheter in the TAP group [23]. And when compared to TEA, intravenous lidocaine appears to be as effective for dynamic pain and bowel recovery [24, 25].

Laparoscopic Surgery

Minimally invasive surgery is a cornerstone in the development of ERAS. The incisions in the abdominal wall are smaller and consequently surgical trauma, and therefore surgical stress response is reduced [26]. This results in less post-operative pain and quicker recovery [27] indicating that adequate analgesia may be achieved by less invasive alternatives to epidural analgesia.

A systematic review in 2010 [28] concluded that although TEA controlled pain better than opioid PCA, other markers of recovery were unchanged. Levy et al. [29] showed in a randomized controlled trial that although pain control was again better when TEA was compared to morphine PCA (but not to intrathecal diamorphine), post-operative pulmonary function and quality of life were unchanged, while bowel recovery and hospital stay were prolonged in the TEA group. In another randomized trial [30] patients experiencing ERAS received either epidural analgesia or PCA morphine for laparoscopic colorectal surgery. Post-operative pain scores were not significantly different throughout recovery, although patients with epidural analgesia suffered significantly more post-operative hypotension requiring vasopressors (27% vs. 4%), more complications (54% vs. 33%) and stayed in the high-dependency unit a day longer than patients receiving PCA. An observational study of nearly 30,000 patients in 300 units in the USA found that TEA for laparoscopic surgery was not associated with an improvement in post-operative complications or death, and found that both hospital stay and costs were increased [5].

The current evidence base indicates that there may be a small analgesic benefit in the use of TEA in laparoscopic colorectal surgery. However, this analgesic benefit may not be clinically significant, and when coupled with the negative impact on a number of post-operative outcomes, this makes it difficult to recommend the routine use of TEA for laparoscopic colorectal surgery. TEA may still be beneficial for patients at high risk of cardiorespiratory disease and could be considered in that subgroup.

Evidence for Outcome Benefit

Major surgery induces a complex neurohumoral cascade that leads to increased secretion of catecholamines and cortisol and a reduction in insulin secretion. The result of this cascade is the peri-operative suppression of the immune system together with increased protein catabolism, oxygen demand and myocardial stress. This stress-mediated immunosuppression is further compounded by other 'anaesthetic' factors that have been shown to depress the immune system, including general anaesthesia, opioids, pain, blood transfusions, hypothermia and hyperglycaemia.

Researchers looking for ways to reduce post-operative morbidity have sought a reduction in this surgical stress response, and this notion has been a cornerstone in the theory of ERAS. TEA has been shown to reduce post-operative adrenaline secretion and improve insulin responsiveness [31, 32] as well as having direct beneficial effects on the cardiac and respiratory systems and the gut. It has been theorised that this blockade of the stress response should lead to a reduction in organ dysfunction and therefore an improvement in peri-operative morbidity [33]. Early meta-analyses appeared to demonstrate this [34].

Mortality

This effect of epidural analgesia has long been a controversial subject, and has generated much debate. Clearly there are plausible mechanisms why epidurals might have an effect on mortality: possible reductions in respiratory failure, cardiac complications, and duration of ventilation will all lead to improvements in patient outcome. However, epidurals are also associated with harm: peri-operative hypotension is common with epidurals and in other studies hypotension has been associated with an increased stroke risk [35]. Epidurals also have a number of rare, but significant complications such as neuraxial abscess formation and respiratory depression, which will have a clear negative effect on outcomes. Additionally, mortality is difficult to estimate. Any rare complication will require a large dataset to estimate its incidence with any accuracy, and the effect of epidurals on mortality is rarely the primary outcome for such studies, therefore the studies are underpowered to detect a mortality difference. Cohort studies and meta-analyses examining mortality tend to include a wide range of studies, and have previously lumped together neuraxial anaesthesia (spinals, thoracic and lumbar epidurals) which may or may not have been performed alongside a general anaesthetic; and for a disparate range of surgical procedures including hip replacements, aortic aneurysm repair and caesarean section, when these are completely separate subsets of patients. Finally, as mentioned previously, peri-operative medicine has changed significantly in recent decades. Therefore, an intervention that was effective in 1985 may not be effective now.

What the Data Tell Us

Rodgers' meta-analysis [34] published in 2000 examined outcomes from 141 trials with a total of 9559 participants. They included trials from many different surgical specialities and variations of regional anaesthesia, including spinal anaesthesia, thoracic and lumbar epidurals, and regional anaesthesia used in combination with general anaesthesia as well as regional anaesthesia alone. They concluded that neuraxial anaesthesia reduced the risk of death by around a third (OR, 0.70; CI, 0.54–0.90). However, after subgroup analysis the results were not quite so straightforward—out of all surgical specialities the confidence intervals crossed the 'line of no effect' in all specialities except orthopaedics, and regional anaesthesia did not reduce mortality when used in combination with general anaesthesia. Additionally, the majority of the included trials were small—around 30 of the 141 trials had 20 or fewer participants—raising questions about the quality of the studies, and included studies dating back to 1971. Again, this is problematic when post-operative management is likely to be considerably different to what we would recognize today, and perioperative mortality was considerably higher.

The MASTER trial [16], published in 2002, is one of the largest RCTs examining epidural outcomes to date and recruited 915 patients undergoing major abdominal surgery to receive either epidural analgesia for 3 days or an opioid infusion. This was a relatively high-risk population: around 30% had two or more significant comorbidities. In contrast to Rodgers' meta-analysis the 30-day mortality was unchanged between the two groups: 5.1% in the epidural group and 4.3% in the control group. However, this study had its issues too, with 50% of the patients included in the epidural arm not fully compliant with the study protocol for a variety of reasons. The epidurals were sited in high lumbar or low thoracic vertebral segments. Epidurals sited in these segments may not have the same effect on preventing complications and death, as epidurals at these lower levels have less impact on cardiac complications than higher-level thoracic epidurals [36]. The only other large RCT examining the effect of epidural on surgical outcomes was the Veterans Affairs Cooperative study [37], and randomised 1021 patients undergoing abdominal surgery to receive either epidural analgesia or parenteral opioid. It could be argued that the trial design is no longer representative of current practice, as only 26% of the control group were given opioids via a PCA device, the rest receiving either intramuscular or intermittent intravenous boluses of either morphine or pethidine, and patients in the epidural group received only epidural morphine without LA, 57% of patients receiving this as intermittent boluses. Nevertheless, investigators found no improvement in mortality with TEA for any type of surgery, and although TEA was associated with a reduction in myocardial infarction in patients undergoing aortic surgery, patients undergoing non-aortic surgery found no improvement in any major complications. Pain scores on day 1 and overall opioid consumption were modestly improved, however this did not translate into improved physical performance or length of hospital stay.

Observational studies have generally supported a reduction in mortality with epidural analgesia. Wu and colleagues [38] took a random sample of Medicare claims data from 1997 to 2001, and out of 12,817 patients undergoing elective colorectal surgery, both 7- and 30-day mortality was reduced (OR 0.52, 95% CI 0.38–0.73, and OR 0.74, 95% CI 0.63–0.88 respectively), although post-operative pneumonia was increased in the epidural group, and overall major morbidity was unchanged, weakening the claim that TEA reduced mortality. Another cohort study examined outcomes in 259,037 patients in Canada over a 10-year period from 1994 to 2004 [39] undergoing vascular, thoracic, colorectal or orthopaedic surgery. Using propensity scoring to case-match the groups receiving, or not receiving, epidurals, the relative risk of mortality was 0.89 for patients receiving epidurals. This, however, translates to a NNT of 477 leading the authors to concede that this reduction in risk was of borderline clinical significance, and did not support the use of epidural analgesia to reduce mortality. The larger effect on mortality was seen in orthopaedic and thoracic surgery, with the effect on mortality in the abdominal surgery group being RR 0.93 (95% CI 0.82–1.06).

It is interesting that these two large datasets generated such different risk calculations for mortality, both taken around the same time period. It is important to note that each study adjusted the data using different techniques, and for different variables. It is important to note that patients with epidurals are more likely to be managed in a High Dependency environment than those managed with opioids alone, meaning closer monitoring, better access to Critical Care physicians, better fluid balance and pain control, and this may lead to outcome bias when datasets are analysed. Additionally, as with all large cohort studies, neither study would be able to adjust for unknown or unmeasurable confounding factors, thus the data must be interpreted with caution.

A Cochrane review was published in 2014 [40] that pooled the studies from previous Cochrane analyses of regional anaesthesia outcomes. The authors concluded that regional anaesthesia when used alone reduced the risk of death by 30 days compared to general anaesthesia (RR, 0.71; 95% CI, 0.53–0.94; n = 1570), however when regional anaesthesia was used in combination with a general anaesthetic, the risk of death was unchanged (n = 1665). However, this review included neuraxial anaesthesia of any type, including intrathecal anaesthesia, and for a wide range of surgeries.

A meta-analysis that was published in 2014 [41, 42] examined mortality as its primary outcome measure. The authors only included studies that examined the effect of epidural analgesia when used in combination with a general anaesthetic, and reported on 125 trials including 9044 patients over a range of surgical procedures. Epidural analgesia appeared to have a benefit on 30-day mortality, with an NNT of 90 to prevent one death. Epidurals appeared to have a clearer mortality benefit when sited in thoracic segments rather than lumbar. Interestingly, peri-operative mortality in this study did not appear to have changed significantly over time, or by year of publication, meaning the outcome may not have been skewed by older studies with higher mortality. What this means in terms of the impact of improvements in peri-operative care on mortality is uncertain.

Bottom Line

There is modest evidence that epidurals may reduce peri-operative mortality. This may only pertain to high-risk patient populations, and may only pertain to neuraxial anaesthesia performed in isolation from a general anaesthetic, meaning any mortality benefit may not apply to patients undergoing abdominal surgery where TEA is not normally used without a general anaesthetic. Data from large RCTs has not shown a reduction in mortality with TEA, which may reflect the fact that these studies are generally underpowered to detect mortality differences, however, the data from large cohort studies that do indicate a mortality benefit are more susceptible to bias and care must be taken when interpreting the data.

Cardiac Complications

Cardiac complications following abdominal surgery are common, more so in the elderly population, occurring in up to 5% of cases [43]. Pain and anxiety leads to sympathetic stress, which increases myocardial workload, while surgery increases metabolic demand resulting in an increased oxygen demand, which in turn may lead to arrhythmias and myocardial ischaemia. Epidurals can have effects on peri-operative cardiac complications via several mechanisms. TEA can ameliorate these effects through both better analgesia, leading to a reduction in sympathetic outflow, and reduction in the surgical stress response. When placed high in the thoracic spine (T2–T4), epidurals appear to have a dual effect on the heart. The resulting segmental anaesthesia leads to sympathetic block that causes negative inotropy [44] and chronotropy [45] thus reducing myocardial oxygen demand along with direct coronary vasodilatation [46] that improves flow in stenotic coronary vessels during sympathetic stress [47]. In one study of TEA for cardiac bypass intra-operative cardiac index and mixed venous oxygen saturations [48] improved. Other investigators have found that following CABG surgery, patients with TEA had significantly lower post-operative troponin [49], reductions in left ventricular dysfunction and cardiac ischaemia, and improved long-term survival [50].

Mid thoracic epidurals result in a sympathectomy, which causes dilatation of splanchnic capacitance vessels. This leads to pooling of blood in the venous systems of abdominal organs [51]. This may be compensated for by constriction of other capacitance vessels, but may result in a reduction in pre-load. Reduction in sympathetic outflow leads to arteriolar vasodilatation and thus a reduction in afterload. Lumbar epidurals cause vasodilatation only in the blocked lumbar and lower thoracic segments, and may even cause a compensatory vasoconstriction in the normally innervated areas above [52].

The sympathetic block that results from thoracic epidural block also causes hypotension [11, 41]. This may result in coronary hypoperfusion and myocardial ischaemia, as well as reducing blood flow to other vital organs such as the brain, kidneys and the colonic anastomosis. As many as 30% of patients receiving epidural anaesthetic infusions require post-operative vasopressor infusions [30], thus prolonging HDU stay, and therefore potentially prolonging recovery.

Regional anaesthesia has been associated with a lower blood loss when compared to general anaesthesia [53], possibly mediated through a reduction in blood pressure. It appears the effect is most pronounced in orthopaedic surgery [54] and there was no association with reduced blood transfusion following abdominal surgery. Additionally it is unclear if epidural analgesia reduces blood loss when used in combination with a general anaesthetic [53, 54].

What the Data Tell Us

A meta-analysis including 14 trials investigating lumbar and thoracic epidurals [55] for abdominal and thoracic surgery found that epidural analgesia significantly reduced the risk of myocardial infarction with 48 epidurals preventing one myocardial infarction (OR, 0.55; 95% CI, 0.37–0.81). Another, later meta-analysis by the same author found that the risks of tachydysrhythmias, heart block and atrial fibrillation were all significantly reduced in patients receiving epidural analgesia [41] but the reduction in myocardial infarction did not reach statistical significance (OR, 0.73; 95% CI, 0.50–1.06). A Cochrane review examining TEA for abdominal aneurysm surgery concluded that TEA leads to a reduction in post-operative myocardial infarction (RR, 0.52), but had no effect on arrhythmias, heart block or heart failure [12].

However not all studies have returned positive results: post-hoc analysis of over 10,000 patients in the POISE-2 randomized trial showed that TEA did not change the rates of myocardial infarction or death. Post-hoc analysis of the POISE-1 trial of 8000 patients found that neuraxial anaesthesia was associated with an increase in cardiovascular complications (OR, 1.24; 95% CI, 1.02–1.49), and this seemed to be most prevalent in patients with TEA undergoing concurrent general anaesthesia, although, in this study, TEA was not associated with significant hypotension, death or stroke [56]. The Veterans Affairs study of 1021 patients [37] found that TEA reduced the risk of myocardial infarction and stroke in patients undergoing aortic surgery, but not those undergoing biliary, gastric or colonic surgery, and the MASTER trial found no difference in cardiovascular outcomes or death [16]. A Cochrane review of TEA for cardiac bypass found that TEA reduced arrhythmias and respiratory complications but not myocardial infarctions or death [57]. Guay's review of epidural outcomes from other Cochrane reviews [40] did not find evidence that epidurals prevent myocardial infarction. A meta-analysis of epidurals used in Enhanced Recovery pathways for colorectal surgery found that epidurals had no effect on cardiac ischaemia [58].

Lumbar epidurals lead to sympathetic blockade in the lower limbs and lower abdomen only, and do not appear to be protective against myocardial infarction. Lumbar epidurals may cause more hypotension than thoracic epidurals [59]. Even in studies that show a reduction in cardiac events with thoracic epidurals, this effect was not seen when lumbar epidurals were used [12, 60].

Bottom Line

The evidence for a reduction in cardiac complications with TEA is conflicting. It is likely that any beneficial effect of epidurals is limited to high-risk groups, such as those undergoing vascular surgery or perhaps patients with existing cardiac disease.

It is often said that the manner in which the epidural is managed post-operatively is important for cardiovascular outcomes [61]. Any beneficial cardiac effects are seen when the cardiac sympathetic innervation is blocked, therefore the epidural must be placed in the mid-high thoracic spine. Blood pressure should be maintained aggressively and attempting to achieve this with intravenous fluids alone may lead to fluid overload. Once normovolaemia is achieved, blood pressure should be supported with vasopressors.

Respiratory Failure

Major surgery predisposes patients to post-operative respiratory insufficiency, and post-operative pneumonia may exceed 10% of major abdominal operations [62]. Uncontrolled pain leads to splinting of respiratory muscles and impairment of the normal excursion of the thoracic cage, which causes atelectasis and impairment of coughing. Opioids depress respiratory drive, and it is suggested that volatile anaesthetics impair mucociliary flow and clearance of sputum [63]. Upper abdominal surgery leads to diaphragmatic dysfunction, via a surgery-induced inhibitory reflex in the phrenic nerve [64], again impairing coughing and deep breathing. This reflex is partially reversed by TEA.

Unsurprisingly post-operative respiratory complications lead to a significant morbidity burden, and prolonged stays in ICU hospital, one study finding that patients undergoing abdominal surgery who developed hospital-acquired pneumonia had an 8.5-fold increase in-hospital mortality (95% CI, 7.94–9.09) and an increase in hospital stay from 6 days (SD, 5.37) to 17 days (SD, 18.66) [62]. TEA has been studied for its impact on post-operative respiratory failure: better dynamic analgesia would allow better coughing, more rigorous chest physiotherapy, improved sputum clearance and reduced atelectasis.

What the Data Tell Us

The MASTER trial in 2002 found that TEA led to a reduction in a composite endpoint of 'respiratory failure', comprising prolonged ventilation, reintubation, hypoxia or hypercapnia, with a NNT of 15. A Cochrane analysis [12] of patients undergoing aortic aneurysm repair found that TEA reduced the duration of ventilation on ICU by 48% but had no effect on the risk of pneumonia. A 2008 meta-analysis [55] also supported this, having examined papers over a 35-year period between 1971 and 2006, finding that TEA led to a reduction in pneumonia. Interestingly this study also found that, over time, the baseline risk of pneumonia had dropped dramatically whilst the rates of pneumonia in the TEA groups remained largely unchanged. In other words, the 'lung protective' effect of epidurals was much less impressive in the 2000s (NNT 25) as it was in the 1970s (NNT 4). Changes in peri-operative care are likely to be behind this improvement in baseline risk: alterations in fluid therapy, physiotherapy and early mobilisation, and avoidance of nasogastric tubes are all commonly practiced now, and are likely to improve post-operative respiratory function and reduce the pneumonia risk.

A Cochrane review [40] concluded that although regional anaesthesia only reduced the risk of post-operative pneumonia when used as the sole anaesthetic modality, the data was inconclusive when regional anaesthesia was used in conjunction with general anaesthesia. Additionally, a subgroup analysis of the MASTER trial [65] examined outcomes in patients deemed to be of high risk of cardiac and respiratory complications. Although they found a reduction in the composite 'respiratory failure' end-point in patients with TEA, the rates of pneumonia, ventilation longer than 24 h, ICU stay, hospital stay and mortality were all unchanged, thus forcing the authors to question the clinical significance of their finding. The effect of TEA on respiratory function in laparoscopic surgery has not been well studied, although one trial [29] found that TEA made no impact on post-operative spirometry. A meta-analysis of TEA studies in patients undergoing open abdominal surgery on an Enhanced Recovery pathway found that TEA did not influence post-operative respiratory complications.

Bottom Line

There is evidence that TEA reduces the risk of pneumonia and respiratory failure in open surgery. However, the strength of this effect is now far less clinically significant compared with a few decades ago, and may only apply to patients in a high-risk group. Improvements in peri-operative medicine may mean that routine use of TEA is no longer clinically justified to prevent respiratory failure. Given the paucity of recent data to support the use of TEA to protect against respiratory failure in open surgery, it is unlikely that TEA use in laparoscopic surgery will have any effect on post-operative respiratory function.

Thromboembolism

It would seem plausible that TEA should reduce the risk of thromboembolism. Attenuation of the surgical stress response leads to enhanced fibrinolysis, alongside the attenuation of the reduction in venous flow within leg veins during surgery by epidural blockade [66]. Local anaesthetic agents themselves may also directly inhibit platelet function [3]. Indeed, in 2000, Rodgers' meta-analysis of the impact of neuraxial blockade on post-operative outcomes examined DVT rates and reported 365 events, although 80% of these were in patients undergoing orthopaedic surgery. The authors concluded that neuraxial blockade was associated with a reduction in the odds of DVT by 44% and PE by 55%, and this purported protection against VTE has found its way into many patient information leaflets and textbooks since. However, the protective effect was much less pronounced on symptomatic DVT than on DVTs found on screening and additionally the majority of studies included in the meta-analysis were performed at a time when VTE chemoprophylaxis was not routinely used. Peri-operative care is now much more focussed on early mobilisation, minimally invasive surgery and VTE chemo- and mechanoprophylaxis, so the relevance of these older studies is uncertain. A more recent meta-analysis failed to find a link between epidural use and a reduction in VTE [41], and an RCT of TEA for open surgery within an ERAS programme found no difference of rates of VTE [58]. It is likely that if any benefit in VTE reduction exists at all with epidural use, it is now far less pronounced than older studies had identified.

Bowel Recovery and Post-operative Ileus

Post-operative ileus (POI) following colorectal surgery is common, affecting 17% of patients undergoing laparoscopic colectomy and 25% of patients undergoing open colectomy [67]. The slow return of bowel function leads to abdominal distension, vomiting, pain and an inability to pass stools and flatus. The impact of this is not insignificant: the ensuing anorexia and vomiting limits energy intake, risking a negative nitrogen balance and muscle loss. Bacterial overgrowth within the gut may lead to bacterial translocation, and nosocomial infections may ensue. Intestinal distension may eventually lead to abdominal compartment syndrome, and the distended bowel is at risk of perforation. The morbidity and economic burden from this is huge: Gan and colleagues estimated that POI led to a 4-day increase in hospital stay, a significant increase in hospital costs, increased 30-day readmission rates from 8.9% to 13.4% [67], and a 2-day increase in ICU stay [68]. The aetiology of POI is multifactorial: sympathetic stress from pain and anxiety as well as the surgical stress response, inflammation, bowel handling, oedema from fluid excess as well as other technical surgical factors all contribute to slower bowel recovery and ileus. Opioid dose also appears to be strongly related to POI in both laparoscopic and open procedures [67, 69]. TEA would therefore seem like a natural choice for reducing ileus: improvements in post-operative pain, reduced opioid consumption, attenuation of inflammation and the surgical stress response, and sympathetic blockade should all improve intestinal motility and therefore reduce POI.

What the Data Tell Us

Studies have consistently found that TEA reduces the time to bowel motion and tolerance of diet for open surgery. A recent Cochrane review of 8754 patients in 128 trials supported this, finding high quality evidence that TEA used for abdominal surgery shortened the time to bowel recovery, as defined as passage of first flatus, by an effect size equivalent to 17 h [70]. Addition of opioid to the epidural local anaesthetic mixture did not affect bowel recovery. Other meta-analyses to date have come to similar conclusions [11, 41]. Moreover the reduction in time to bowel recovery allowed a significant increase in oral diet, in terms of both protein and overall energy intake [13].

Surgical pathways have evolved rapidly since then: reduction in pre-operative fasting, targeted fluid therapy and opioid sparing analgesic regimens are now commonplace. Intravenous lidocaine, which has been shown to reduce the duration of ileus, through multiple mechanisms including opioid-sparing (see Chap. 6), is now finding favour. So, does TEA still have the same positive impact on bowel recovery in the context of modern Enhanced Recovery pathways and all the aforementioned interventions? A meta-analysis in 2007 [11] examined the rate of ileus in patients undergoing surgery either on ERAS or traditional pathways, predominantly in open surgery. The authors found that TEA reduced the duration of ileus in all but one study, both in ERAS and traditional groups, by an average of 36 h. A more recent systematic review [58] found that TEA used within an Enhanced Recovery context for open abdominal surgery still led to reductions in time to first bowel movement in four of the six studies. However, this reduction in ileus does not appear to translate into a reduction in hospital stay [11, 22].

Laparoscopic surgery is well known for reducing POI [67] through limitation in surgical trauma, leading to reductions in post-operative pain, attenuated stress response and minimised bowel handling. One might then theorise that the positive effect of TEA on reducing the time to bowel recovery would be weaker. One randomised study found that the time to bowel recovery in patients having a laparoscopic colectomy was longer in those managed with TEA compared to those randomised to IV lidocaine or IV PCA, and TEA was associated with an increase in vomiting and belching [29]. Another RCT found that TEA prolonged the time to 'sufficient oral intake' by 1 day in patients undergoing laparoscopic colectomy [30]. A meta-analysis of studies comparing epidurals to IV PCA for laparoscopic surgery found that TEA reduced time to first bowel movement (WMD −0.6d) but did not affect time to flatus or return to diet [71]. The effect of TEA on the development of ileus may be specific to surgical site: one observational study found that TEA was associated with faster bowel recovery in patients undergoing laparoscopic anterior resection, but not laparoscopic right hemicolectomy [72].

The Bottom Line

There is high quality evidence that TEA reduces the time to return of gut function, and this benefit still exists in patients undergoing surgery on Enhanced Recovery Pathways. The evidence supporting TEA to reduce POI in laparoscopic surgery is mixed. TEA may reduce the time to return of bowel function, but the effect is likely to be small, and it is difficult to make a case for using TEA for laparoscopic surgery with the primary aim of reducing the time to bowel recovery.

Cancer Recurrence Rates

During surgery for cancer, handling of cancer-containing tissues results in the release of cancer cells into the circulation and this may lead to the formation of micrometastases. Whether or not these circulating cancer cells become metastases is determined by the balance between the immune systems attempts to destroy cancer cells and the tendency of cancer cells to disseminate via blood and lymph-borne spread, invasively grow locally and angiogenesis. Failure of this balance leads to clinical metastases. Therefore, any peri-operative interventions that impair the immune system may lead to an increase in post-operative cancer recurrence. Regional anaesthesia has shown promise for reducing the risk of peri-operative micrometastases, and investigators have found links between regional anaesthesia and reduced cancer recurrence in breast [73], gastrooesophageal [74] and prostate cancer surgery. The mechanism behind this effect isn't entirely clear. Opioids have been shown to reduce the immune response through suppression of natural killer cell function and promote angiogenesis [75], so perhaps TEA may improve immune function by reducing opioid dosage. TEA-induced attenuation of the surgical stress response may improve NK cell function [76] and TEA allows a reduction in volatile anaesthetic concentrations, which have been shown to be immunosuppressive in their own right [77]. Perhaps local anaesthetic agents have a direct cytotoxic effect on the cancer cells themselves, mediated via sodium channel blockade as cancer cells express voltage-gated sodium channels in high concentrations [77], indeed ropivacaine and lidocaine have been found to be directly cytotoxic to in-vitro breast cancer cells, and this effect was not seen with bupivacaine [78].

What Data Tell Us

Studies showing a reduction in cancer recurrence have tended to be cohort studies but the results of randomized studies are less promising. Post-hoc analysis of long-term cancer survival in the MASTER trial found that the median time to cancer recurrence was unchanged in patients with TEA, a finding that was supported by a meta-analysis of cancer outcome studies [79]. A Cochrane review in 2014 [80] found the evidence to support TEA improving cancer free survival was inadequate, and retrospective studies specifically examining colorectal cancer have also tended to find no impact of TEA on cancer recurrence [81]. Observational data from 42,000 patients undergoing surgery for colorectal cancer, in which 22% received epidural analgesia, found that TEA use was associated with an improved 5-year survival (hazard ratio, 0.91) but cancer recurrence was not changed [82].

Bottom Line

Whatever the purported mechanism of action, a definitive link between regional anaesthesia and improved cancer survival has yet to be identified.

Anatomy (See Chap. 2)

The epidural space is found between the ligamentum flavum posteriorly and the posterior ligament of the vertebral bodies anteriorly, and envelops the spinal cord wrapped in its dura mater. It runs the length of the vertebral canal, from the foramen magnum at the skull base down to the hiatus of the sacrum, and its lateral borders are formed by the vertebral pedicles. The epidural space is not the empty canal that we imagine it to be. Nerve roots span the epidural space as they leave the cord and go on to form terminal nerves. The epidural space contains large amounts of epidural fat and connective tissue. The volume of epidural fat appears to be determined by body habitus and appears to be non-uniform in distribution, tending to lie in bands within the epidural space. Within the epidural space lies a rich venous plexus, known as Bateson's venous plexus, which drains blood supply from the spinal cord into the iliac veins, and hemiazygous and azygous veins. Fortunately, this plexus is found predominantly in the epidural space anterior to the spinal canal, although veins can still be found in the posterior epidural space and are therefore prone to injury from the epidural needle or even inadvertent cannulation by the epidural catheter. The venous system is valveless, meaning that increased pressure in abdominal or thoracic compartments may translate to increased pressure and engorgement of epidural veins.

The anterior dura has a dense sensory innervation. The posterior dura is also innervated but more sparingly so than the anterior dura. The spinal periosteum also receives sensory innervation, though the ligamentum flavum and other spinal ligaments are asensate. This is fortunate for the anaesthetist—a midline needle pass that avoids bony structures should be relatively painless.

Epidural Insertion Technique

Identifying the Epidural Space

'Loss of resistance' is a commonly employed method of identifying the epidural space, and usually uses either saline or air in the syringe. This technique relies on the needle tip advancing from vertebral ligaments to the epidural space, whereby the resistance felt on attempting to inject sudden falls as the ligamentum flavum is breached. Insertion technique depends on loss of resistance medium used: with loss of resistance to air, the syringe plunger is 'bounced' as the needle is inserted, whereas using saline allows the epidural needle to be advanced through continuous pressure along the syringe plunger, meaning the needle stops moving once the epidural space is encountered. Although the latter was the preferred technique in one survey of UK anaesthetists [83] neither technique seems to be superior in terms of either success or complications [84, 85]; however, one study concluded that the complication rates were lowest when the clinicians' 'preferred technique' was used, whichever this was, although more needle passes were required when using loss of resistance to air [86].

The hanging drop technique has also been described: a drop of sterile liquid, such as saline, is placed on the end of the epidural needle, and when the negative-pressure epidural space is encountered the drop is sucked into the space and disappears. The popularity of the hanging drop technique has dwindled: in a recent survey of UK obstetric anaesthetists, only 2% used the hanging drop routinely [87]. This technique appears to be less reliable for identifying the epidural space [87, 88] and the needle placement with the hanging drop technique is deeper than if loss of resistance is used [87, 89]. This, in theory at least, may increase the risk of inadvertent dural puncture.

Patient Positioning

The way the patient is positioned for epidural insertion affects both the position and shape of the spinal canal, and the position of the spinal cord within the canal itself. In the sitting position, the patient's back tends to be more flexed, therefore opening the spaces in between the spinous processes and facilitating needle placement [86]. Epidural placement has been found to be faster in the sitting position [90] and is associated with less difficulty in passing the epidural catheter. The distance to the epidural space is also shorter in the flexed sitting position, but increases when the patient moves to a neutral spine position again, for example on lying down. This means that an epidural catheter that is fixed at the skin may be pulled out of the epidural space by a short distance when the patient is repositioned following epidural insertion [91]. This may lead to displacement of the epidural catheter if only a short distance of catheter is placed within the epidural space. The sitting position also leads to engorgement of the epidural venous plexus, and epidurals placed in the lateral position appear to have a lower rate of bloody tap or epidural venous cannulation than in the sitting position (OR, 0.53; 95% CI, 0.32–0.86) [92]. The hanging drop technique relies on sub-atmospheric pressure within the epidural space, and pressure within the epidural space is lower in the sitting position than lateral. The sitting position is therefore the favoured position when using the hanging drop technique.

Midline Versus Paramedian Approach

The epidural space may either be approached in the midline of the spine, or from a paramedian approach. The midline approach has the advantages of being an easy technique to learn, and structures in the midline tend to have minimal sensory innervation meaning it is generally well tolerated by the patient. In a paramedian approach the needle is inserted 1–2 cm off the midline and directed medially toward the spinal canal. Once the needle makes contact with the vertebral lamina it is 'walked' cranially off the lamina and into the epidural space. In the lower thoracic spine this paramedian approach may be advantageous as the vertebral spinous processes are angulated steeply downwards and lie close together, which may make the midline approach technically difficult or even impossible. The paramedian approach aims to direct the needle around the side of the spinous process and take a more direct route to the epidural space. This has the advantages of requiring a less steeply angulated approach to the epidural space, and allowing a larger target window in the ligamentum flavum, therefore this approach is less dependent upon spine flexion and patient positioning [93]. Additionally, the ligamentum flavum is known to have gaps in the midline that may make feedback through the needle subtler during a midline approach, and the endpoint is therefore less obvious. One study has suggested that the paramedian approach reduces the incidence of paraesthesia during epidural insertion, and reduces the risk of dural puncture [94].

Vertebral Level for Insertion

Epidural analgesia produces a segmental block for a number of dermatomes cranio-caudally either side of the epidural insertion point, therefore the level of epidural insertion is an important determinant of the final segmental block. If the insertion point is wrong, then there is a risk that the blocked segment will not encompass the entire surgical field and the patient will experience pain. Unfortunately, estimation of vertebral interspaces is difficult and often wrong, especially in those patients where bony landmarks are difficult to locate, such as the obese. Additionally, the spread of anaesthetic within the spinal canal tends to vary between patients, meaning that the blocked segment may differ even when the same interspace and same volume of anaesthetic is used [95]. The direction of local anaesthetic flow varies with level of epidural insertion, and below the level of high thoracic vertebrae the spread of injectate is predominantly cranial rather than caudal [96]. See Table 8.1 for levels of insertion by operation type.

Ultrasound-Guided Insertion

The standard means of epidural insertion remains essentially a blind procedure, and the anaesthetist uses tactile feedback through the Tuohy needle to aid needle advancement and redirections toward the epidural space. Epidural insertion is not always straightforward, and factors such as obesity, prior back surgery and spinal conditions such as kyphoscoliosis and ankylosing spondylitis can make epidural insertion considerably more difficult. Ultrasound (US) has found favour recently for aiding epidural insertion, and the structures that can be identified on ultrasonic examination of the spine can be seen in Figs. 8.1 and 8.2. A pre-procedural 'scouting scan' can give vital information to assist the anaesthetist: a transverse scan of the spinal column is useful in identifying spinous processes and the midline, and may give some hint to the degree of vertebral rotation in the scoliotic spine (Table 8.2). A longitudinal scan in a paramedian approach can view the vertebral laminae in successive segments, and on occasion the ligamentum flavum and dura mater are visible as separate entities thus allowing the epidural space itself to be visualised. This longitudinal scan is useful for estimating the vertebral level and distance to the ligamentum flavum (although this doesn't correlate well with needle length because the soft tissues are compressed with the US probe, and the needle may take a less perpendicular approach toward the spine). US can also be used to locate a sonographic 'window' to confirm that epidural placement is possible at that level. The insertion point can then be marked, and the Tuohy needle inserted along

Table 8.1 Levels of insertion by operation type

Type of surgery	Examples	Level of epidural insertion
Upper abdominal surgery	Hepatic resection Gastrectomy	T4–6
Abdominal surgery through midline incision	Small bowel resection Right hemicolectomy Laparotomy	T6–9
Lower abdominal surgery	Anterior resection Abdomino-perineal resection	T9–T12

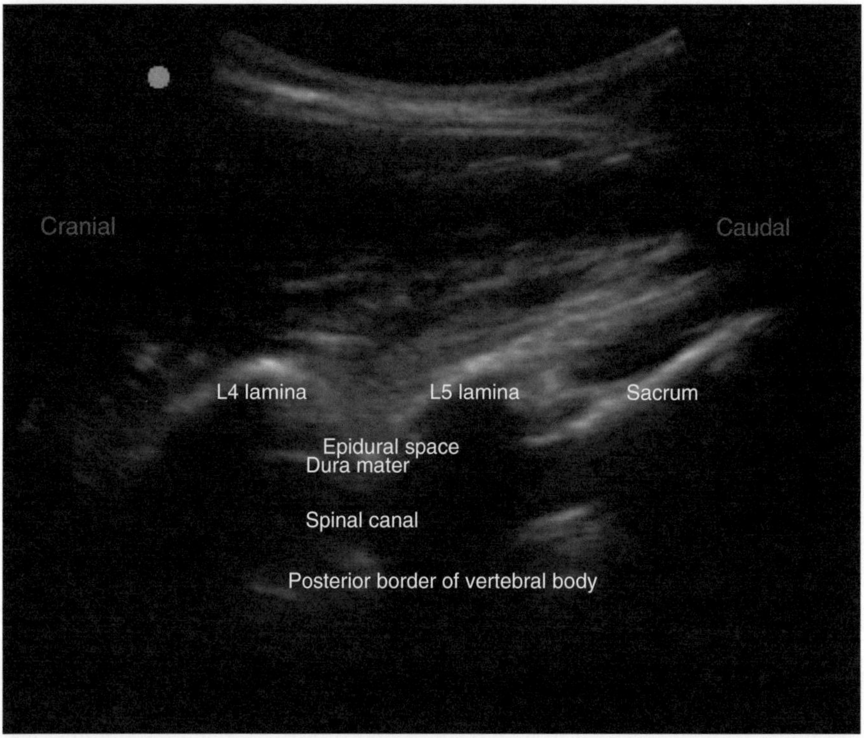

Fig. 8.1 Longitudinal paramedian ultrasound scan of vertebral canal. (1) Sacrum. (2) L5 lamina. (3) L4 lamina. (4) Dura mater. (5) Epidural space. (6) Spinal canal. (7) Posterior border of vertebral body

the same angle as the US probe/beam. A systematic review of studies comparing ultrasound guided epidural insertion to traditional techniques concluded that ultrasound guidance reduced the number of failed procedures (risk ratio, 0.23; 95% CI, 0.09–0.60), traumatic procedures (risk ratio, 0.27; 95% CI, 0.11–0.67) and number of insertion attempts (mean difference −0.44 (−0.64 to −0.24)) [97].

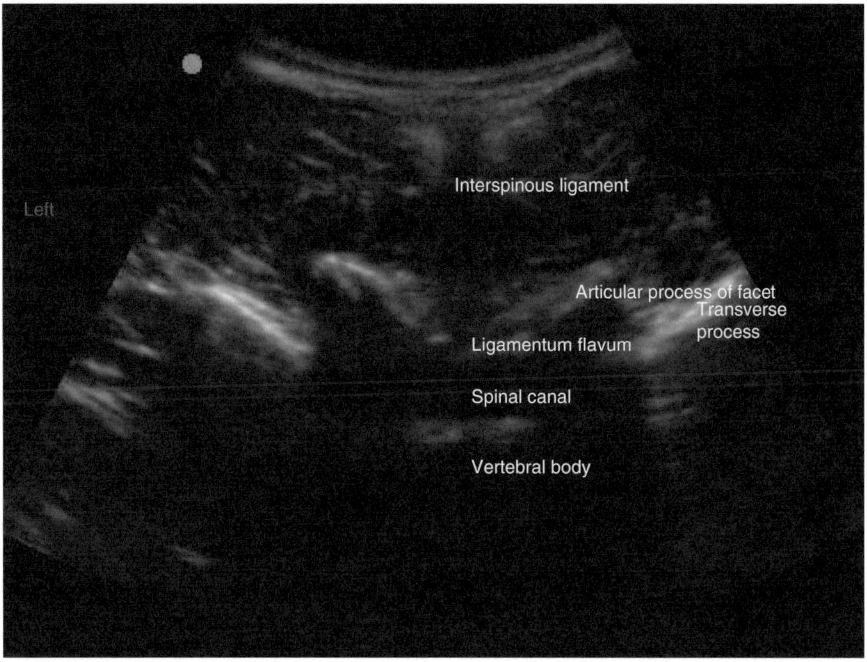

Fig. 8.2 Transverse ultrasound scan of vertebral canal at L3/4 interspace. (1) Interspinous ligament. (2) Articular process of facet. (3) Transverse process. (4) Ligamentum flavum. (5) Spinal canal. (6) Vertebral body

Ultrasound has also been used for real-time visualised epidural insertion. However, it is technically difficult: the angle of needle insertion is steep meaning the needle is not well visualised, and needle placement may be hindered by the size of the ultrasound probe face. With the currently available technology, this technique of visualised needle insertion is difficult to recommend for routine use.

Epidural Drugs

Local anaesthetic (LA) agents provide the mainstay of the analgesic benefit from epidurals, and during the early years of post-operative epidural analgesia, the use of local anaesthetics alone was common. Increasing concentration, and thus dose, of LA leads to motor block in a dose-dependent manner and dose finding studies have suggested the optimal balance of analgesia to motor block occurs with 0.2% ropivacaine [98]. When LA solutions are used in isolation, high doses are required to optimise analgesia, and this increases the incidence of hypotension. However plain LA infusions may be desirable under circumstances where opioids are to be avoided, such as uncontrolled obstructive sleep apnoea or severe vomiting [99].

Table 8.2 Information derived from pre-procedural ultrasound scan of vertebral column

Transverse scan	Longitudinal scan
Localisation of midline	Level of vertebral interspaces
Estimation of depth of spinal canal	Estimation of depth of spinal canal
Estimation of placement and angle of needle required when midline insertion technique is used	Estimation of placement and angle of needle required when paramedian technique is used
Degree and direction of vertebral rotation in the scoliotic spine	

The addition of opioids to the LA improves the quality of analgesia [100, 101] although dose related side effects occur according the opioid used. This improvement in analgesia allows a reduction in the dose of LA used, which in turn may reduce motor block and hypotension. Lipophilic opioids, such as fentanyl, are taken up into epidural fat, and therefore remain in the epidural space for a longer period than hydrophilic opioids [102]. Hydrophilic opioids, such as morphine, readily diffuse across the dura and into the CSF. This increases the risk of respiratory depression, which may follow a biphasic pattern. The first peak is seen 30–90 min post injection and probably relates to systemic absorption. The second peak is seen 6–18 h later and relates to rostral spread of opioid within the CSF [103]. Opioids appear to treat pain more effectively and may cause less respiratory depression when the same dose is given via the epidural route, compared to the intravenous route [104]. Opioids themselves appear to be largely equally effective in terms of analgesia when compared to each other, however morphine appears to cause more nausea than fentanyl [105]. The use of epidural opioids alone has the advantage of reducing epidural related hypotension. However epidural opioids alone are much less effective than opioid/local anaesthetic combinations, especially for dynamic pain [9].

Clinicians have theorized that intermittent bolusing of an epidural may allow better spread of injectate within the epidural space and therefore provide more consistent analgesia. Patient-controlled intermittent bolus epidural analgesia (PCEA) has been popularized in obstetric anaesthesia as it allows less motor blockade and lower risk of instrumented delivery [106]. This use of PCEA has now transferred to peri-operative care, although comparison of PCEA to continuous epidural infusion has not well been studied in surgical patients. One meta-analysis suggested that in fact PCEA was associated with worse analgesia than continuous epidural infusion [10] possibly because patients using PCEA commonly use less LA [107]. Whether this reduced dose of LA translates into less hypotension is not known.

Epidural Failure

Why epidurals fail is the subject of many excellent review papers [86, 108] and the causes are listed in Table 8.3. Epidural failure is not well defined, though studies often define failure as severe pain necessitating further analgesic interventions, loss or removal or replacement of the epidural catheter, or cessation of epidural infusion earlier than the intended duration. The latter definition has the advantage over the former that it includes intended epidural cessation because of side effects such as hypotension or motor block.

Primary epidural failure refers to the epidural that has never worked, and is due to either misplacement of the epidural catheter into pleural or intravascular spaces, or a catheter which exits the epidural space through an intervertebral foramen. Additionally, synechiae and fat depositions exist within the epidural space which may impede spread of LA and therefore lead to a patchy block [109]. Secondary epidural failure refers to an epidural which worked following insertion and then failed some time later, and is commonly due to insufficient LA or catheter migration. One of the commonest causes of secondary epidural failure appears to be inadvertent removal of the epidural catheter [110], the next most common cause appearing to be migration of the epidural catheter out of the epidural space. Interestingly, in one study, 9 of 20 patients who suffered epidural failure had normal symmetrical spread of radiological contrast within the epidural space [110]. When an epidural catheter is fixed at the skin and the patient moves or changes position, the patient's skin and subcutaneous tissue is moved relative to the vertebral column underneath, and therefore the catheter migrates slowly out of the space, and an epidural catheter may be displaced by a considerable distance just through this action [86]. Leaving an adequate length of epidural catheter within the epidural space can mimimize this risk of natural catheter migration. The epidural must not be inserted so far that a unilateral block ensues, although withdrawing the epidural catheter a short distance can rectify a unilateral block whereas a catheter that has migrated out of the epidural space must be replaced. A catheter length of 5 cm within the epidural

Table 8.3 Contraindications to epidural insertion

	Examples
Absolute contraindications	
Patient refusal	
Allergy to local anaesthetics	Urticaria with bupivacaine
Uncontrolled coagulopathy	Disseminated intravascular coagulation
Uncontrolled systemic sepsis	Peritonitis with sepsis
Infection at the site of insertion	Local cellulitis
Relative contraindications	
Fixed cardiac output states	Severe aortic stenosis
Mild derangement of coagulation	INR 1.5–2.0 Platelet count 80–100
Anatomical abnormality	Severe kyphoscoliosis Ankylosing spondylitis
Previous spinal surgery at the level of insertion	Laminectomy Correction of scoliosis
Raised intracranial pressure	Cerebral oedema
Hypovolaemia	

space has been suggested as adequate [86, 111] and is the author's current practice.

Many studies suggest a failure rate of 10–20%, and some as high as 30–40% [16, 86]. In the MASTER study, only 225 patients out of 447 randomized to receive epidural analgesia actually received epidural analgesia for the intended duration, and an observational study of 1286 patients undergoing Caesarean section under epidural anaesthesia found an overall epidural failure rate of 24% [112]. This failure rate has significant implications. The epidural provides the mainstay of the post-operative analgesia. Any delay between the epidural failing and actions to rectify this may result in the patient experiencing severe pain and then much of the benefits of TEA, which are thought to derive from good quality analgesia and opioid sparing as well as from sympathetic block, are lost. Consequently, epidural failure has been associated with an increase in peri-operative complications—both nonsurgical and at the operative site [113] (Table 8.4).

Timely management of the failed epidural is critical. They should be managed aggressively in order to minimize the duration of severe pain and the amount of systemic opioids. This may require boluses of local anaesthetic with or without adjunct epidural analgesics, or catheter manipulation followed by further epidural boluses. Replacement of failed epidurals may significantly improve overall analgesic control [114] but this may be complicated by other factors such as timing of administration of anticoagulants for VTE prophylaxis. Clearly this management is time and resource consuming, and a specialist acute pain service can provide the dedicated input required to maximize the analgesic benefit from epidural infusions.

Safety

A meta-analysis of ERAS trials found no difference between TEA and PCA in composite complication rates [58] and an observational study of nearly 28,000 patients found no difference in complication rates for laparoscopic surgery [5]. However urinary retention and hypotension are common with epidural analgesia. Urinary retention is more common with epidural analgesia than other forms of pain relief [10] and it is generally considered best practice to retain a urinary catheter for the duration of the epidural infusion. The vasoplegia that results from TEA leads to hypotension (OR, 13.5; 95% CI, 4.0–57.7) [11], and virtually all studies to date indicate that the risk of hypotension is greater with TEA than with systemic opioids and any of the truncal blocks. This, in theory, risks myocardial ischaemia and splanchic hypoperfusion. However, hypotension related to epidurals is easily treatable with vasopressors, so TEA-related hypotension should never translate to anastomotic failure or myocardial ischaemia. Unfortunately, this results in many patients with TEA requiring additional days in higher care areas solely due to their dependency on vasopressor infusions. Epidural infusions that include opioids lead to an increased risk of pruritis [10, 41], which is even greater than from systemic opioids, with NNH 21 (95% CI 13–53) [41]. It is easy to dismiss pruritus; however, this symptom can be very

Table 8.4 Peri-operative epidural management

For surgery
• Insert the epidural at the appropriate level for the operation, leaving at least 4 cm catheter in the epidural space
• A test dose of 3–5 ml 2% lidocaine with adrenaline may help to differentiate epidural catheter placement from inadvertent intrathecal or intravascular placement
• Establish a block prior to induction of anaesthesia using 5 ml aliquots of 0.25%. This allows assessment that the epidural is functioning correctly prior to surgery
• During surgery, further local anaesthetic may be required and should be titrated to anticipated pain and cardiovascular indices
• Epidural opioid improves post-operative pain control and should be used unless contraindication exists. Suggestions include fentanyl 50–100 μg or diamorphine 3 mg given as a bolus near the start of surgery
After surgery
• The patient should be nursed in an environment where the appropriate nursing and medical input is at hand. The patient should have easy access to vasopressors and expertise in fluid management. Some units require patients with epidurals to be managed in a high-dependency or critical care environment whereas other units have wards with increased staffing
• Regular nursing observations should include pain score and level of motor block, and monitoring for respiratory depression. A pain score (0–10) of >3 on movement or coughing should be addressed and treated promptly. Motor block out of keeping with epidural insertion level and dose of anaesthetic may signify spinal cord ischaemia and should prompt immediate action
• Maintain the epidural block with an infusion of local anaesthetic with opioid. The local anaesthetic solution should be of low concentration to minimise the risk of motor block and hypotension. The author uses 0.1% levobupivacaine +2 μg/ml fentanyl, though ropivacaine, sufentanyl, and hydromorphone are all appropriate choices
• The epidural solution may be given either by infusion (CEI) or by patient controlled epidural boluses (PCEA). Appropriate starting rates would be 6 ml/h by infusion or patient controlled boluses of 8 ml at 30 min lock-out with 4 ml/h background infusion
• The patient with an epidural should be managed after surgery by an Acute Pain Service, and the patient should ideally be reviewed at least every 12 h whilst the epidural is running. These reviews should focus on the adequacy of analgesia balanced against complications, and can troubleshoot the epidural if necessary. The Acute Pain Service can also assist with stepping down the epidural onto systemic opioids
• Hypotension should be managed promptly. Intravenous fluid boluses should be given until hypovolaemia is no longer suspected, and goal-directed fluid therapy may assist with this. If hypotension persists then an infusion of vasoconstrictor may be required to maintain an adequate MAP. It is essential to avoid excess fluid, and it is a common pitfall to try to treat hypotension related to epidurals with IVF. Avoid reducing the epidural infusion rate unless the block is extensive or denser than clinically warranted as this may lead to worsening of pain control
• The patient should be able to cooperate with physiotherapy and rehabilitation with a working epidural, and this should be actively encouraged. For example patients may be hoisted into a chair for periods of time during the day. Motor blockade in the legs is minimal when a high thoracic epidural is used, which may allow active mobilisation of the patient. This is advantageous in reducing the risks of venous thrombosis and improving post-operative respiratory function, and is seen as a recovery goal of many ERPs

(continued)

Table 8.4 (continued)

• The epidural infusion should be continued until the morning of post-operative day 3, although the infusion can be continued for longer if the patient has severe cardiorespiratory disease or is at high risk of ileus
• After this the epidural can be discontinued, and either oral analgesia or systemic opioids (such as intravenous PCA or transdermal opioid patches) can be used in its place depending on whether normal gut function has resumed

distressing for patients, and has the same impact on quality of life as pain [115]. Treat the pruritus by reducing, or removing, the opioid from the epidural local anaesthetic solution, or by using small doses of a mu antagonist such as naloxone.

Neuraxial Complications

Even though the risk of permanent harm is small neuraxial complications associated with epidurals can have a catastrophic effect on the patient's quality of life. This is of particular relevance when epidurals are considered for low risk patients in whom there is unlikely to be any outcome benefit.

The NAP3 project [116] assessed the outcomes of over 707,000 neuraxial procedures, of which 98,000 were peri-operative epidurals. Although the incidence of harm was higher in the peri-operative group (27 cases, of which 16 suffered permanent injury) than in any other, the incidence of harm was low. This accounted for 80% of all complications in less than half of all neuraxial procedures (see Table 8.5). The outcomes for patients who developed an epidural haematoma or spinal cord ischaemia were poor (only one in ten made a full recovery) and diagnosis was often delayed. Seven out of eight patients who developed a vertebral column haematoma had received drugs which interfered with blood clotting around either the time of the insertion of epidural, or at the time of the removal of the epidural catheter; most cases occurring in elderly patients undergoing high risk surgery. Patients should be monitored closely for the classic signs of back pain and neurological deficits in the legs, including leg weakness out of proportion to the epidural infusion. These signs should prompt urgent imaging and decompression of the haematoma. Most patients will receive chemoprophylaxis for prevention of venous thrombosis after surgery, and here timing of administration is critical around both insertion of epidural and removal of epidural catheter to reduce the risk of epidural haematoma. Horlocker and colleagues [117] have published guidance on the safe performance of neuraxial anaesthesia in patients taking anticoagulant drugs (see Table 8.6).

The formation of an epidural abscess is associated with either a source of infection or a disordered immune response. In the NAP3 audit [116], presenting features of vertebral canal abscesses were vague, with only 9 of 17 patients complaining of back pain, and only nine showing features of infection. Also striking was that in many cases presentation was delayed, with more than half presenting later than 7 days from epidural insertion. Staphylococcus aureus was the commonest infective organism.

Table 8.5 Causes of epidural failure: primary epidural failure—epidural does not work from the outset. Secondary epidural failure: working block initially, followed by subsequent epidural failure

Causes of primary epidural failure
Pharmacological
Inadequate mass (volume or concentration) of local anaesthetic agent
Technical
Catheter inserted at inappropriate vertebral level for surgical site
Catheter inserted but not in epidural space
Catheter migration through intervertebral foramen
Catheter placed in epidural vein
Catheter inserted too far into epidural space (>5 cm)
Anatomical
Failure to site epidural
Epidural synechiae preventing spread of local anaesthetic
Causes of secondary epidural failure
Inadequate mass/infusion rate of local anaesthetic
Catheter migration out of epidural space
Failure or disconnection of infusion device

Anastomotic Leak

The use of TEA for colonic surgery has been controversial due to concerns regarding anastomotic leakage. TEA may result in a reduction in splanchnic vascular resistance and therefore improve blood flow, due to sympathetic blockade (T5–T11) of the gut supply, as well as beneficial effects on the gut microcirculation [118]. However, the increase in peristalsis resulting from the unopposed parasympathetic tone has led to concerns that this may lead to the much-feared complication of anastomotic breakdown. Additionally, splanchnic blood flow is pressure dependent rather than flow dependent; TEA is strongly associated with post-operative hypotension, and this hypotension leads to a fall in colonic blood flow. This reduction in perfusion is not improved with intravenous fluids, and vasopressors may be required for restoration of flow [119]. Despite these potential risks studies to date have either shown no association between TEA and anastomotic leak [11, 41, 120] or have in fact shown a reduction in anastomotic leak.

Epidurals and their Role in Enhanced Recovery Pathways

Enhanced Recovery After Surgery (ERAS) combines multiple strategies into a pathway aimed at improving recovery after surgery and reducing complications. This results in an earlier discharge from hospital than traditional surgical models. This early discharge poses a problem for clinicians wishing to use TEA as older trials aimed to continue epidural infusions for 72 h post-operatively [16]. However, within an ERAS pathway, patients can be expected to mobilize much earlier than this, and on many units patient will have been discharged by 72 h following surgery [121–123]. Clearly extending an epidural infusion in this patient group for 72 h

Table 8.6 Recommendations for performance of neuraxial anaesthesia in anticoagulated patients

Drug	Recommendation
Warfarin	Discontinue chronic warfarin therapy 4–5 days before spinal procedure and evaluate INR. INR should be within the normal range at the time of procedure to ensure adequate levels of all vitamin K-dependent factors. After operation, daily INR assessment with catheter removal occurring with INR, 1.5
Antiplatelet medications	No contraindications with aspirin or other NSAIDs. Thienopyridine derivatives (clopidogrel and prasugrel) should be discontinued clopidogrel 5–7 days, prasugreal 7 days, and ticlopidine 14 days before procedure. GP IIb/IIIa inhibitors should be discontinued to allow recovery of platelet function before procedure (8 h for tirofiban and eptifibatide, 24–48 h for abciximab)
Thrombolytics/ fibrinolytics	There are no available data to suggest a safe interval between procedure and initiation or discontinuation of these medications. Follow fibrinogen level and observe for signs of neural compression
LMWH	Delay procedure at least 12 h from the last dose of thromboprophylaxis LMWH dose. For 'treatment' dosing of LMWH, at least 24 h should elapse before procedure. LMWH should not be administered within 24 h after the procedure. Indwelling epidural catheters should be maintained only with once daily dosing of LMWH and strict avoidance of additional haemostasis altering medications, including NSAIDs
Unfractionated s.c. heparin	There are no contraindications to a neuraxial procedure if total daily dose is <10,000 units. For higher dosing regimens, increase neurological monitoring and cautiously co-administer antiplatelet medications
Unfractionated i.v. heparin	Delay needle/catheter placement 2–4 h after last dose, document normal aPTT. Heparin may be restarted 1 h after procedure. Sustained heparinization with an indwelling neuraxial catheter associated with increased risk; monitor neurological status aggressively
Dabigatran	Discontinue 7 days before procedure; for shorter time periods, document normal TT. First post-operative dose 24 h after needle placement and 6 h post-catheter removal (whichever is later)

Data from Horlocker et al. [117]

will delay discharge. However, if the infusion duration is reduced many of the other benefits of TEA such as bowel recovery and attenuation of the surgical stress response may be realized.

Borzellini et al. [124] published a meta-analysis of studies examining outcomes in patients undergoing laparoscopy surgery on an ERP, and found that patients receiving TEA stayed in hospital a day longer than those who received less invasive analgesic techniques (WMD, 1.07 d; 95% CI, 0.06–2.08), and the rates of complications and hospital readmissions were unchanged.

Hughes meta-analysis of studies including patients undergoing open surgery on an ERAS pathway found that epidurals did not shorten LOS. One observational study of 231 patients undergoing open colorectal surgery on an ERP found than epidurals were associated with prolonged LOS, but also found that patients that had an epidural infusion for <24 h post-operatively were more likely to go have a shorter LOS than those whose epidurals were run for longer than 48 h [123] and an epidural infusion run for 2 days after hepatectomy allowed a shorter LOS than infusions run for 4 days [122].

What does this mean for clinicians designing peri-operative pathways for abdominal surgery? It is likely that for most patients undergoing laparoscopic surgery, the disadvantages of TEA outweigh the benefits, and outside of special circumstances, other modalities of effective analgesia that allow earlier rehabilitation should be sought. In patients undergoing open surgery it appears that TEA may have some benefits, chiefly analgesia and enhancing return of bowel function, and may have respiratory and cardiac benefits in the right patients. Which patient groups will benefit is still a matter of debate, although healthy patients undergoing uncomplicated open surgery on an ERP may well be ideally managed with multimodal analgesia including less invasive trunk blocks or intravenous lidocaine. In more complex patients and surgery, TEA may be beneficial but must be used in such a way that allows early mobilization and physiotherapy, and must involve acute pain teams who can troubleshoot and manage the patient's pain where necessary. Running the epidural for 48–72 h is probably ideal—any shorter means the patient is unlikely to see the intended outcome benefit, and routinely running epidurals for longer will undoubtedly prolong hospital stay.

Conclusion

Although the role of TEA in laparoscopic surgery is unclear, it remains the single most effective modality of analgesia for open abdominal surgery, and reduces the time to return of bowel function. It may also limit post-operative morbidity and possibly mortality in the right patients. The recent popularity of ERAS has led to the development of standardized anaesthetic pathways, where the focus has been to standardise the analgesic regimen so that every patient receives the same analgesia for every operation subtype. However, there is a great deal of difference between a healthy 50-year-old patient undergoing a laparoscopic right hemicolectomy, where an epidural may slow down mobilisation, and an elderly patient with multiple co-morbidities undergoing an open anterior resection of the rectum, where an epidural may have tangible benefits. Additionally, there are patient-specific or surgery-specific factors which may make TEA an ideal option for analgesia, such as the patient with chronic pain or opioid intolerance, or patients undergoing painful procedures such as oesophagogastrectomy. We now have many analgesic modalities at our fingertips, and the indications for each will be different, depending on the patient and the operation. In a peri-operative pathway, our goal should be for excellent analgesia while avoiding high dose systemic opiates, rather than the blanket use of a single analgesic technique. Epidural analgesia still has a role in post-operative analgesia, with the proviso of appropriate patient selection and epidural management.

References

1. Carli F, Kehlet H, Baldini G, Steel A, McRae K, Slinger P, et al. Evidence basis for regional anesthesia in multidisciplinary fast-track surgical care pathways. Reg Anesth Pain Med. 2011;36(1):63–72.
2. Varadhan KK, Neal KR, Dejong CHC, Fearon KCH, Ljungqvist O, Lobo DN. The enhanced recovery after surgery (ERAS) pathway for patients undergoing major elective open

colorectal surgery: a meta-analysis of randomized controlled trials. Clin Nutr. 2010;29(4): 434–40.
3. Kettner SC, Willschke H, Marhofer P. Does regional anaesthesia really improve outcome? Br J Anaesth. 2011;107(suppl 1):i90–5.
4. Rawal N. Epidural technique for postoperative pain. Reg Anesth Pain Med. 2012;37(3):310–7.
5. da Silva M, Lomelin D, Tsui J, Klinginsmith M, Tadaki C, Langenfeld S. Pain control for laparoscopic colectomy: an analysis of the incidence and utility of epidural analgesia compared to conventional analgesia. Tech Coloproctol. 2015;19(9):515–20.
6. Power GE, Warden B, Cooke K. Changing patterns in the acute pain service: epidural versus patient-controlled analgesia. Anaesth Intensive Care. 2005;33:501–5.
7. Low J, Johnston N, Morris C. Epidural analgesia: first do no harm. Anaesthesia. 2008;63(1):1–3.
8. Garimella V, Cellini C. Postoperative pain control. Clin Colon Rectal Surg. 2013;26(03): 191–6.
9. DAHL JB, Rosenberg J, Hansen BL, Hjortsø NC, Kehlet H. Differential analgesic effects of low-dose epidural morphine and morphine-bupivacaine at rest and during mobilization after major abdominal surgery. Anesth Analg. 1992;74(3):362–5.
10. Wu CL, Cohen SR, Richman JM, Rowlingson AJ, Courpas GE, Cheung K, et al. Efficacy of postoperative patient-controlled and continuous infusion epidural analgesia versus intravenous patient-controlled analgesia with opioids: a meta-analysis. Anesthesiology. 2005;103(5):1079–88. quiz 1109–10
11. Marret E, Remy C, Bonnet F. The postoperative pain forum group. Meta-analysis of epidural analgesia versus parenteral opioid analgesia after colorectal surgery. Br J Surg. 2007;94(6):665–73.
12. Nishimori M, Low JHS, Zheng H, Ballantyne JC. Epidural pain relief versus systemic opioid-based pain relief for abdominal aortic surgery. Cochrane Database Syst Rev. 2012;7:CD005059.
13. Carli F, Mayo N, Klubien K, Schricker T, Trudel J, Belliveau P. Epidural analgesia enhances functional exercise capacity and health-related quality of life after colonic surgery: results of a randomized trial. Anesthesiology. 2002;97(3):540.
14. Farrar JT, Berlin JA, Strom BL. Clinically important changes in acute pain outcome measures. J Pain Symptom Manag. 2003;25(5):406–11.
15. Olsen MF, Bjerre E, Hansen MD, Hilden J, Landler NE, Tendal B, Hróbjartsson A. Pain relief that matters to patients: systematic review of empirical studies assessing the minimum clinically important difference in acute pain. BMC Med. 2017;15(1):35.
16. Rigg JRA, Jamrozik K, Myles PS, Silbert BS, Peyton PJ, Parsons RW, et al. Epidural anaesthesia and analgesia and outcome of major surgery: a randomised trial. Lancet. 2002;359(9314):1276–82.
17. Mann C, Pouzeratte Y, Boccara G, Peccoux C, Vergne C, Brunat G, et al. Comparison of intravenous or epidural patient-controlled analgesia in the elderly after major abdominal surgery. Anesthesiology. 2000;92(2):433–41.
18. Albrecht E, Kirkham KR, Liu SS, Brull R. Peri-operative intravenous administration of magnesium sulphate and postoperative pain: a meta-analysis. Anaesthesia. 2012;68(1):79–90.
19. Ventham NT, Hughes M, O'Neill S, Johns N, Brady RR, Wigmore SJ. Systematic review and meta-analysis of continuous local anaesthetic wound infiltration versus epidural analgesia for postoperative pain following abdominal surgery. Br J Surg. 2013;100(10):1280–9.
20. Bell R, Pandanaboyana S, Prasad KR. Epidural versus local anaesthetic infiltration via wound catheters in open liver resection: a meta-analysis. ANZ J Surg. 2015;85(1–2):16–21.
21. Mungroop TH, Veelo DP, Busch OR. Continuous wound infiltration versus epidural analgesia after hepato-pancreato-biliary surgery (POP-UP): a randomised controlled, open-label, non-inferiority trial. Lancet. 2016;1:105–13.
22. Hughes MJ, Harrison EM, Peel NJ, Stutchfield B, McNally S, Beattie C, Wigmore SJ. Randomized clinical trial of perioperative nerve block and continuous local anaesthetic infiltration via wound catheter versus epidural analgesia in open liver resection (LIVER 2 trial). Br J Surg. 2015;102(13):1619–28.
23. Niraj G, Kelkar A, Hart E, Horst C, Malik D, Yeow C, et al. Comparison of analgesic efficacy of four-quadrant transversus abdominis plane (TAP) block and continuous posterior TAP

analgesia with epidural analgesia in patients undergoing laparoscopic colorectal surgery: an open-label, randomised, non-inferiority trial. Anaesthesia. 2014;69(4):348–55.
24. Kuo CP, Jao SW, Chen KM, Wong CS, Yeh CC, Sheen MJ, Wu CT. Comparison of the effects of thoracic epidural analgesia and i.v. infusion with lidocaine on cytokine response, postoperative pain and bowel function in patients undergoing colonic surgery. Br J Anaesth. 2006;97(5):640–6.
25. Swenson BR, Gottschalk A, Wells LT, Rowlingson JC, Thompson PW, Barclay M, et al. Intravenous lidocaine is as effective as epidural bupivacaine in reducing ileus duration, hospital stay, and pain after open colon resection: a randomized clinical trial. Reg Anesth Pain Med. 2010;35(4):370–6.
26. Veenhof AAFA, Vlug MS, van der Pas MHGM, Sietses C, van der Peet DL, de Lange-de Klerk ESM, et al. Surgical stress response and postoperative immune function after laparoscopy or open surgery with fast track or standard perioperative care. Ann Surg. 2012;255(2):216–21.
27. Schwenk W, Haase O, Neudecker J, Müller JM. Short term benefits for laparoscopic colorectal resection. Cochrane Database Syst Rev. 2005;3:CD003145.
28. Levy BF, Tilney HS, Dowson HMP, Rockall TA. A systematic review of postoperative analgesia following laparoscopic colorectal surgery. Colorect Dis. 2010;12(1):5–15.
29. Levy BF, Scott MJ, Fawcett W, Fry C, Rockall TA. Randomized clinical trial of epidural, spinal or patient-controlled analgesia for patients undergoing laparoscopic colorectal surgery. Br J Surg. 2011;98(8):1068–78.
30. Hübner M, Blanc C, Roulin D, Winiker M, Gander S, Demartines N. Randomized clinical trial on epidural versus patient-controlled analgesia for laparoscopic colorectal surgery within an enhanced recovery pathway. Ann Surg. 2015;261(4):648–53.
31. Barr J, Boulind C, Foster JD, Ewings P, Reid J, Jenkins JT, et al. Impact of analgesic modality on stress response following laparoscopic colorectal surgery: a post-hoc analysis of a randomised controlled trial. Tech Coloproctol. 2015;19(4):231–9.
32. Ahlers O, Nachtigall I, Lenze J, Goldmann A, Schulte E, Höhne C, et al. Intraoperative thoracic epidural anaesthesia attenuates stress-induced immunosuppression in patients undergoing major abdominal surgery. Br J Anaesth. 2008;101(6):781–7.
33. Kehlet H, Wilmore DW. Evidence-based surgical care and the evolution of fast-track surgery. Ann Surg. 2008;248(2):189–98.
34. Rodgers A, Walker N, Schug S, McKee A, Kehlet H, van Zundert A, et al. Reduction of postoperative mortality and morbidity with epidural or spinal anaesthesia: results from overview of randomised trials. BMJ. 2000;321(7275):1493.
35. POISE Study Group, Devereaux PJ, Yang H, Yusuf S, Guyatt G, Leslie K, et al. Effects of extended-release metoprolol succinate in patients undergoing non-cardiac surgery (POISE trial): a randomised controlled trial. Lancet. 2008;371(9627):1839–47.
36. Meissner A, Rolf N, Van Aken H. Thoracic epidural anesthesia and the patient with heart disease: benefits, risks, and controversies. Anesth Analg. 1997;85(3):517–28.
37. Park WY, Thompson JS, Lee KK. Effect of epidural anesthesia and analgesia on perioperative outcome: a randomized, controlled Veterans Affairs cooperative study. Ann Surg. 2001;234(4):560–9. discussion 569–71
38. WU C, HURLEY R, ANDERSON G, HERBERT R, ROWLINGSON A, FLEISHER L. Effect of postoperative epidural analgesia on morbidity and mortality following surgery in medicare patients. Reg Anesth Pain Med. 2004;29(6):525–33.
39. Wijeysundera DN, Beattie WS, Austin PC, Hux JE, Laupacis A. Epidural anaesthesia and survival after intermediate-to-high risk non-cardiac surgery: a population-based cohort study. Lancet. 2008;372(9638):562–9.
40. Guay J, Choi P, Suresh S, Albert N, Kopp S, Pace NL. Neuraxial blockade for the prevention of postoperative mortality and major morbidity: an overview of Cochrane systematic reviews. Cochrane Database Syst Rev. 2014;1:CD010108.
41. Pöpping DM, Elia N, Van Aken HK, Marret E, Schug SA, Kranke P, et al. Impact of epidural analgesia on mortality and morbidity after surgery. Ann Surg. 2014;259(6):1056–67.
42. Pöpping DM, Elia N, Van Aken HK, Marret E, Schug SA, Kranke P, et al. Impact of epidural analgesia on mortality and morbidity after surgery, supplementary Fig. C, supplemental digital

content Fig. C. Ann Surg. 2014;259(6):1056–67. http://links.lww.com/SLA/A469. Accessed Apr 2017
43. Grosso G, Biondi A, Marventano S, Mistretta A, Calabrese G, Basile F. Major postoperative complications and survival for colon cancer elderly patients. BMC Surg. 2012;12(Suppl 1):S20.
44. Reiz S. Circulatory effects of epidural anesthesia in patients with cardiac disease. Acta Anaesthesiol Belg. 1988;39(3 Suppl 2):21–7.
45. Goertz AW, Seeling W, Heinrich H, Lindner KH, Schirmir U. Influence of high thoracic epidural anesthesia on left ventricular contractility assessed using the end-systolic pressure-length relationship. Acta Anaesthesiol Scand. 1993;37(1):38–44.
46. Chaney MA. Intrathecal and epidural anesthesia and analgesia for cardiac surgery. Anesth Analg. 2006;102(1):45–64.
47. Nygard E. Effects of high thoracic epidural analgesia on myocardial blood flow in patients with ischemic heart disease. Circulation. 2005;111(17):2165–70.
48. Gurses E, Berk D, Sungurtekin H, Mete A. Effects of high thoracic epidural anesthesia on mixed venous oxygen saturation in coronary artery bypass grafting surgery. Med Sci Monit. 2013;19:222–9.
49. Loick HM, Schmidt C, Van Aken H, Junker R, Erren M, Berendes E, et al. High thoracic epidural anesthesia, but not clonidine, attenuates the perioperative stress response via sympatholysis and reduces the release of troponin T in patients undergoing coronary artery bypass grafting. Anesth Analg. 1999;88(4):701–9.
50. Berendes E, Schmidt C, Van Aken H. Reversible cardiac sympathectomy by high thoracic epidural anesthesia improves regional left ventricular function in patients undergoing coronary artery bypass grafting. Arch Surg. 2003;138:1283–90.
51. Hainsworth R. Vascular capacitance: its control and importance. Rev Physiol Biochem Pharmacol. 1986;105:101–73.
52. Baron JF, Payen D, Coriat P, Edouard A. Forearm vascular tone and reactivity during lumbar epidural anesthesia. Anesth Analg. 1988;67:1065–70.
53. Richman JM, Rowlingson AJ, Maine DN, Courpas GE, Weller JF, Wu CL. Does neuraxial anesthesia reduce intraoperative blood loss? A meta-analysis. J Clin Anesth. 2006;18(6):427–35.
54. Guay J. The effect of neuraxial blocks on surgical blood loss and blood transfusion requirements: a meta-analysis. J Clin Anesth. 2006;18(2):124–8.
55. Pöpping DM, Zahn PK, Van Aken HK, Dasch B, Boche R, Pogatzki-Zahn EM. Effectiveness and safety of postoperative pain management: a survey of 18 925 consecutive patients between 1998 and 2006 (2nd revision): a database analysis of prospectively raised data. Br J Anaesth. 2008;101(6):832–40.
56. Leslie K, Myles P, Devereaux P, Williamson E, Rao-Melancini P, Forbes A, et al. Neuraxial block, death and serious cardiovascular morbidity in the POISE trial. Br J Anaesth. 2013;111(3):382–90.
57. Svircevic V, Passier MM, Nierich AP, van Dijk D, Kalkman CJ, van der Heijden GJ. Epidural analgesia for cardiac surgery. Cochrane Database Syst Rev. 2013;6:CD006715.
58. Hughes MJ, Ventham NT, McNally S, Harrison E, Wigmore S. Analgesia after open abdominal surgery in the setting of enhanced recovery surgery: a systematic review and meta-analysis. JAMA Surg. 2014;149(12):1224–30.
59. Sagiroglu G, Meydan B, Copuroglu E, Baysal A, Yoruk Y, Altemur Karamustafaoglu Y, Huseyin S. A comparison of thoracic or lumbar patient-controlled epidural analgesia methods after thoracic surgery. World J Surg Oncol. 2014;12(1):96.
60. Beattie WS, Badner NH, Choi P. Epidural analgesia reduces postoperative myocardial infarction: a meta-analysis. Anesth Analg. 2001;93(4):853–8.
61. Popping DM, Van Aken HK, Brodner G, Wenk M. It is not the epidural that is dangerous, but the person who gives it (letter). Br J Anaesth. 2014;112(2):392–3.
62. Thompson DA, Makary MA, Dorman T, Pronovost PJ. Clinical and economic outcomes of hospital acquired pneumonia in intra-abdominal surgery patients. Ann Surg. 2006;243(4):547–52.
63. Ledowski T, Paech MJ, Patel B, Schug SA. Bronchial mucus transport velocity in patients receiving propofol and remifentanil versus sevoflurane and remifentanil anesthesia. Anesth Analg. 2006;102(5):1427–30.

64. Manikian B, Cantineau JP, Bertrand M, Kieffer E, Sartene R, Viars P. Improvement of diaphragmatic function by a thoracic extradural block after upper abdominal surgery. Anesthesiology. 1988;68(3):379–86.
65. Peyton PJ, Myles PS, Silbert BS, Rigg JA, Jamrozik K, Parsons R. Perioperative epidural analgesia and outcome after major abdominal surgery in high-risk patients. Anesth Analg. 2003;96(2):548.
66. N S, Yuzbasioglu MF, Oksuz H, Yildiz H, Dogan Z, Bulbuloglu E, Goksu M, Gisi G. Effects of epidural-and-general anesthesia combined versus general anesthesia alone on femoral venous flow during laparoscopic cholecystectomy. J Laparoendosc Adv Surg Tech A. 2010;20(3):219–23.
67. Gan TJ, Robinson SB, Oderda GM, Scranton R, Pepin J, Ramamoorthy S. Impact of postsurgical opioid use and ileus on economic outcomes in gastrointestinal surgeries. Curr Med Res Opin. 2015;31(4):677–86.
68. Kuruba R, Fayard N, Snyder D. Epidural analgesia and laparoscopic technique do not reduce incidence of prolonged ileus in elective colon resections. Am J Surg. 2012;204(5):613–8.
69. Barletta JF, Asgeirsson T, Senagore AJ. Influence of intravenous opioid dose on postoperative ileus. Ann Pharmacother. 2011;45(7–8):916–23.
70. Guay J, Nishimori M, Kopp S. Epidural local anaesthetics versus opioid-based analgesic regimens for postoperative gastrointestinal paralysis, vomiting and pain after abdominal surgery. Cochrane Database Syst Rev. 2016;7:CD001893.
71. Khan SA, Khokhar HA, Nasr ARH, Carton E, El-Masry S. Effect of epidural analgesia on bowel function in laparoscopic colorectal surgery: a systematic review and meta-analysis. Surg Endosc. 2013;27(7):2581–91.
72. Kamiński JP, Pai A, Ailabouni L, Park JJ, Marecik SJ, Prasad LM, et al. Role of epidural and patient-controlled analgesia in site-specific laparoscopic colorectal surgery. JSLS. 2014;18(4):e2014.00207.
73. Exadaktylos AK, Buggy DJ, Moriarty DC, Mascha E, Sessler DI. Can anesthetic technique for primary breast cancer surgery affect recurrence or metastasis? Anesthesiology. 2006;105(4):660–4.
74. JG HILLER, MB HACKING, EK LINK, KL WESSELS, BJ RIEDEL. Perioperative epidural analgesia reduces cancer recurrence after gastro-oesophageal surgery. Acta Anaesthesiol Scand. 2014;58(3):281–90.
75. Gupta K, Kshirsagar S, Chang L, Schwartz R, Law PY. Morphine stimulates angiogenesis by activating proangiogenic and survival-promoting signaling and promotes breast tumor growth. Cancer Res. 2002;62:4491–8.
76. Koltun WA, Bloomer MM, Tilberg AF, Seaton JF. Awake epidural anesthesia is associated with improved natural killer cell cytotoxicity and a reduced stress response. Am J Surg. 1996;171:68–73.
77. Mao L, Lin S, Lin J. The effects of anesthetics on tumor progression. Int J Physiol Pathophysiol Pharmacol. 2013;5(1):1–10.
78. Lirk P, Hollmann MW, Fleischer M, Weber NC, Fiegl H. Lidocaine and ropivacaine, but not bupivacaine, demethylate deoxyribonucleic acid in breast cancer cells in vitro. Br J Anaesth. 2014;113(suppl 1):i32–8.
79. Sun Y, Li T, Gan TJ. The effects of perioperative regional anesthesia and analgesia on cancer recurrence and survival after oncology surgery. Reg Anesth Pain Med. 2015;40(5):589–98.
80. Cakmakkaya OS, Kolodzie K, Apfel CC. Anaesthetic techniques for risk of malignant tumour recurrence. Cochrane Database Syst Rev. 2014;11:Art. No.: CD008877.
81. Day A, Smith R, Jourdan I, Fawcett W, Scott M, Rockall T. Retrospective analysis of the effect of postoperative analgesia on survival in patients after laparoscopic resection of colorectal cancer. Br J Anaesth. 2012;109(2):185–90.
82. Cummings KC, Xu F, Cummings LC, Cooper GS. A comparison of epidural analgesia and traditional pain management effects on survival and cancer recurrence after colectomy: a population-based study. Anesthesiology. 2012;116(4):797–806.
83. Wantman A, Hancox N, Howell PR. Techniques for identifying the epidural space: a survey of practice amongst anaesthetists in the UK. Anaesthesia. 2006;61(4):370–5.

84. Schier R, Guerra D, Aguilar J, Pratt GF, Hernandez M, Boddu K, et al. Epidural space identification: a meta-analysis of complications after air versus liquid as the medium for loss of resistance. Anesth Analg. 2009;109(6):2012–21.
85. Antibas PL, do Nascimento Junior P, Braz LG, Vitor Pereira Doles J, NSP M, Dib El R. Air versus saline in the loss of resistance technique for identification of the epidural space. Cochrane Database Syst Rev. 2014;7:CD008938.
86. Hermanides J, Hollmann MW, Stevens MF, Lirk P. Failed epidural: causes and management. Br J Anaesth. 2012 Jul;109(2):144–54.
87. Todorov L, VadeBoncouer T. Etiology and use of the "hanging drop" technique: a review. Pain Res Treat. 2014;2014(4):1–10.
88. Bonica JJ, Backup PH, Anderson CE, HADFIELD D, Crepps WF, Monk BF. Peridural block: analysis of 3,637 cases and a review. Anesthesiology. 1957;18(5):723–84.
89. Hoffmann VL, Vercauteren MP, Vreugde JP, Hans GH, Coppejans HC, Adriaensen HA. Posterior epidural space depth: safety of the loss of resistance and hanging drop techniques. Br J Anaesth. 1999;83(5):807–9.
90. Stone PA, Kilpatrick AW, Thorburn J. Posture and epidural catheter insertion. The relationship between skill, experience and maternal posture on the outcome of epidural catheter insertion. Anaesthesia. 1990;45(11):920–3.
91. Hamilton CL, Riley ET, Cohen SE. Changes in the position of epidural catheters associated with patient movement. Anesthesiology. 1997;86(4):778–84. discussion 29A
92. Mhyre JM, Greenfield MLVH, Tsen LC, Polley LS. A systematic review of randomized controlled trials that evaluate strategies to avoid epidural vein cannulation during obstetric epidural catheter placement. Anesth Analg. 2009;108(4):1232–42.
93. Podder S, Kumar N, Yaddanapudi LN, Chari P. Paramedian lumbar epidural catheter insertion with patients in the sitting position is equally successful in the flexed and unflexed spine. Anesth Analg. 2002;99:1829–32.
94. Leeda M, Stienstra R, Arbous MS, et al. Lumbar epidural catheter insertion: the midline vs. the paramedian approach. Eur J Anaesthesiol. 2005;22:839–42.
95. Visser WA, Liem TH, van Egmond J, Gielen MJM. Extension of sensory blockade after thoracic administration of a test dose of lidocaine at three different levels. Anesth Analg. 1998;86:332–5.
96. Yokoyama M, Hanazaki M, Fujii H, Mizobuchi S, Nakatsuka H, Takahashi T, Matsumi M, Takeuchi M, Morita K. Correlation between the distribution of contrast medium and the extent of blockade during epidural anesthesia. Anesthesiology. 2004;100:1504–10.
97. Shaikh F, Brzezinski J, Alexander S, Arzola C, Carvalho JCA, Beyene J, et al. Ultrasound imaging for lumbar punctures and epidural catheterisations: systematic review and meta-analysis. BMJ. 2013;346:f1720.
98. Scott DA, Chamley DM, Mooney PH. Epidural ropivacaine infusion for postoperative analgesia after major lower abdominal surgery—a dose finding study. Anesth Analg. 1995;81:982–6.
99. Manion SC, Brennan TJ. Thoracic epidural analgesia and acute pain management. Anesthesiology. 2011;115(1):181–8.
100. Hjortsø NC, Lund C, Mogensen T, Bigler D, Kehlet H. Epidural morphine improves pain relief and maintains sensory analgesia during continuous epidural bupivacaine after abdominal surgery. Anesth Analg. 1986;65(10):1033–6.
101. Bromage PR, Camporesi E, Chestnut D. Epidural narcotics for postoperative analgesia. Anesth Analg. 1980;59(7):473–80.
102. Ummenhofer WC, Arends RH. Comparative spinal distribution and clearance kinetics of intrathecally administered morphine, fentanyl, alfentanil, and sufentanil. Anesthesiology. 2000;92:739–53.
103. Carvalho B. Respiratory depression after neuraxial opioids in the obstetric setting. Anesth Analg. 2008;107(3):956–61.
104. Kabon B, Fleischmann E, Treschan T, Taguchi A, Kapral S, Kurz A. Thoracic epidural anesthesia increases tissue oxygenation during major abdominal surgery. Anesth Analg. 2003;97(6):1812–7.

105. Youssef N, Orlov D, Alie T, Chong M, Cheng J, Thabane L, et al. What epidural opioid results in the best analgesia outcomes and fewest side effects after surgery? Anesth Analg. 2014;119(4):965–77.
106. Capogna G, Camorcia M, Stirparo S, Farcomeni A. Programmed intermittent epidural bolus versus continuous epidural infusion for labor analgesia. Anesth Analg. 2011;113(4):826–31.
107. Vallejo MC, Ramesh V, Phelps AL, Sah N. Epidural labour analgesia: continuous infusion versus patient-controlled epidural analgesia with background infusion versus without background infusion. J Pain. 2007;8:970–5.
108. Arendt K, Segal S. Why epidurals do not always work. Rev Obstet Gynecol. 2008;1(2):49–55.
109. Hogan QH. Epidural anatomy: new observations. Can J Anesth. 1998;45:R40–8.
110. Motamed C, Farhat F, R m rand F, St phanazzi J, Laplanche AS, Jayr C. An analysis of postoperative epidural analgesia failure by computed tomography epidurography. Anesth Analg. 2006;103(4):1026–32.
111. Afshan G, Chohan U, Khan FA, Chaudhry N, Khan ZE, Khan AA. Appropriate length of epidural catheter in the epidural space for postoperative analgesia: evaluation by epidurography. Anaesthesia. 2011;66(10):913–8.
112. Kinsella SM. A prospective audit of regional anaesthesia failure in 5080 Caesarean sections. Anaesthesia. 2008;63:822–32.
113. Sugimoto M, Nesbit L, Barton JG, Traverso LW. Epidural anesthesia dysfunction is associated with postoperative complications after pancreatectomy. J Hepatobiliary Pancreat Sci. 2016;23(2):102–9.
114. Pan PH, Bogard TD, Owen MD. Incidence and characteristics of failures in obstetric neuraxial analgesia and anesthesia: a retrospective analysis of 19,259 deliveries. Int J Obstet Anesth. 2004;13(4):227–33.
115. Kini SP. The impact of pruritus on quality of life. Arch Dermatol. 2011;147(10):1153.
116. Cook TM, Counsell D, Wildsmith JAW, On Behalf of The Royal College of Anaesthetists Third National Audit Project. Major complications of central neuraxial block: report on the Third National Audit Project of the Royal College of Anaesthetists. Br J Anaesth. 2009;102(2):179–90. https://academic.oup.com/bja/article-lookup/doi/10.1093/bja/aen360
117. Horlocker TT. Regional anaesthesia in the patient receiving antithrombotic and antiplatelet therapy. Br J Anaesth. 2011;107(Suppl 1):i96–106.
118. Siniscalchi A. Thoracic epidural anesthesia: effects on splanchnic circulation and implications in anesthesia and intensive care. World J Crit Care Med. 2015;4(1):89.
119. Gould T, Grace K, Thome G. Effect of thoracic epidural anaesthesia on colonic blood flow. Br J Anaesth. 2002;89(3):446–51.
120. Piccioni F, Mariani L, Negri M, Casiraghi C, Belli F, Leo E, et al. Epidural analgesia does not influence anastomotic leakage incidence after open colorectal surgery for cancer: a retrospective study on 1,474 patients. J Surg Oncol. 2015;112(2):225–30.
121. Lovely JK, Maxson PM, Jacob AK, Cima RR, Horlocker TT, Hebl JR, et al. Case-matched series of enhanced versus standard recovery pathway in minimally invasive colorectal surgery. Br J Surg. 2011;99(1):120–6.
122. Ntinas A, Kardassis D, Konstantinopoulos I, Kottos P, Manias A, Kyritsi M, et al. Duration of the thoracic epidural catheter in a fast-track recovery protocol may decrease the length of stay after a major hepatectomy: a case control study. Int J Surg. 2013;11(9):882–5.
123. Ahmed J, Lim M, Khan S, McNaught C, MacFie J. Predictors of length of stay in patients having elective colorectal surgery within an enhanced recovery protocol. Int J Surg. 2010;8(8):628–32.
124. Borzellino G, Francis NK, Chapuis O, Krastinova E, VXR D, Genna M. Review article. Role of epidural analgesia within an ERAS program after laparoscopic colorectal surgery: a review and meta-analysis of randomised controlled studies. Surg Res Pract. 2016;2016:7543684.

Truncal Blocks: Thoracic Paravertebral Blocks

9

Kevin King

Key Points

1. Paravertebral blocks have regained popularity due to the increased safety of ultrasound assisted or live-time needle guided paravertebral blockade with or without catheter placement.
2. Efficacious for both thoraco-abdominal and abdominal surgery, and may have the same potency as thoracic epidural analgesia with greater haemodynamic stability.
3. It can be unilaterally or bilaterally inserted; single-shot or continuously administered. Bilateral continuous blocks are required for open abdominal surgery.
4. Pneumothoax and potential vascular injury are the most serious potential complications.
5. Limiting catheter insertion to less than 3 cm within the paravertebral space reduces misplacement.

Introduction and Historical Perspective

The history of regional and neuraxial anaesthesia is characterized by the search for the safest and most effective methods to relieve pain during and after surgical procedures. As a regional and paraneuraxial technique, paravertebral blockade (PVB) has, for over 110 years since its initial description, gone through cycles of frequent use and obscurity depending on the perceived balance of risk and benefit. The initial and subsequent descriptions of PVB for surgical anaesthesia of the thoraco-abdominal region have been revisited recently in peer-reviewed journals and well-known trade

K. King
Department of Anesthesiology and Perioperative Medicine, University of Pittsburgh Medical Center, Passavant Hospital, Pittsburgh, PA, USA

A. Krige, M. J. P. Scott (eds.), *Analgesia in Major Abdominal Surgery*,
https://doi.org/10.1007/978-3-319-94482-1_9

journals [1–3]. PVB was first described in the early part of the twentieth century primarily as surgical anaesthetic while needle and syringe technology was in its infancy. PVB was utilized due to its relative safety (hemodynamic stability and less narcosis) compared to spinal and general anesthesia in those years which predated advanced monitoring, resuscitation by intravenous (IV) fluid therapy and safe human-to-human transfusion, the latter of which was developed during World War I. Plastic over-the-needle IV catheters, without which our practices of medicine would be very different, were not introduced until the 1950s [4]. As increased monitoring and airway instrumentation capabilities made spinal and general anesthesia safer, the likely perception was that risks associated with PVB for surgical anesthesia were unnecessary, leading to decreased utilization of the technique.

One of the early mid-twentieth century practitioners of PVB for abdominal surgery recognized both the risks and the broad utility of PVB; "if a true paravertebral block is performed in the manner originally suggested by Sellheim in 1905 and perfected by Labat (1922) then the rami communicantes and the sympathetic nerves are blocked as well as the intercostal nerves" [4]. He realized the risks of injecting relatively high volumes, unwittingly, into the "prolongations of the subarachnoid space" when the needle insertion point was medial and close to the vertebral body. Indeed, PVB was regarded as requiring a significant amount of skill. In order to avoid the risk of a high spinal blockade, as well as the alternative of general anesthesia, in high-risk patients presenting with an acute abdomen, he advised a modified multiple-injection technique. This consisted of bilateral injections of ribs six through twelve, 6 cm from the midline (intercostal) instead of a more medial PVB location [5]. Interestingly, he advocated 8 ml of local anaesthetic (LA) (1% Novocaine with adrenaline) at each level along with a 30–40 ml splanchnic block bilaterally, using up to 200 ml in total. This technique likely traded the risk of high dose intrathecal injection (leading to high/total spinal anesthesia) for the risk of LA systemic toxicity (LAST), which was not well recognized until the 1970s.

Due to the increased safety of modern general anesthesia, the purpose of performing PVB has largely shifted from surgical anesthesia to post-operative analgesia. When Eason and Wyatt reintroduced thoracic PVB into medical literature after decades of barely being mentioned, they presented case reports of continuous and single-shot use primarily as a modality for post-operative analgesia and post-traumatic analgesia (rib fractures) [6]. Though risk cannot be eliminated, the high level of training and the medical advances of the twenty-first century should lead to consideration of PVB as a relatively safe and extremely effective modality to relieve post-operative pain [7–11].

Evidence for Efficacy

Abdominal Surgery

Although the majority of recent literature on PVB focuses on thoracic surgery and comparisons to epidural analgesia, there is some evidence for PVB in abdominal surgery. When this is considered within the context of the total body of scientific knowledge on the topic, it is a reasonable conclusion that PVB is advantageous for all types surgery from the apex of the thoracic cage to the pelvic floor. Of additional interest in historic literature, PVB was even used to relieve chronic angina pectoris and to reverse ischemic electrocardiographic changes in a time that predated our current era of percutaneous coronary interventions [12]. Indeed, the reduction in sympatholytic activity that in turn decreased myocardial strain in the previously mentioned case exemplifies the breadth of the utility of paravertebral LA injection.

Recently, PVB has been validated as a safe and effective analgesic for abdominoplasty, hepatectomy, hepatic radiofrequency ablation (RFA), gynaecological surgery and urological surgery. Bilateral thoracic PVB has been described in a case series as an excellent post-operative analgesic modality for in-patient and outpatient abdominoplasty procedures, wherein no patients experienced PONV and none required post-operative opioid administration [13]. Pre-operatively placed, right unilateral single shot thoracic PVB at T6–10 have proven to be effective for anaesthesia and post-operative analgesia for patients undergoing percutaneous RFA [14]. PVB performed at T10 level has also been compared to transversus abdominis plane (TAP) block recently and found to be marginally superior for analgesia following midline laparotomy for gynaecological cancer [15]. While single shot PVB are useful for less invasive surgeries such as RFA, patients undergoing more invasive surgeries like right-lobe hepatectomy, which involve a subcostal incision, will benefit from better pain control with a continuous PVB technique [16].

Oesophagectomy

Perhaps the most difficult post-operative recovery of all abdominal or thoraco-abdominal surgeries is that following Ivor-Lewis Oesophagectomy (ILO) due to the thoracic and abdominal incisions. ILO is a debilitating open surgical approach for oesophagectomy but is slowly becoming less common due to the emergence of minimally invasive oesophagectomy (MIO). Length of stay (LOS) for ILO patients was shortened from 13 to 10 days in an enhanced recovery after surgery (ERAS) clinical pathway, which utilized PVB as the cornerstone of the multi-modal acute pain regimen [17].

Though, MIO does not involve the invasiveness of a large open technique, including extensive cutting of respiratory/abdominal muscle, it is the combination of a video-assisted thoracic surgery with the addition of abdominal laparoscopy. VATS is typically performed on the right side, and a right-sided chest tube is left in place for several days after surgery. Another name for one of the MIO approaches in surgical literature is combined thoracoscopic-laparoscopic oesophagectomy (TLO). Recently, it was found that even single shot PVB performed pre-operatively had a significant beneficial effect during and after surgery. Specifically, less opioid was administered intra-operatively and post-operative patient-controlled analgesia (PCA) demands were reduced. Also, patient reported pain scores were lower, and post-operative pulmonary function tests were better when measured at the third post-operative day. Additionally, patients undergoing TLO who received PVB had earlier hospital discharge [18].

Anatomy

That anatomical target for PVB and also catheter placement is the small triangular-shaped PVS (Figs. 9.1 and 9.2). The PVS in the thoracic region is contiguous between vertebral levels and is bounded posteriorly by the anterior surface of the transverse processes, rib head and neck, and the superior costo-transverse ligaments and innermost intercostal membrane complex. The antero-lateral border is the parietal pleura, and the medial boundary contacts the lateral intervertebral neuroforamina, intervertebral discs, and the vertebral bodies. The anatomic contents of the paravertebral space (PVS) consist of loose adipose and connective tissue, including the endothoracic fascia, which divides the PVS into an anterior and posterior compartment. The anterior compartment of the PVS communicates with the prevertebral fascia and prevertebral space [10]. At the neuroforamen, the dorsal and ventral rami combine to form each spinal nerve entering the PVS. The spinal nerve

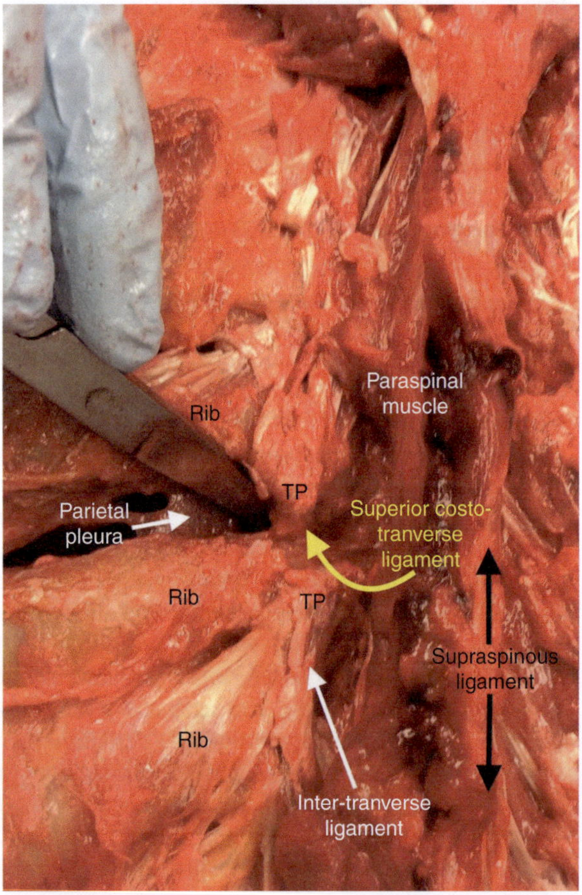

Fig. 9.1 Cadaveric dissection of Paravertebral Space (the metal instrument is positioned deep to the transverse process and superficial to the parietal pleura of the thoracic cavity)

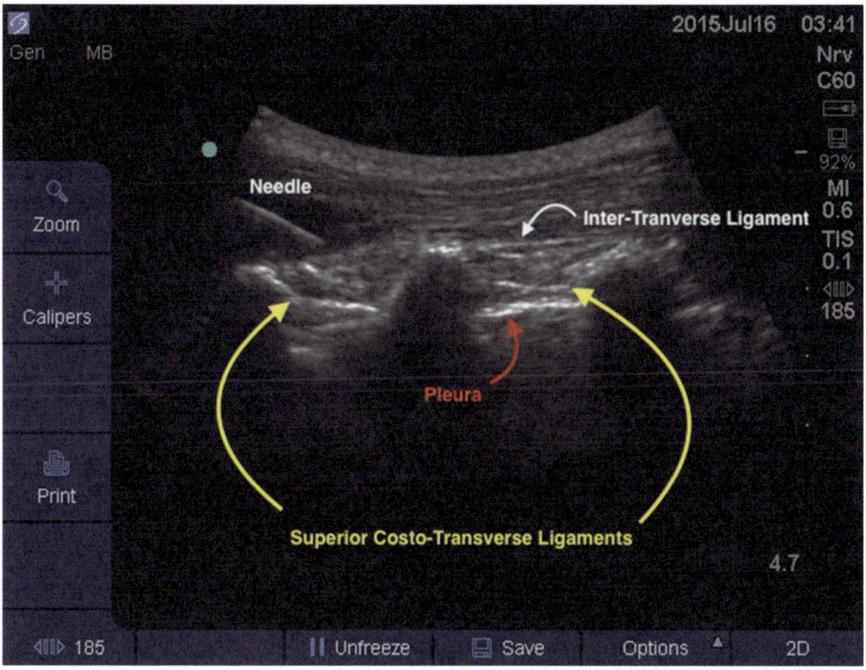

Fig. 9.2 Typical sonographic image when orienting the curvilinear probe in a parasaggital plane (parallel to the longitudinal axis of the spinal column). This image can be obtained with patient positioned in either the classic sitting pisition or the lateral recumbent position

immediately branches into somatic nerves and sympathetic nerves, and it is this anatomic fact that accounts for the higher quality blockade with PVB compared to intercostal block (ICB). However, many experts believe that the superior analgesic quality of PVB is due, at least partially, to segmental epidural spread through intervertebral foramina, which has been shown in cadaveric dye studies to occur in as much as 40% of injections with volumes of 20 ml (single injections) and even dual injections of 10 ml [11]. Additionally PVB catheter tips may be located in either the epidural space, the PVS or the intercostal space.

Ultrasound-Guided Paravertebral Block Techniques

Assess the following factors in order to determine the optimal USG PVB technique (Fig. 9.2) to employ:

1. Determine the type of PVB: single shot versus continuous and unilateral versus bilateral.
2. Optimize patient positioning: sitting, lateral decubitus or prone (Figs. 9.3, 9.4, 9.5, and 9.6).

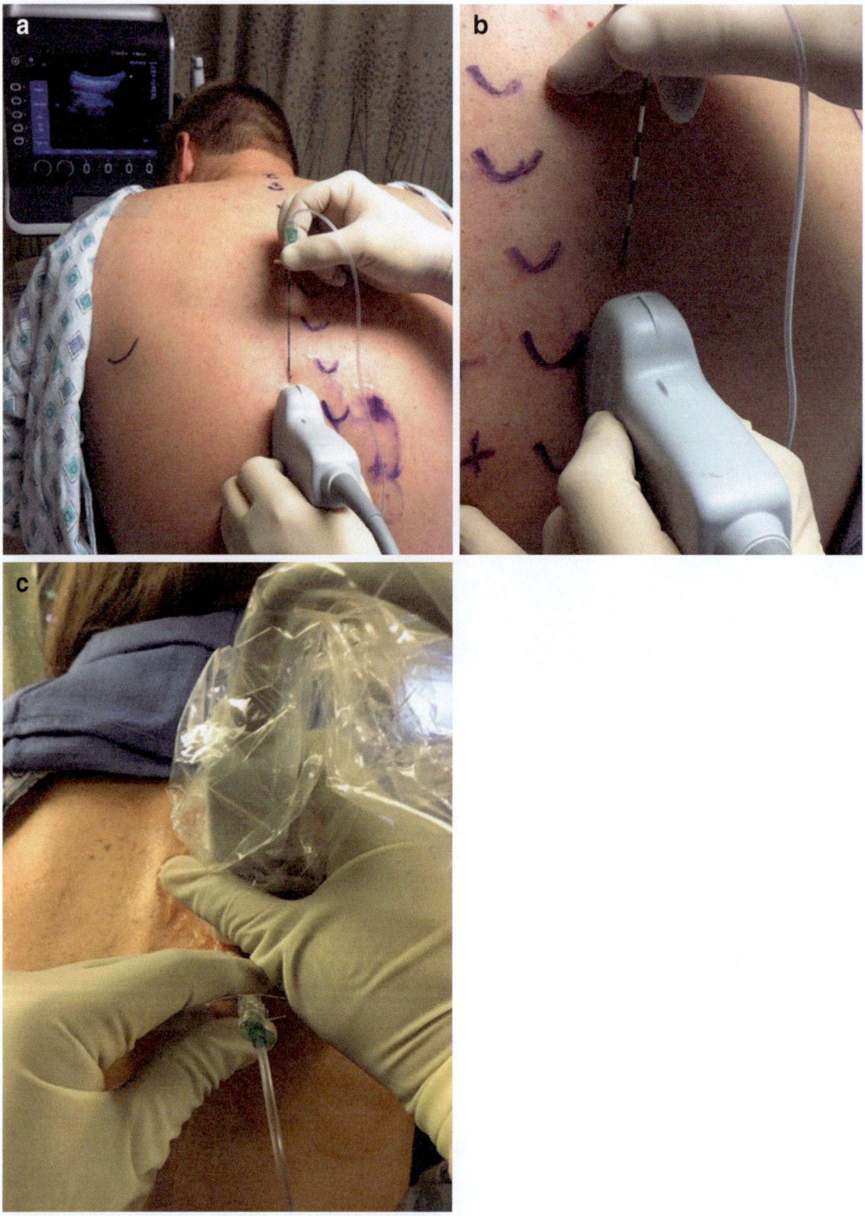

Fig. 9.3 (**a**) Classic sitting position with parasaggital probe orientation. (**b**) Needle cephalic to probe approach and Probe midline guide used to ensure a needle in-plane approach. (**c**) Needle caudad to Probe with parasaggital orientation

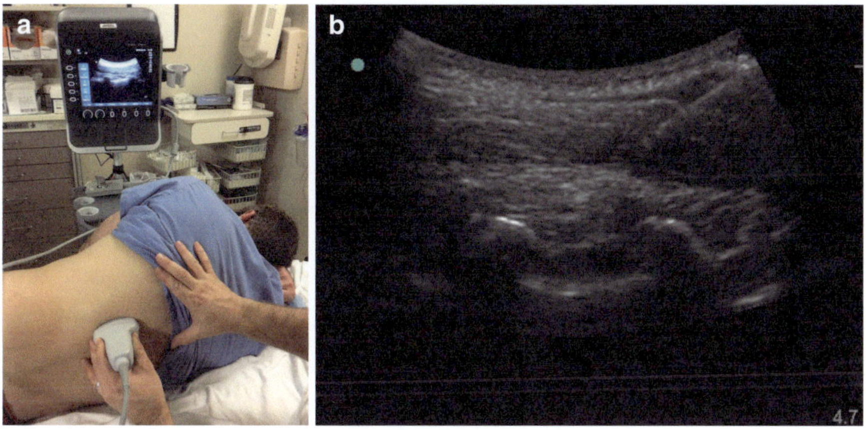

Fig. 9.4 (**a**) Lateral patient positioning with a parasaggital probe orientation. (**b**) Typical sonographic image when orienting the curvilinear probe in a parasaggital plane (parallel to the longitudinal axis of the spinal column). This image can be obtained with patient in the classical sitting position or in the lateral recumbent position

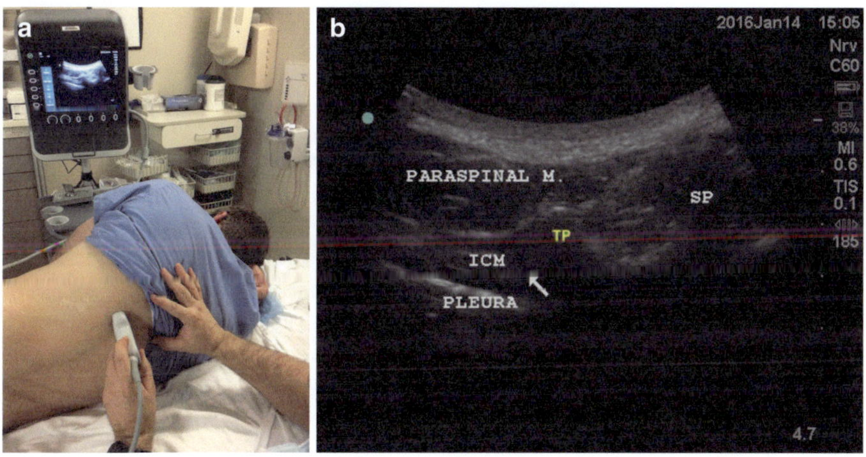

Fig. 9.5 (**a**) Lateral patient positioning (a common PVB position for ipsilateral rib fractures, unilateral surgery e.g. inguinal herniorrhaphy, or for post-operative PVB). (**b**) Correlating sonographic image of the PVS using a horizontal probe orientation

3. Perform a pre-procedural scan to determine optimum probe position: parasagittal (parallel to spine, *see* Figs. 9.2, 9.3, and 9.4), horizontal/transverse (perpendicular to spine, *see* Fig. 9.5) or oblique/diagonal.
4. Choose Live-time needle USG versus Ultrasound Assisted [UA] method (see below).

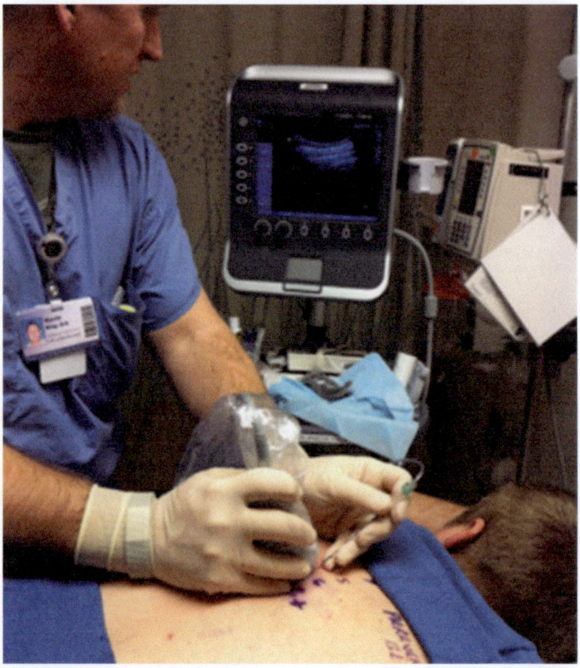

Fig. 9.6 Prone patient positioning for PVB (may reduce the frequency of vagal induced hypotensive episodes during block performance)

5. In-plane (long-axis, *see* Fig. 9.3) versus Out of plane (short axis) for live-time needle guidance. (Note: Most fellowships and the American Society of Regional Anesthesia recommends using In-plane live time guidance whenever possible [19].)

The decision whether to administer a single shot or a continuous technique should be based on the patient's analgesic needs and the invasiveness of the surgery as well as whether bilateral PVBs will be necessary. Typically, bilateral blocks are advised for abdominal surgery, and unilateral blocks are advised for thoracotomy, VATS, and the treatment of pain secondary to unilateral rib fractures.

The decisions about these factors will then influence the position in which the patient is placed for optimal comfort, stability, and ease of performance of the procedure.

Pre-procedural US scanning of the relevant bony anatomy and soft tissues near the target PVS(s) is recommended prior to creating the aseptic field. This aids determination of the best needle trajectory. For example, scanning may reveal the transverse processes to be relatively close as is common in children and small stature adults. Generally the upper and mid-thoracic intervertebral spaces and intertransverse spaces are smaller than in the lower thoracic and lumbar levels as those lower, weight-bearing vertebrae, are subsequently larger in the caudal direction. In smaller patients and in the upper or mid-thoracic spaces, the horizontal probe orientation and in-plane needle advancement can usually be performed with less technical difficulty than a parasagittal approach.

Although parasagittal and horizontal probe positions are the most often utilized, other modifications have been developed which enable the placement of the needle tip and thereby, the catheter, into the PVS. Regional anaesthetists often place the target PVS in the middle of the viewing screen and attempt to approach the PVS with an in-plane technique using a low angle of insonation (<35°). One recently published modification of the parasagittal probe placement technique is to move the probe caudad so that the inferior transverse process (TP) moves out of the US image thus no longer presenting an obstruction to the needle path. By moving the probe caudally the target PVS moves closer to the needle-insertion side of the viewing screen. This overcomes what is called the "double fulcrum" effect often noted in the USG parasagittal approach. Transducer pressure is used to upwardly deflect the needle tip when the needle is passing over a TP. The TP creates the second fulcrum [20].

The benefit of such parasagittal probe positions is that the needle is not directed medially toward the neuraxial structures and should thereby reduce the risk of epidural spread of injectate, epidural hematoma, and cord injury. However, when the optimal techniques are not working, a slight oblique position of the probe or an out-of-plane technique may also move an obstructing bony structure out of the needle trajectory.

Out-of-plane techniques have been described and may also be safe in skilled hands. Such techniques have been studied in cadavers and have shown to reliably deposit local anesthetic in the PVS, as long as the needle tip is advanced deep to the articular processes near the intervertebral foramen and the antero-medial surface of the parietal pleura [21].

An oblique probe positioning with in-plane needle insertion at the caudal end of the probe introduces a slight medial needle direction, but it accomplishes two tasks; it avoids the bony obstruction on the inferior end of the viewing screen and it keeps the targeted PVS at the mid-superior end of the screen, thus allowing continuous in-plane needle advancement with the desired low angle of insonation. To obtain this view, first visualize the PVS using a parasagittal probe position with a planned needle insertion site inferior to the probe (Fig. 9.3c). Afterward, the operator rotates the caudal end of the probe counter-clockwise, keeping the superior end of the probe at a fixed point in order to move the inferior TP out of the needle trajectory.

The UA technique enhances the ability of the physician to determine the underlying anatomical characteristics prior to needle insertion so that fewer needle passes or re-directions are necessary to enter the PVS. A possible advantage is that it may aid the physician in the performance of a PVB by allowing direction of the needle with two hands instead of one. The proceduralist can focus on needle advancement and controlling the depth of insertion using both hands while focusing on the patient's back instead of the ultrasound image. The pre-procedural scanning process allows the determination of skin-to-target depths for the TP, the costo-transverse ligament (CTL), and the parietal and visceral pleura so that close attention can be paid to the depth markings on the needle as the needle is inferiorly "walked off" the transverse process and advanced a predetermined distance (Figs. 9.3 and 9.4).

The approximate vertebral level is chosen and marked on the skin by the physician based upon the surgeon's planned or reported approach to the abdomen and/or thorax. The ultrasound can be used to precisely triangulate the location of the lateral tip of the TP correlating to the vertebral level planned for insertion of the PVB. This triangulation is accomplished by marking the location of the lateral extent of the underlying TP on the skin with the probe in two different positions. With the probe in parasagittal orientation and placed slightly lateral to the palpated midline spinous processes (Figs. 9.3 and 9.4), the superficial lamina and facet joints can be appreciated (represented by a wavy line of continuous hyper-echoic bone), after which, the probe is slowly moved more laterally (Figs. 9.3 and 9.4), revealing interrupted soft tissue and bone. The bone cortices with underlying acoustic shadows represent the TPs. It is at this position that marks are made just superior and inferior to the probe to denote that the needle should not be placed any more medial than the line connecting these dots. Adjusting the probe in this same plane, the preferred target TP should be placed in the middle of the ultrasound image and a correlating mark made immediately lateral to the midpoint of the probe, denoting the location of the underlying TP. Then the TP may be confirmed by turning the probe 90° to find the classic horizontal or transverse image of the TP, and again position the lateral edge of the TP in the middle of the ultrasound image to denote the lateral tip of the underlying TP. The practitioner should then have two dots on the skin in close proximity along the long horizontal axis of the underlying TP.

Ultrasound-Guided Paravertebral Catheter Placement

A recently published review of USG PVBs with PVS catheterization confirmed the efficacy and safety of USG techniques, and that US should afford similar benefits as US studied in other regional anaesthesia blocks. Some of those benefits are faster onset, longer duration of single shot blockade, improved block quality, fewer needle passes through tissue and fewer complications [21].

Within the last decade, several descriptions of USG PVB techniques have been validated with cadaver injection and subsequent dissection or radiologic evaluation, then clinically applied to live patients [11, 22]. A study in 2009 showed that even when the needle is visualized clearly in-plane to enter the thoracic PVS, a catheter advanced 5 cm past the tip of the needle will often not remain in the PVS [23]. In a cadaver study, only 11 of 20 paravertebral catheters yielded a paravertebral spread with contrast dye. The other nine (45%) were either in the epidural space (6), intrapleural (1), or prevertebral (2). The same author showed that USG single shot PVBs in cadavers displayed no pleural punctures via contrast spread evaluated under CT scan.

As mentioned earlier, a 20 ml single injection PVB has been compared with 10 ml dual-injections (two-level) technique. The single and dual injection techniques were compared in a cadaver study counting the number of paravertebral/intercostal segments covered with dye after USG injection and anatomic dissection. Transverse probe orientation with in-plane needle advancement was used.

Interestingly, this study used a 4 cm insertion distance past the Touhy needle tip. The results showed that single injection covers a mean of 4.5 vertebral levels, whereas dual injection covers six levels with the same total volume. Additionally, the study showed that the catheters and dye injections are located in non-ideal locations (epidural, intercostal, and pre-vertebral) [11]. The authors of that study concluded that the PVS is in continuity with the epidural space and PVB should have the same indications and contraindications as epidural analgesia.

In contrast to those studies with catheter insertion depths of 4 or 5 cm, a 2010 study using a transverse/oblique, in-plane technique (parallel to the ribs) threaded the catheters only 2 cm past the needle and had remarkably different results. There were 36 patients and 100% had correct placement confirmed by dye injection and antero-posterior chest radiograph [24]. Considering this evidence, one might conclude that the orientation of the probe and entry point of the needle in USG continuous PVB are not as important to success as the distance the catheter is inserted past the needle tip. It is intuitive that a catheter inserted a greater distance than the dimensions of the paravertebral space width or depth encourages misplacement into unintended locations.

Safety Considerations

Similar to all regional anaesthesia techniques, PVB carries the relatively low-incidence risks of skin infection, bleeding, nerve injury, and LAST secondary to intravascular injection or absorption. However, PVB has some unique risks due to the close proximity of vital structures to the anatomic target (see anatomy section and Fig. 9.2).

Of all the possible complications, the most feared is a pneumothorax. The risks involved with needle advancement with or without ultrasound guidance (USG) include puncture of the parietal pleura or worse, injury of the visceral pleura. While a visceral pleura injury would release inspired air into the sub-atmospheric pleural space, resulting in clinical or subclinical pneumothorax, a puncture of the parietal pleura may only cause an uncomfortable sensation, and is unlikely to be transformed into a pneumothorax if the practitioner is taking precautions to avoid allowing the communication of ambient pressure with the typically sub-atmospheric intra-thoracic pressure. This author recommends using a continuous circuit consisting of Touhy needle, extension tubing, and a syringe containing the LA agent, while advancing the needle under live-time guidance with ultrasound to minimize the incidence of pneumothorax.

The vascular structures at risk include the vessels contained in the paraspinal muscles, the segmental intercostal artery and vein, and the azygous vein anteriorly on the right side.

At the author's institution, we have occasionally noted blood in the 27 g catheter after advancing it through the Touhy needle and into the PVS. This flow of blood may be due to capillary action as the tip of the catheter enters a haematoma caused by the advancing needle or by the pressure present in a vessel, which the catheter

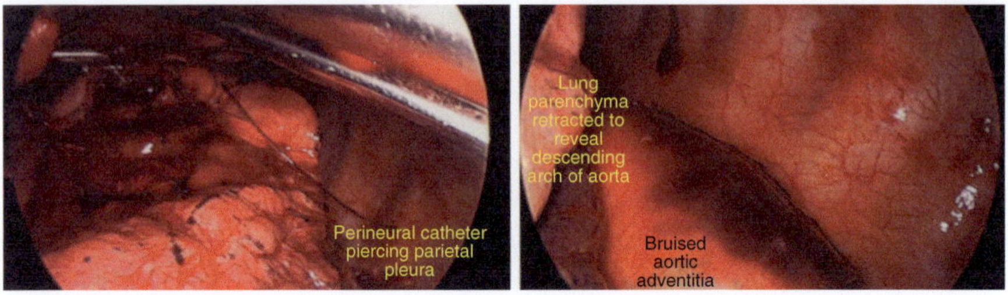

Fig. 9.7 Perineural catheters have the potential to damage intrathoracic vascular structures—a video thoracoscopic view of an over-inserted PVB catheter resulting in a bruised aorta

may inadvertently enter. If this occurs, it is prudent to remove the catheter and place it at another vertebral level. Otherwise, a bolus of LA delivered through the catheter could theoretically lead to symptoms of LAST.

Although, there are no major vascular injuries reported in the literature due to PVB, there is a theoretical risk to major vascular structures including the aorta. This is possible if a stiff catheter tip were to be unintentionally inserted through structures such as vessel walls or the parietal pleura. In a recent case report a surgeon observed the uncommon finding of bruising to the adventitial lining of the aorta along with the presence of an intrathoracic perineural catheter while placing a thoracoscope through the chest (Fig. 9.7). Presumably either the Touhy needle tip was unknowingly advanced through the pleura into the intrathoracic space or the paravertebral catheter itself pierced the parietal pleura. Though there was no harm to the patient, we presume that the stiff perineural catheter caused this minor vascular injury [7]. Furthermore, the catheter may have pierced the pleura and then made contact with the aorta upon advancing. At the author's institution, the acute pain and regional anaesthesia service has recognized that the few intra-pleural catheters which have been verified by thoracoscope, and the few cases of unintentional epidural extension have occurred when the perineural catheter was inserted more than 5 cm past the needle tip. Just as epidural catheters can puncture a weak spot in the dura mater when the Touhy needle is correctly placed within the epidural space, it is likely that these semi-rigid catheters may also puncture parietal pleura when the needle is correctly placed. Avoiding advancement of the catheter more than 3 cm past the needle tip is now the author's recommendation.

Conclusions

As ultrasound technology continues to improve, clinicians will endeavor to make improvements in the performance and efficacy of PVB. This is likely the case because those who regularly employ PVB experientially know that there is no other block that has the same high efficacy and low side-effect profile. Indeed, a recent study also supports this assertion, reporting better hemodynamic stability and equivalent pain control when compared to thoracic epidural analgesia (TEA) [25]. PVB has the potency of epidural anesthesia yet may likely avoid many of the potential problems associated with epidural/extradural catheterization. A para-laminar USG approach has recently been described which advocated a live time view of walking the needle off the lateral edge or "cliff" of the lamina between TPs [26].

The posterior approach to the transversus abdominus plane (TAP) (see Chap. 11), now typically called a quadratus lumborum block or QL block (see Chap. 10), which has been more recently described as an alternative regional anaesthesia technique for abdominal surgery, seems to owe its efficacy and extended duration to the fact that retrograde or posterior flow of local anaesthetic occurs, and blocks nerves found in the paravertebral space [27, 28].

Finally, it is worth mentioning a few other positive findings for the use of PVB in abdominal surgery. First, an extensive review of the evidence for truncal (thoracic and abdominal) blocks from 2009 to 2015 revealed that PVB continues to be a high interest area for clinical researchers, and only the TAP block has been studied with the same frequency. The review summarized that USG may increase success rates of single-injection PVB, but there is currently no evidence that USG improves success of continuous PVB [29]. Newer studies have also confirmed USG PVB as more hemodynamically stable than TEA [30]. Additionally, a surgical journal has published a study that compared intra-operative surgeon-administered intercostal blocks for thoracic surgery to USG PVBs administered by anesthesiologists pre-operatively, and the answer is clear: Pre-operative USG PVBs are superior for post-operative analgesia, and the objective findings of improved pulmonary function were also quantified. Forced expiratory volume at 1 sec and forced expiratory flow 25–75% were significantly higher in the PVB group [31]. Just as the para-neuraxial PVB is superior to the more distally placed intercostal blocks in thoracic surgery, it is likely that PVB is also superior to more distal or peripheral blocks for the abdomen.

References

1. Richardson J. Bilateral thoracic paravertebral block: potential and practice. Br J Anaesth. 2011;106(2):164–71.
2. King K. Paravertebral blocks: the evolution of a standard of care. Anesthesiol News. New York, NY: McMahon Publishing; 2012.
3. Richardson J. Thoracic paravertebral block. Br J Anaesth. 1998;81:230–8.
4. Rivera AM. The history of peripheral intravenous catheters: how little plastic tubes revolutionized medicine. Acta Anaesthesiol Belg. 2005;56:271–82.
5. James NR. An improved method of regional anaesthesia in acute abdominal surgery. Br Med J. 1941;2(4225):906–8.
6. Eason MJ, Wyatt R. Paravertebral thoracic block-a reappraisal. Anaesthesia. 1979;34(7):638–42.
7. Thangada S, King K. Understanding the risks of continuous paravertebral nerve blocks (CPVB): classical approach versus ultrasound guided; a case report poster board presented at American Society of Anesthesiologists annual scientific meeting, 2012.
8. Pace MM. Ultrasound-guided thoracic paravertebral blockade: a retrospective study of the incidence of complications. Anesth Analg. 2016 Apr;122(4):1186–91.
9. Merman R. Hypotensive bradycardic events and paravertebral blocks in the sitting position. Anesth Analg. 2006;(102):S134.

10. Karmakar MK. Thoracic paravertebral block: radiological evidence of contralateral spread anterior to the vertebral bodies. Br J Anaesth. 2000;84:263–5.
11. Cowie B. Ultrasound guided thoracic paravertebral blockade: a cadaveric study. Anesth Analg. 2010;110:1735–9.
12. Braun K. Paravertebral block and the electrocardiogram in angina pectoris. Br Heart J. 1946;8(1):47–52.
13. Rudkin GE. Bilateral thoracic paravertebral block for abdominoplasty. J Clin Anesth. 2008;20:54–6.
14. Ning MC. Right thoracic paravertebral anaesthesia for percutaneous radiofrequency ablation of liver tumours. Br J Radiol. 2011;84:785–9.
15. Melnikov A. Thoracic paravertebral block versus transversus abdominis plane block in major gynecological surgery: a prospective, randomized, controlled, observer-blinded study. Local Reg Anesth. 2012;5:55–61.
16. Chen H. Continuous right thoracic paravertebral block following bolus initiation reduced postoperative pain after right-lobe hepatectomy. Reg Anesth Pain Med. 2014;39:506–12.
17. Ford SJ. The implementation and effectiveness of an enhanced recovery programme after oesophago-gastrectomy: A prospective cohort study. The International Journal of Surgery 2014;12(4):320-324.
18. Zhang W. Single-dose bilateral paravertebral block plus intravenous sufentanil analgesia in patients with esophageal cancer undergoing combined throracoscopic-laparoscopic esophagectomy: a safe and effective alternative. J Cardiothorac Vasc Anesth. 2014;28(4):966–72.
19. Sites BD, Chan VW, Neal JM, et al. The American Society of Regional Anesthesia and Pain Medicine (ASRA) and The European Society of Regional Anesthesia and Pain Therapy (ESRA) joint committee recommendations for education and training in ultrasound-guided regional anesthesia. Reg Anesth Pain Med. 2009;34:40–6.
20. Abdallah F, Brull R. Off Side! A simple modification to the parasagittal in-plane approach for paravertebral block. Reg Anesth Pain Med. 2014;39:240–2.
21. Vogt A. Review about ultrasounds in paravertebral blocks. Eur J Pain. 2011;S5:489–94.
22. O Riain S, Donnel B. Thoracic paravertebral block using real-time ultrasound guidance. Anesth Analg. 2010;110:248–51.
23. Luyet C. Ultrasound-guided paravertebral puncture and placement of catheters in human cadavers: an imaging study. Br J Anaesth. 2009;102:534–9.
24. Renes SH. In-plane ultrasound-guided thoracic paravertebral block: a preliminary report of 36 cases with radiologic confirmation of catheter position. Reg Anesth Pain Med. 2010;35(2):212–6.
25. Pintaric T. Comparison of continuous thoracic epidural with paravertebral block on perioperative analgesia and hemodynamic stability in patients having open lung surgery. Reg Anesth Pain Med. 2011;36:256–60.
26. Taketa Y. A novel paralaminar in-plane approach for ultrasound-guided paravertebral block using microconvex array transducer. Reg Anesth Pain Med. 2015;40(4):390.
27. Carney J. Studies on the spread of local anaesthetic solution in transversus abdominis plane blocks. Anaesthesia. 2011;66:1023–30.
28. Abdallah FW. Duration of analgesic effectiveness after the posterior and lateral transversus abdominis plane block techniques for transverse lower abdominal incisions: a meta-analysis. Br J Anaesth. 2013;111(5):721–35.
29. Abrahams M. Update of ultrasound for truncal blocks. Reg Anesth Pain Med. 2016;41:275–88.
30. Okajima H. Ultrasound-guided continuous thoracic paravertebral block provides comparable analgesia and fewer episodes of hypotension than continuous epidural after lung surgery. J Anesth. 2015;29(3):373–8.
31. Maytal R. Preemptive ultrasound-guided paravertebral block and immediate postoperative lung function. General Thorac Cardiovasc Surg. 2015;63:43–8.

Truncal Blocks: Quadratus Lumborum Blocks

10

Rafael Blanco and Jens Børglum

Key Points

1. The Quadratus Lumborum Block (QLB) involves deposition of local anaesthetic (LA) at various points around the quadratus lumborum (QL) muscle.
2. This leads to spread of LA to the paravertebral space analagous to the landmark based and the USG posterior TAP blocks.
3. There are three common approaches: QLB type 1 (antero-lateral), QLB type 2 (posterior) and the transmuscular approach.
4. Spread to the paravertebral space results in both somatic nerve block as well as the sympathetic nerves, which provide visceral innervation, thereby eliminating the need for any additional opiate analgesia.
5. Due to the complete blockade of the abdominal wall and viscera any abdominal surgery can be undertaken with this technique.
6. To date there have been no adverse events reported.

Introduction

The ultrasonography-guided quadratus lumborum block (QLB) was first reported in 2007 by Blanco and presented at the ESRA (GB and I) Annual Scientific Meeting in Exeter, UK, when we described the infiltration of local anaesthetic (LA) solution adjacent to the anterolateral aspect of the quadratus lumborum (QL) muscle [1]. This location is close to the final position of the needle tip for the landmark based TAP block. In fact, the original concept for the QLB arose from

R. Blanco (✉)
Department of Anaesthesia & Intensive Care Medicine, King's College Hospital, Dubai, UAE

J. Børglum
Department of Anesthesiology & Intensive Care Medicine, Zealand University Hospital, University of Copenhagen, Roskilde, Denmark

A. Krige, M. J. P. Scott (eds.), *Analgesia in Major Abdominal Surgery*, https://doi.org/10.1007/978-3-319-94482-1_10

the observation that, due to the spread of LA to the paravertebral space, the duration of analgesia is prolonged with more posterior approaches to the TAP block (see Chap. 11). This technique has been constantly refined in parallel with the successful development of the transversus abdominis plane block (TAP block) as part of the multimodal approach to pain relief for abdominal operations [2]. In 2011 Carney et al. showed that the spread of the LA after QLB could reach the thoracic paravertebral space. In contrast, anterior spread of the LA solution into the TAP plane was observed after mid-axillary and anterior subcostal ultrasonography-guided approaches (see Chap. 11) [3]. In a recent double blind clinical trial, Telnes et al. compared TAP block to wound infiltration with LA. In that study, TAP blocks did not reduce cumulative morphine consumption following caesarean section, compared to the control group, and were associated with more pronounced sedation [4]. This suggests that blocking somatic fibres alone is insufficient, and including blockade of the visceral fibres may be more likely to provide adequate analgesia [5].

The objective of the QLB is to reach the paravertebral space with different optimal points of injection and locations around the quadratus lumborum (QL) muscle. Since it's original description, various approaches have been described and the three most popular are: the QLB type 1 in the anterolateral side of the QL muscle in the space formed by the internal oblique (IO), the transversus abdominis (TA) and QL muscles; the QLB type 2 in the posterior side of the QL muscle (between latissimus dorsi, QL and erector spinae) [6] and the transmuscular approach (TQL block) described by Børglum (between the QL and the psoas muscles) [7]. The idea for the transmuscular approach (the TQL block) was formulated when investigating a new ultrasound-guided approach to block the lumbar plexus with the Shamrock technique [8]. This approach allows for optimal visualization of the QL muscle and the psoas muscle. The three approaches are depicted in Fig. 10.1.

We performed contrast enhanced MRI studies (unpublished data) of QLB type 1 at the anterolateral side of the QL muscle (Fig. 10.2) and QLB type 2, at the posterior aspect of the muscle (Fig. 10.3) and examined the spread of contrast within the fascial planes. The MRI images showed that moving the point of injection to the posterior border of the QL muscle might provide a more predictable spread of LA into the paravertebral space, although the mechanism for the rapid and long-lasting analgesia now appears to be due to the blockade of sympathetic fibres in the thoracolumbar fascia. The advantage of using a more superficial point of injection is that we obtain a better ultrasonographic resolution and a potentially safer injection. When injecting posterior to the QL muscle (QLB type 2) the needle tip position is separated from the peritoneum, thus reducing the risk of intraperitoneal injection and bowel injury. This is a characteristic that the TAP block is unable to fulfill. In fact the distance to puncture intra-abdominal contents with TAP blocks is on average only five millimetres. We describe this QLB point of injection as the "six airbags approach" because it is surrounded by the following muscles: external oblique, internal oblique, psoas, QL, latissimus dorsi and the erector spinae muscles.

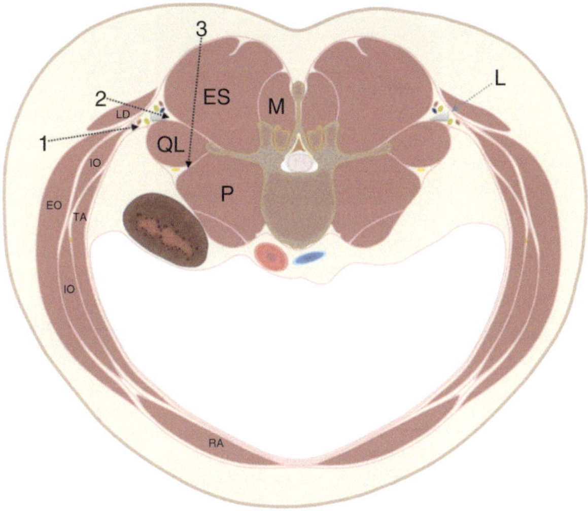

Fig. 10.1 Cross section of anatomical references together with different optimal points of injection for the QLB. Point of injection for the QLB I (1), QLBII (2) and the transmuscular QLB (3). Muscular references: multifidus (M), erector spine (ES), quadratus lumborum (QL), psoas (P), latissimus dorsi (LD), external oblique (EO), internal oblique (IO), transversus abdominis (TA) and rectus abdominis muscles (RA). There is a triangular connective tissue reinforcement called lumbar interfacial triangle (L). It is also called LIFT. (image with permission of Maria Fernandez Rojas)

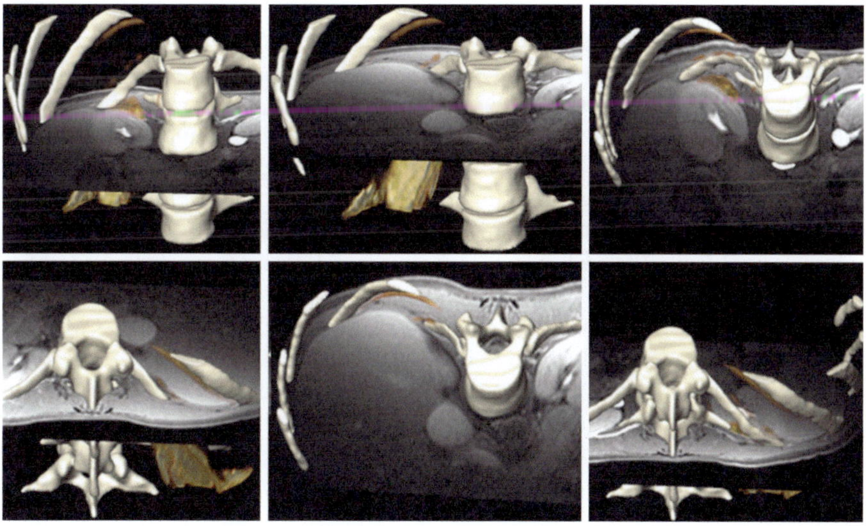

Fig. 10.2 MRI reconstructions of the spread of LA when the point of injection is anterolateral to the QL muscle (QLB type 1)

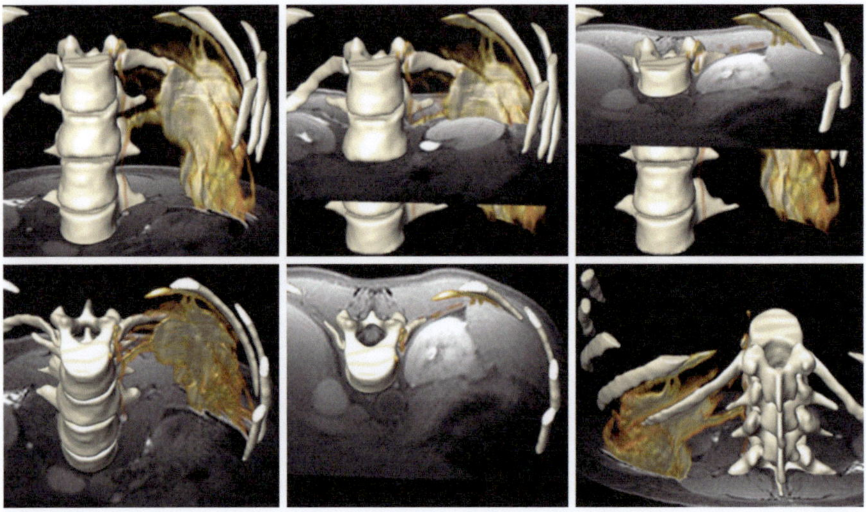

Fig. 10.3 MRI reconstructions of the spread of LA when the point of injection is behind the QL muscle (QLB II)

Evidence for Efficacy

Several case reports have shown that LA injection around the QL is effective in providing pain relief after various abdominal operations and in patients with chronic pain [9–12]. Abdallah et al. reported their meta-analysis of twelve RCTs, including 641 patients, in 2013 [13]. Four studies examined the posterior TAP block technique (which we can consider analogous to the QLB) and eight assessed the lateral TAP block technique (this is the widely recognized ultrasound-guided TAP block with injection between internal oblique and transversus abdominus muscles). Compared with the control groups, the posterior TAP block reduced the post-operative morphine consumption during the 12- to 24-h and 24- to 48-h intervals by 9.1 mg (95% CI, −16.83, −1.45; $P = 0.02$) and 5 mg (95% CI, −9.54, −0.52; $P = 0.03$), respectively. The conclusion of this meta-analysis recommended a RCT comparing the two techniques to confirm these findings. In 2015 we published the first randomized, controlled, double-blinded study to evaluate the analgesic efficacy of QLB after caesarean section. The results demonstrated statistically better morphine consumption and morphine demands in the QLB group compared to the control group [14]. In the same year we conducted a second RCT comparing QLB to TAP blocks [15]. We found that the QLB obtains a statistically more prolonged effect up to 48 h, reinforcing the message that this is a valuable block to perform for abdominal wall operations.

Mechanisms of Action

Recent evidence suggests that blockade of autonomic transmission as a result of the QLB may enhance the quality of analgesia of this technique by providing analgesia for visceral, as well as somatic pain [5, 13]. In their MRI studies, Carney et al. compared various ultrasound (USG) approaches with their original landmark-based technique at the triangle of Petit [3]. These studies illustrated that anterior subcostal and mid-axillary USG techniques result in a predominantly anterior spread of the injected solution within the TAP, whereas more posterior approaches result in predominantly posterior spread of the injected solution around the QL muscle extending to the paravertebral space. Carney and McDonnell found that there was a non-contiguous paravertebral, epidural and lymphatic contrast enhancement at T5–T10 in one subject, and similarly contrast at T6–T10 in two other subjects with the posterior US approach.

The QLB anaesthetizes both the lateral and anterior cutaneous branches from T7 to L1 but, in addition, also appears to result in cranial spread of LA into the thoracic paravertebral space. Injection of LA between the psoas muscle and QL muscle (as it is described with the so-called Transmuscular Quadratus Lumborum (TQL) block) leads to cranial spread into the thoracic paravertebral space as recently described for the first time by Dam et al. [16]. This study also describes the pathways involved and which nerves are directly affected. This is due to both muscles having their embryonic origin and insertion within the thoracic cage. This paravertebral extension of LA agent after the TQL block may be responsible for the extent of analgesia and prolonged duration of pain relief after the various quadratus lumborum block techniques in comparison with the more anterior approach [13]. As a result, the QLB may be seen as a lumbar approach to the thoracic paravertebral space [16–18].

Indications

Any unilateral or bilateral surgery for upper and lower abdominal procedures e.g. laparoscopic cholecystectomies, gastric sleeves, nephrectomies, colostomies, Hartmann's procedures, myomectomies, hysterectomies, caesarean sections, inguinal and peri-umbilical hernias (including chronic pain post-herniorrhaphy) and hip surgery.

Anatomy

The QL muscle is found lateral to the lumbar spine and connects the ilium to the 12th rib and to the lumbar vertebrae. Phillips et al. [19] studied the anatomy of QL by dissection of six cadavers. They reported the following principal types of QL fascicles as defined by their osseus attachments: iliocostal, iliolumbar, iliothoracic, and lumbocostal. The QL originates from the iliac crest and inserts into the transverse processes of L1 to L4 and the inferior surface of the 12th rib. Occasionally, fascicles arise from the iliolumbar ligament instead of the iliac crest.

The QL muscle is lateral to the transverse processes of T12–L5. The TA muscle provides the lateral border and the psoas major muscle overlaps it medially. It thickens inferiorly and so is visualized best on ultrasound at the L4 transverse process. At this level it is related to the psoas muscle anteriorly, the erector spinae muscle posteriorly and the transverse process of L4 medially.

One anatomical model describes the QL muscle being invested by the thoracolumbar fascia (three-layer model), which is a continuation of the common aponeurosis formed by the continuation of the fascia surrounding the internal oblique (IO) and the TA muscles after these muscles taper off [18, 19]. Another anatomical model (two-layer model) describes that the anterior layer of the thoracolumbar fascia separates the QL muscle from the erector spinae muscles (Willard et al.), and that the transversalis fascia covers the investing fascias of the QL muscle and the psoas major muscle [20]. What is clear though, is the fact that the thoracolumbar fascia is a complex of several layers that separate the paraspinal muscles from the muscles of the posterior abdominal wall, i.e. the QL muscle and the psoas major muscle. At the level of the diaphragm, the transversalis fascia splits in two. One sheet becomes the inferior diaphragmatic fascia. The second passes superior to the diaphragm to blend with the endothoracic fascia. This creates a potential route for spread of LA to the thoracic paravertebral space following the TQL block, although current thinking is that this spread may instead be to the thoracolumbar fascia resulting in blockade of sympathetic fibres in this space [20].

The anterolateral abdominal wall is supplied by the somatic nervous system via the branches of the anterior rami of the thoracolumbar spinal nerves T6–L1; namely the intercostal nerves (T6–T11), the subcostal nerve (T12), the IHN and IIN (L1) [18–20]. In addition, the T6–T12 nerves provide motor innervation to the pyramidalis and rectus muscles in the anterior abdomen, and the T6–L1 nerves innervate the intercostal muscles, the external oblique (EO) and IO muscles, the TA muscles and the parietal peritoneum [18–20]. The thoracolumbar nerves with their accompanying blood vessels branch and communicate within the neurovascular plane called the transversus abdominis plane, forming nerve plexuses [18–20]. The intercostal plexus (T6–T9) in the epigastric area travels antero-laterally, the lower TAP plexus (T10–L1) in the hypogastric area accompanies the deep circumflex iliac artery and the rectus sheath plexus (T6–L1) accompanies the deep inferior epigastric artery. Segmental nerves T6–T9 emerge from the costal margin to enter the TAP between the midline and the anterior axillary line. T6 enters the TAP immediately lateral to the linea alba, while T7–T9 emerge from the costal margin at increasingly lateral positions. T9 emerges from the costal margin either medial or lateral to the anterior axillary line [18–20].

In addition to somatic innervation, the parasympathetic nervous system, via the vagus nerve, and the sympathetic system via the splanchnic nerves, contribute to the nerve supply of the viscera. The splanchnic nerves carry both visceral efferent and afferent nerve fibres.

Thus the QLB aims to act at two different levels: a direct effect over the thoracolumbar fascia by spreading cranio/caudally thereby blocking the sympathetic fibres that cover the entire fascia, and an indirect effect by communicating with the paravertebral space thereby reaching the sympathetic chain [18–20].

Insertion Technique

There are three different approaches to consider depending on patient position and the type of ultrasound probe used i.e. anterior, lateral or posterior.

Anterior Approach

With the patient supine a low frequency probe is placed at the level of the anterior superior iliac spine and moved cranially until the three abdominal wall muscles can be clearly identified. The EO muscle is followed postero-laterally until its posterior border is visualised ("hook sign"), leaving the IO muscle underneath, like a roof over the QL muscle. The probe is tilted down to identify a bright hyperechoic line that corresponds with the thoracolumbar fascia (Fig. 10.4). The needle (a 21-G 100 mm) is inserted in plane from anteromedial to posterolateral. The optimal point of injection is determined using hydrodissection (QLB 2).

It is advisable to tilt the probe upwards to visualise the lower pole of the kidney as a reference, and also to identify the QL muscle, if it is not clear. This muscle is found behind the kidney, at the level of the lower pole of the kidney, and can be tracked up and down. It is not advisable to use the vertebral body as a reference with the anterior approach unless the patients are thin or small. The latissimus

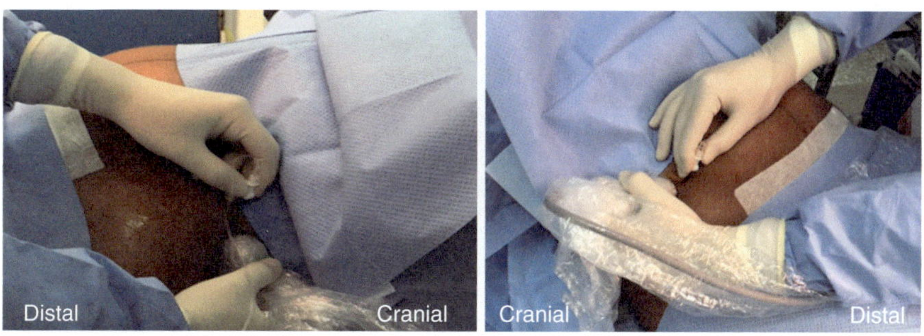

Fig. 10.4 Probe position for an anterior approach for the QLB type 2 with a convex probe

dorsi fascial planes are seen as bright lines posterior and anterior. With the anterior approach the optimal point of injection is in the anterior fascial plane of the latissimus dorsi, as close as possible to the "hook sign" made by the EO folding anteriorly.

Lateral Approach

The lateral approach is commonly used when the patient is able to lie on their side. A slight wedge of the body facilitates the probe position and the needle orientation. In this approach a linear probe is sufficient, but with larger patients a convex probe will demonstrate all the muscular and bony sono landmarks. For a QLB type 1 the aim is for the spread of LA to the anterolateral side of the QL muscle (Figs. 10.5 and 10.6).

For a QLB type 2 the aim is for the spread of LA to the posterior side of the QL muscle (Fig. 10.7). This technique is a modification of the QLB type 1 in which the needle is passed through the latissimus dorsi muscle. LA is injected posterior to the QL muscle outside the fascia. As the injection point is more superficial, the ultrasound images obtained are of higher quality, which may make the QLB type 2 safer and more reliable than the QLB type 1.

The use of a convex probe will allow use of the vertebrae and the aorta as references. The sequence can start from the abdominal muscles postero-laterally, until the transverse process and vertebral body can be seen (Fig. 10.8).

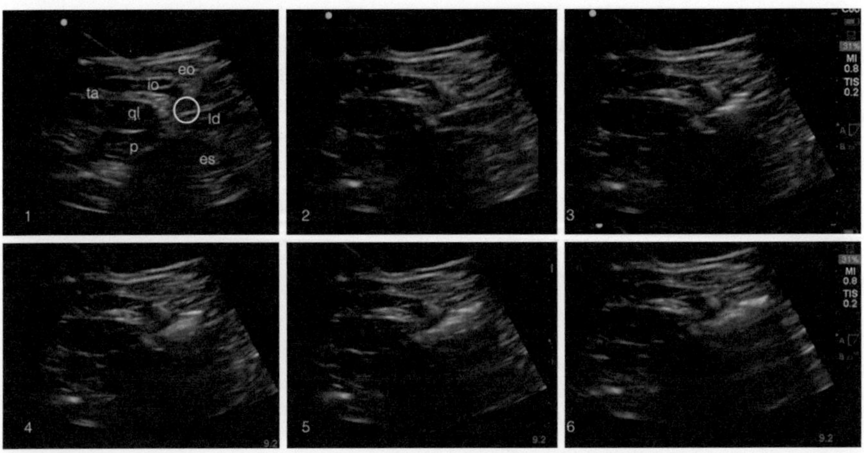

Fig. 10.5 Sonogram for an anterior approach for the QLB type 2 with a convex probe. The "six airbags" sign (eo, io, ql, p, es, ld) and the "hook sign" (the external oblique folding over the quadratus lumborum) can be seen. The sequence 1–6 shows the infiltration of LA at the level of the thoracolumbar fascia. External oblique (eo), internal oblique (io), quadratus lumborum (ql), psoas (p), erector spine (es) and latissimus dorsi (ld) muscles. Tranversus abdominis (ta)

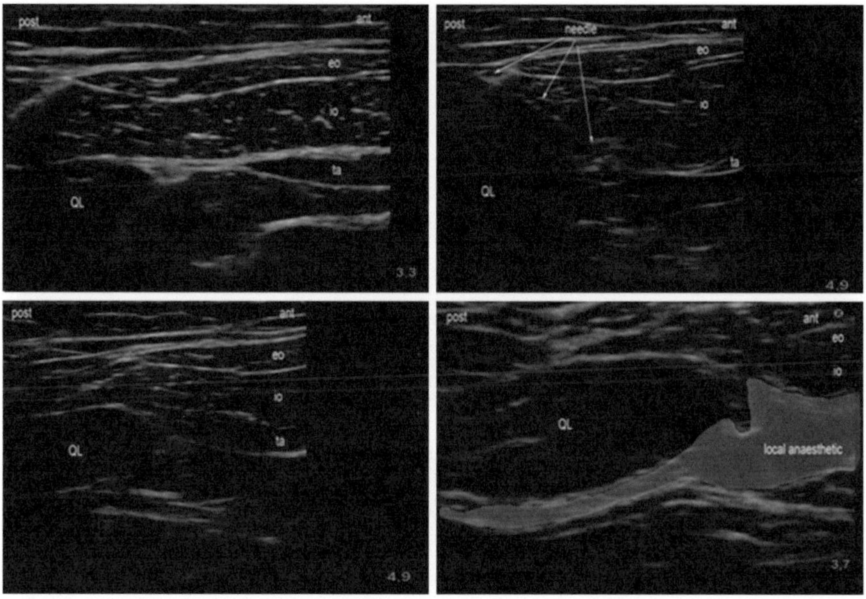

Fig. 10.6 Sonogram for a lateral approach for the QLB type 1 with a linear probe. The needle path is easily seen (top right quadrant)

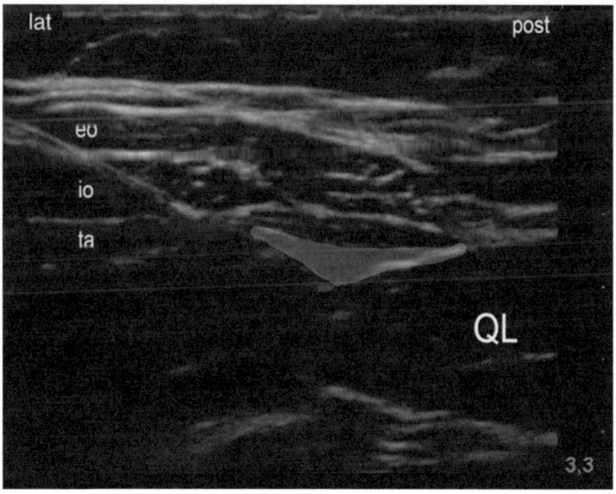

Fig. 10.7 Sonogram for a lateral approach for the QLB type 2 with a linear probe. The LA clearly distributes along the posterior border of the QL muscle

Posterior Approach

This is termed the transmuscular quadratus lumborum (TQL) block and was described by Børglum et al. [7]. LA is deposited anterior to the QL muscle in the plane between the QL and the psoas major muscles. The patient is placed in the lateral position, and a curvilinear probe is placed transversely on the flank just superior

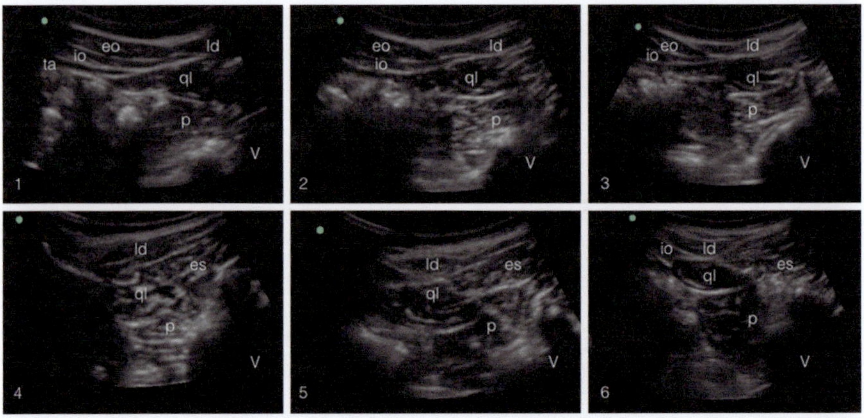

Fig. 10.8 Sonogram for a lateral approach with a convex probe. The sequence 1–6 shows the muscles variation at the level of the second vertebrae. External oblique (eo, internal oblique (io), tranversus abdominis (ta), quadratus lumborum (ql), psoas (p), erector spine (es), latissimus dorsi (ld) muscles and vertebrae (V)

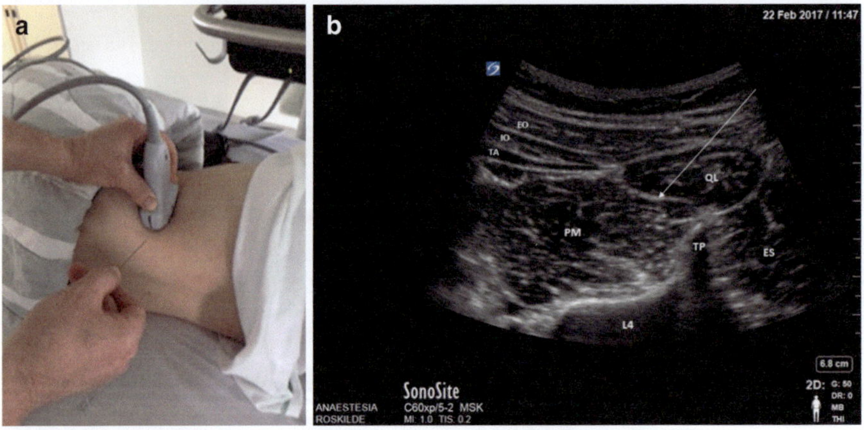

Fig. 10.9 The transmuscular quadratus lumborum (TQL) block. (**a**) Patient is in the lateral position. The curved arrary transducer is positioned transversely in the posterior axillary line just above the iliac crest. The needle is inserted in plane to the transducer. (**b**) The end-point of the injection is in the plane between the quadratus lumborum (QL) and psoas major (PM) muscles. *EO* external oblique, *IO* internal oblique, *TA* transversus abdominis, *TP* transverse process, *ES* erector spinae muscles, *L4* vertebral body of L4

to the iliac crest (Fig. 10.9a). The probe is moved posteriorly until the QL muscle is identified with its attachment to the L4 transverse process. At this point the 'Shamrock' sign can be identified [8]. The L4 transverse process is the stem of the clover, while the psoas muscle anteriorly, erector spinae muscle posteriorly and the QL muscles attached to the transverse process are the leaves. The needle is advanced in-plane from the lateral aspect of the probe (which is placed approximately over the mid-axillary line) through the QL muscle. The ventral fascia of the QL muscle is pierced and LA is injected in the plane between the QL and the psoas muscle (Fig. 10.9b). The TQL block does not result in redundant antero-lateral spread of the injectate as can occur with other techniques [16, 17]. Futhermore, by utilizing the posterior approach the TQL block is considered a somewhat safer block by some. This is because the tip of the needle is kept separated from the peritoneal recess that is often visualised lateral to the QL and psoas muscles [7, 8].

Local Anaesthetic

The QLB is a field block with a mechanism based on the spread and distribution of LA over the posterior abdominal wall reaching the paravertebral space. The use of 0.2 mL/kg of 0.125% Laevobupivacaine is the volume and concentration of choice regarding the QLB 1 and 2 blocks. With the TQL block the preferred volume is 30 mL of 0.375% ropivacaine for a unilateral block.

Practical Considerations

- With the anterior approach displace the abdomen to the contralateral side if distended.
- Tense the skin to facilitate an easier puncture.
- Identify kidney and liver and try to make them disappear from the sonographic image.
- Always use low concentrations and high volumes of LA.
- Do not look at the sonographic image until you have punctured the skin and dropped your needle to the shallowest angle.
- Aspirate before injecting LA, there are blood vessels in the fascial planes.

Role Within ERAS

The original QLBs (and the TQL block variation) are retroperitoneal fascial plane blocks. The spread of LA posteriorly and cranially into the thoracic paravertebral space provides visceral analgesia in addition to the somatic analgesia seen with more traditional anterior approaches to the abdominal wall blocks. It provides analgesia along lower thoracic and upper lumbar dermatomes. It may become an important part of multimodal analgesic strategies for selected abdominal surgeries due to the long duration of effect from a single injection [21]. This allows avoidance of pumps and attachments, as well as the absence of hypotension seen with epidural blockade, and the need for systemic opiate seen with other truncal blocks. All of these hamper early mobilization in ERAS and therefore the QLB may be well suited to abdominal surgery in the context of ERAS.

However, more randomized controlled studies are required to further elucidate the spread of LA beyond the anterior border of the QL muscle into thoracic and lumbar paravertebral spaces, as well as its efficacy and potential complications. Recent studies have begun to look at the potential of this block outside the scope of the abdominal wall. In Dr. Blanco's most recent publication, the QLB was demonstrated to have beneficial effects in patients with fractured neck of femurs [15].

References

1. Blanco R. Tap block under ultrasound guidance: the description of a 'no pops' technique [abstract]. Reg Anesth Pain Med. 2007;32(S1):130.
2. McDonnell JG, O'Donnell B, Curley G, Hefferman A, Power C, Laffey JG. The analgesic efficacy of transversus abdominis plane block after abdominal surgery: a prospective randomized controlled trial. Anesth Analg. 2007;104(1):193–7.
3. Carney J, Finnerty O, Rauf J, Bergin D, Laffey JG, Mc Donnell JG. Studies on the spread of local anaesthetic solution in transversus abdominis plane blocks. Anaesthesia. 2011;66:1023–30.
4. Telnes A, Skogvoll E, Lonnee H. Transversus abdominis plane block vs. wound infiltration in Caesarean section: a randomised controlled trial. Acta Anaesthesiol Scand. 2015;59:496–504.
5. Bantel C, Trapp S. The role of the autonomic nervous system in acute surgical pain processing – what do we know? Anaesthesia. 2011;66:541–4.
6. Blanco R, McDonnell JG. Optimal point of injection: the quadrates lumborum type I and II blocks. http://www.respond2articles.com/ANA/forums/post/1550.aspx. Accessed 10 Jan 2014.
7. Børglum J, Moriggl B, Jensen K, Lunquist PA, Christensen AF, Sauter A, Bendtsen TF Ultrasound-guided transmuscular quadratus lumborum blockade. Br J Anaesth. 2013. Published 25 Mar 2013, Online ISSN 1471–6771-Print ISSN 0007–0912. http://bja.oxfordjournals.org/forum/topic/brjana_el%3b9919. Accessed 4 Mar 2014.
8. Sauter AR, Ullensvang K, Niemi G, Lorentsen HT, Bendtsen TF, Borglum J, Pripp AH, Romundstad L. The Shamrock lumbar plexus block: a dose-finding study. Eur J Anaesthesiol. 2015;32(11):764–70.
9. Kadam VR. Ultrasound-guided quadratus lumborum block as a postoperative analgesic technique for laparotomy. J Anaesthesiol Clin Pharmacol. 2013;29:550–2.
10. Carvalho R, Segura E, Loureiro MD, Assuncao JP. Quadratus lumborum block in chronic pain after abdominal hernia repair: case report. Braz J Anesthesiol. 2017;67(1):107–9.
11. Visoiu M, Yakovleva N. Continuous postoperative analgesia via quadratus lumborum block – an alternative to transversus abdominis plane block. Paediatr Anaesth. 2013;23:959–61.
12. Chakraborty A, Goswami J, Patro V. Ultrasound-guided continuous quadratus lumborum block for postoperative analgesia in a paediatric patient. Anesth Analg Case Rep. 2015;4:34–6.
13. Abdallah FW, Laffey JG, Halpern SH, Brull R. Duration of analgesic effectiveness after the posterior and lateral transversus abdominis plane block techniques for transverse lower abdominal incisions: a meta-analysis. Br J Anaesth. 2013;111:721–35.
14. Blanco R, Ansari T, Girgis E. Quadratus lumborum block for postoperative pain after caesarean section: a randomised controlled trial. Eur J Anesthesiol. 2015;32(11):812–8.
15. Parras T, Blanco R. Randomised trial comparing the transversus abdominis plane block posterior approach or quadratus lumborum block type 1 with femoral block for postoperative analgesia in femoral neck fracture, both ultrasound-guided. Rev Esp Anestesiol Reanim. 2015;PMID:26302669.
16. Dam M, Moriggl B, Hansen CK, Hoermann R, Bendtsen TF, Børglum J. The pathway of injectate spread with the transmuscular quadratus lumborum (TQL) block – a cadaver study. Anesth Analg. 2017;125(1):303–12.

17. Hansen CK, Dam M, Bendtsen TF, Børglum J. Ultrasound-guided quadratus lumborum blocks: definition of the clinical relevant endpoint of injection and safest approach. Anesth Analg Case Rep. 2016;6(2):39.
18. Schuenke MD, Vleeming A, Van Hoof T, Willard FH. A description of the lumbar interfascial triangle and its relation with the lateral raphe: anatomical constituents of load transfer through the lateral margin of the thoracolumbar fascia. J Anat. 2012;221(6):568–76.
19. Willard FH, Vleeming A, Schuenke MD, Danneels L, Schleip R. The thoracolumbar fascia: anatomy, function and clinical considerations. J Anat. 2012;221(6):507–36.
20. Phillips S, Mercer S, Bogduk N. Anatomy and biomechanics of quadratus lumborum. Proc Inst Mech Eng H. 2008;222(2):151–9.
21. Børglum J, Jensen K. Abdominal surgery: advances in the use of ultrasound-guided truncal blocks for perioperative pain management. In: Derbel F, editor. Abdominal surgery. London: InTech; 2012. p. 69–94.

Truncal Blocks: Transversus Abdominis Plane Blocks and Derivatives

11

Aisling McMahon, John G. McDonnell, and Jens Børglum

Key Points

1. Transversus Abdominis Plane (TAP) block, Transversalis Fascia Plane (TFP) block and Iliiohypogastric/Ilioinguinal blocks are discussed.
2. There are landmark-based and ultrasound-based insertion techniques described for each block with differences in efficacy and duration of effect.
3. TAP approaches include subcostal oblique (anaesthesia above the umbilicus), mid-axillary (anaesthesia below the umbilicus), posterior (anaesthesia below the umbilicus) and the bilateral dual (complete abdominal wall anaesthesia).
4. The TFP block provide anaesthesia of the L1 and L2 distribution and can provide analgesia for iliac crest bone grafting, open inguinal hernia repair and open appendicectomy. The subcostal nerve T12 will also be anaesthetized. Thus, the TFP block can also be used to anaesthetize the lateral cutaneous branches innervating the skin area from the iliac crest distal to the major trochanter and can be used for analgesia following hip repair.
5. Iliohypogastric/ilioinguinal nerve blocks are primarily used for inguinal hernia repair surgery and can be landmark based as well as ultrasound guided.

A. McMahon
Department of Anaesthesia, The Clinical Sciences Institute, National University of Ireland, Galway, Ireland

J. G. McDonnell (✉)
Department of Anaesthesia, The Clinical Sciences Institute, National University of Ireland, Galway, Ireland

Department of Anaesthesia and Intensive Care Medicine, Galway University Hospitals, Galway, Ireland

J. Børglum
Department of Anesthesiology and Intensive Care Medicine, Zealand University Hospital, University of Copenhagen, Roskilde, Denmark

A. Krige, M. J. P. Scott (eds.), *Analgesia in Major Abdominal Surgery*,
https://doi.org/10.1007/978-3-319-94482-1_11

Introduction

Post-operative somatic pain following abdominal wall incision and distention of the abdominal wall with laparoscopic surgery can cause substantial distress and impede patient recovery. Abdominal wall blocks have long been included in the armamentarium of the regional anaesthetist but it is only more recently that their application and clinical utility has been appreciated. When used appropriately, they can contribute significantly to post-operative analgesia, reduction in opioid consumption, early ambulation and discharge from hospital.

In this chapter, we provide an overview of the transversus abdominis plane (TAP) block, its derivative the transversalis fascia plane block, and the Ilioinguinal/Iliohypogastric block. Thoracic paravertebral blocks, quadratus lumborum (QLB) blocks (including the variant of this initial block called the transmuscular quadratus lumborum [TQL] block) and rectus sheath blocks are covered in separate dedicated chapters. For each we will describe the anatomy, sonoanatomy and the method for performing the block, including both landmark and ultrasound guided techniques. We will also discuss the efficacy and clinical outcomes of each, along with pharmacological considerations and safety concerns to be aware of for the various blocks.

Anatomy of the Anterior Abdominal Wall

The anterior abdominal wall is bounded by the costal margin and xiphoid process of the sternum superiorly, the inguinal ligament and pelvic bone inferiorly, and the mid-axillary line laterally [1]. It is made up of skin, adipose tissue and a musculo-aponeurotic layer in which each muscle is enveloped by an anterior and posterior fascia. These give support to the trunk and abdominal contents.

Musculature

Within the abdominal wall there are three muscle layers. From superficial to deep these are the external oblique (EO), internal oblique (IO) and transversus abdominis (TA). Each is invested in its own fascial sheath. A fourth muscle, the paired rectus abdomini, form a layer either side of the midline. It is separated in the midline by the linea alba and enclosed in the rectus sheath. This sheath is deficient posteriorly in the lower abdomen from a point located one third of the way from the umbilicus to the pubic crest. This is known as the arcuate line [1].

Innervation

The abdominal wall is supplied by the lower six thoracic and upper two lumbar sensory nerves [2]. The anterior rami of these nerves are contained within a neurovascular plane that traverses between IO and TA muscles. The thoracic nerves

T6–T11 enter this plane at the costal margin and traverse it to eventually pierce the posterior wall of the rectus sheath as anterior cutaneous branches supplying the over-lying skin. The T7–T9 nerves emerge to supply the skin superior to the umbilicus, T10 supplies the umbilicus, while T11, the cutaneous branch of the subcostal T12, the iliohypogastric nerve (IHN) and the ilioinguinal nerve (IIN) supply the skin inferior to the umbilicus.

The IIN and IHN are both derived from the L1 nerve root and are the first two branches of the lumbar plexus. On emerging from the psoas muscle, they cross anterolaterally over the quadratus lumborum (QL) muscle towards the iliac crest. The IIN is found inferior to the IHN and it runs medially in a plane deep to the IHN. The nerves then follow a path between the transversalis fascia and TA for a variable distance until above the iliac crest, and close to the anterior superior iliac spine (ASIS), they pierce the TA muscle to run between it and the IO in the neurovascular (TAP) plane. After a variable distance, at a point below the ASIS the nerves pierce the IO to course between it and the EO. They continue anteromedially and become superficial as they terminate in branches to skin and muscles of the inguinal region.

The IIN provides innervation to the upper medial thigh, anterior scrotum, labia majora and root of the penis. The genito-femoral nerve is also found in this area with its origins from the L1–2 segments of the lumbar plexus [3].

Blood Supply

Knowledge of the vasculature of the anterior abdominal wall is also essential for safe performance of truncal blocks. The primary blood vessels of the abdominal wall are the superior and inferior epigastric arteries. The superior epigastric artery enters the posterior aspect of the rectus abdominus (RA) superiorly to run inferiorly and anastomose with the inferior epigastric artery. This vessel originates from the external iliac artery, and initially runs upwards in the transversalis fascia before entering the RA at the arcuate line. A second branch of the external iliac artery, the deep cirumflex, runs parallel to the inguinal ligament between the IO and TA muscles. The superficial circumflex iliac artery, a branch of the femoral, loops up from below the inguinal ligament to run towards the umbilicus and can also be encountered in blocks of the abdominal wall [1].

Transversus Abdominis Plane Block

Introduction

The transversus abdominis plane (TAP) block, first described by Rafi in 2001 [4], is a relatively new abdominal wall block. The aim of the technique is to deposit local anaesthetic (LA) in the plane between the IO and TA muscles to block the somatic nerves supplying the anterior and lateral abdominal wall. It does not provide analgesia for visceral pain. Originally performed as a landmark based technique, a number of ultrasound-guided approaches have now been described. Both will be discussed below. The TAP block can be considered as part of a multimodal approach to analgesia following colorectal, urological, gynaecological and obstetric procedures. Bilateral TAP blocks may also be an option in those for whom epidural analgesia is not an option.

Historical Perspective

The original landmark technique for the TAP block involved identifying the triangle of 'Petit', and injecting through this site. The concept was a development of a similar block by Prof. B. Dalens, who was injecting LA agents into the TAP between the umbilicus and the anterior superior iliac spine in a pediatric population undergoing appendicectomy. The original approach involved inserting a blunted regional anaesthesia needle through the lumbar triangle of 'Petit', which resulted in a 'pop' sensation as it passed through what was supposed to be the fascial extensions of both EO and IO muscles to leave the needle tip within the TAP. The initial concept was that the LA solution instilled would bathe the extensions of the intercostal nerves that coursed through the TAP. The lumbar triangle of Petit was decided as the entry point into the TAP, as firstly, it was posterior to the mid-axillary line and therefore would also block the lateral cutaneous branches of the nerves that emerge from the TAP at the level of the mid-axillary line theoretically providing enhanced analgesic efficacy as compared to Prof. B. Dalens approach. Secondly, it was conjectured that the lumbar triangle of 'Petit' was a constant feature that was easily palpated allowing this technique to be a readily reproducible and predicable block. However, the landmark based block has a significant learning curve [5] and so with the advent of ultrasound, the ability to visualize the muscle layers has superseded the requirement to palpate the triangle of petit. Indeed, the ultrasonic appearance of this area can be quite confusing and difficult to interpret. Because of this the probe position on the abdominal wall was dramatically altered resulting in the mid-axillary and sub-costal approaches being adopted as the de facto techniques and optimal end points of needle-tip placement. These new approaches altered the dynamics of the block and the analgesic profile differs from that produced with the original landmark based approach, both in reported extent and duration.

The randomized controlled trials using the landmark based technique report statistically significant analgesic benefits up to 48 h post-operatively, when used as part of a multi-modal analgesic technique. Randomized controlled trials investigating the landmark-based technique have shown benefits in terms of duration and quality of analgesia [6, 7]. The change in dynamics of the block most probably relate to the distribution of the LA solution, with the original and newer posterior approaches resulting in spread of LA solution to the thoracic paravertebral space [8]. The anterior abdominal wall blocks are constrained to the duration of somatic nerve blockade by the specific LA agents [9].

Landmark-Based Technique

With the patient in the supine position, the lumbar triangle of Petit is identified. This is the area bounded by the posterior border of the EO anteriorly, anterior border of latissimus dorsi posteriorly, and the iliac crest inferiorly (see Figs. 11.3b and 11.4b for sonoanatomy depiction of the likely needle endpoint). Using a blunt regional anaesthesia needle the skin is pierced towards the apex of the triangle. The needle is advanced at right angles to the skin in the coronal plane through the subcutaneous tissue. With gentle advancement a pop or loss of resistance is appreciated indicating that the needle tip has entered the plane between the EO and IO muscles. Further advancement results in a second pop as the needle advances into the TAP. After careful aspiration to exclude vascular puncture, LA solution is injected with repeated aspirations. The technique is repeated on the contralateral side for incisions encompassing the mid-line. This block requires large volumes of LA solution in order for the extension to the paravertebral space to be achieved. It is recommended that approximately 0.4 mL/kg be used each side. With this in mind, care must be exercised to ensure that the dosage of drug administered does not approach or exceed recommended doses.

Ultrasound-Guided Technique

There are four main approaches to the TAP block with ultrasound [10–13]. These are the mid-axillary, anterior oblique subcostal, posterior and bilateral dual TAP approach. The transducer position for each is as follows:

- **Anterior Oblique Subcostal** (Fig. 11.1): the probe is placed under the costal margin close to the midline. Here the TA muscle is seen deep to RA. The needle is inserted from the medial side of the transducer and final location of the tip is between the posterior rectus sheath and TA.
- **Mid-Axillary** (Figs. 11.2 and 11.3): in the mid-axillary line, the ultrasound probe is placed in a transverse orientation to the lateral abdominal wall between the lower costal margin and iliac crest (*see* Fig. 11.1).
- **Posterior** (Fig. 11.4): place the probe transversely on the anterior abdominal wall between the costal margin and iliac crest. Identify the three muscle layers and the slide the probe laterally/posteriorly to the point where the TA begins to tail off (see Fig. 11.2).
- **Bilateral dual (BD) TAP**: a four-point single shot approach is taken to target nerves of both the upper (T6–9) and lower (T10–12) abdominal wall. This is a combination of the Mid-axillary and Anterior Oblique Subcostal approaches described above. The probe is first placed between the costal margin and iliac crest with the needle insertion point at the anterior axillary line. This is repeated on the opposite side to target the lower abdominal nerves using the classic mid-axillary TAP block. For the upper abdominal nerves, the probe is placed caudad to the xiphoid process identifying the linea alba. The probe is then moved laterally following the costal margin until the TA muscle is identified below the rectus sheath. The local anaesthetic is deposited between these two structures bilaterally.

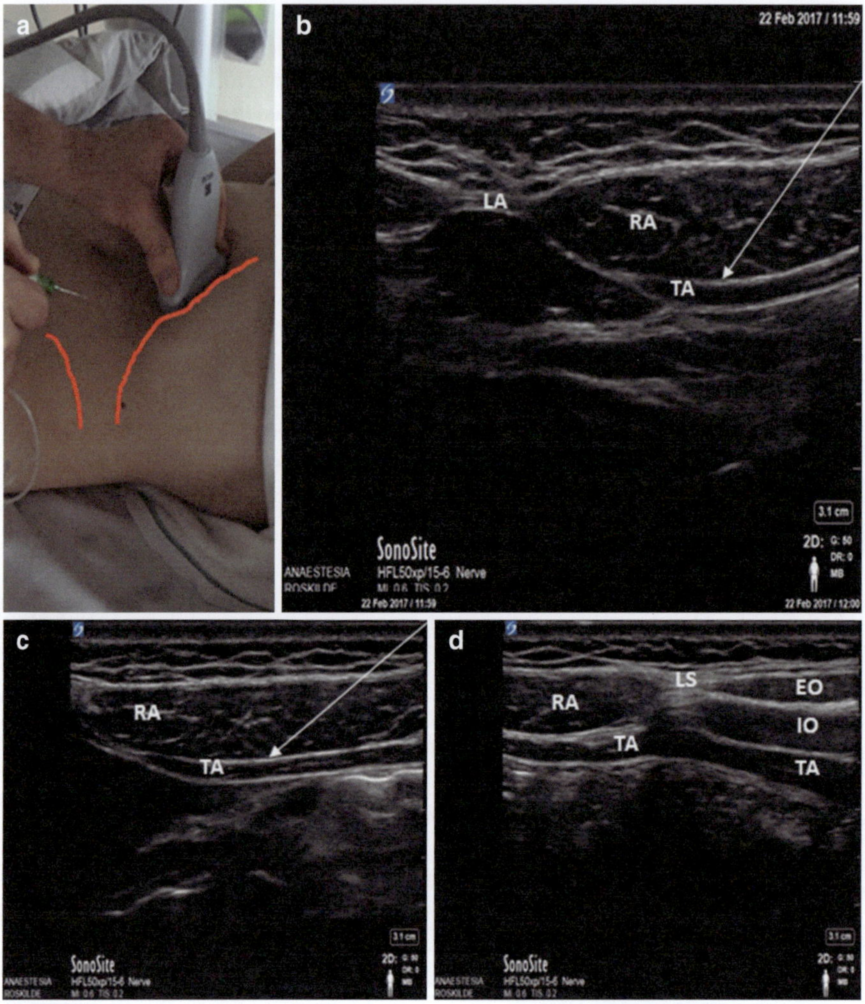

Fig. 11.1 (**a**) Upper intercostal TAP block in the epigastric area (model photo). The patient is placed in the supine position. The linear transducer is positioned along the costal cuvature (close to the subcostal angle). The needle can be inserted in plane to the probes lateral edge (as shown) or at the medial edge (depending on preference). The end-point is in the neurovascular plane between the rectus abdominis (RA) and transversus abdominis (TA) muscles. (**b**) Sonoanatomy. The linea alba (LA) is identified at the most medial position of the ultrasound probe. Lateral to the LA the RA and TA muscles are identified. White arrow indicates needle trajectory. (**c**) Sonoanatomy. The transducer can be alligned gradually more lateral along the costal cuverture if necessary. White arrow indicates needle trajectory. (**d**) Sonoanatomy. If necessary, the transducer can be aligned even more lateral to identify the linea semilunaris (LS). Lateral to the LS the three abdominal wall muscles of the hypogastric area can be visualized; i.e. *EO* external oblique, *IE* internal oblique and TA

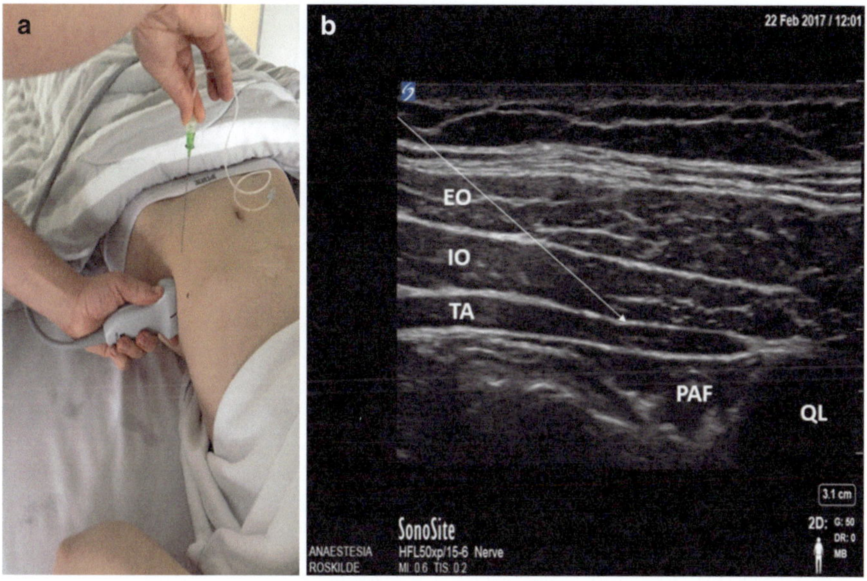

Fig. 11.2 (**a**) Ultrasound-guided midaxillary approach to the TAP block (supine position). In the hypogastric area, a linear placed is placed in a transverse plane in the mid axillary position. (**b**) Sonoanatomy. The needle is inserted in plane to the transducer with the endpoint in the neurovascular plane between the internal oblique (IO) and transversus abdominis (TA) muscles. *EO* external oblique, *PAF* pararenal fat, *QL* quadratus lumborum muscle

These approaches require the identification of the three abdominal muscles (see Figs. 11.1, 11.2, 11.3, and 11.4): the EO and IO and the TA muscles. The TAP is approached using an in-plane technique. The needle is visualised as it passes through the subcutaneous tissue and the body of both IO and EO muscles. On passing through the deep aspect of the IO muscles, the needle tip passes into the TAP. The space is hydro-dissected with 10 mL of 0.9% saline. After aspiration to exclude vascular puncture, LA solution is injected with repeated aspirations. The use of ultrasound allows visualization of correct needle placement and allows the operator to observe the expansion of LA solution within the TAP.

Evidence for Efficacy

Thanks to a multitude of recent studies much is known of this block in terms of its distribution, sensory anaesthesia and clinical efficacy for specific procedures. The original landmark based approach to the TAP block has being shown in randomized, controlled trials to offer analgesic benefit in patients undergoing abdominal and pelvic surgery when compared to placebo in both adult and paediatric populations [14–16].

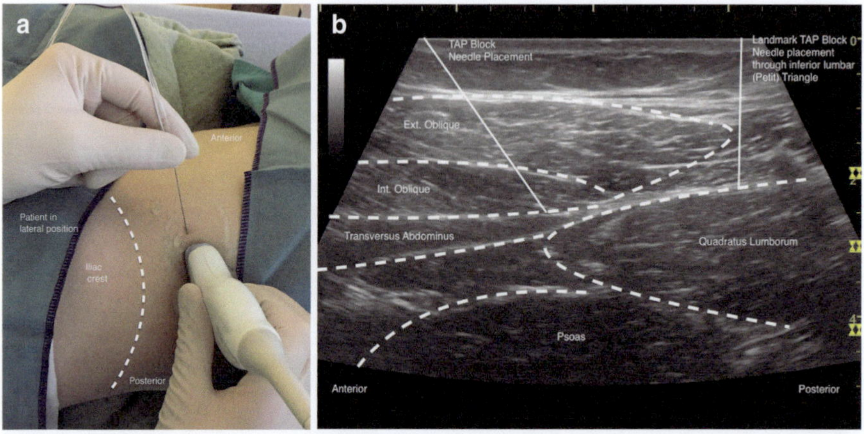

Fig. 11.3 (**a**) Ultrasound-guided midaxillary approach to the TAP block (lateral position). This image has the patient in a right lateral position. The probe is placed in the axial plane. The needle is introduced in an anterior to posterior manner with an in-plane technique. Should only require identification of the internal, external oblique and the transversus abdominis muscles. (**b**) Midaxillary approach sonoanatomy (including depiction of landmark technique target). With the patient in the lateral position or with the pelvis tilted with the aid of a wedge the image can be generated with a linear array probe in the axial plane. The relevant lateral abdominal muscles can be readily identified and their relationship to the quadratus lumborum appreciated. The needle is introduced in an anterior to posterior manner and passes through the substance of skin, subcutaneous tissue, the external and internal oblique muscles. As it passes into the plane between the internal oblique and the transversus abdominis muscles, the anterograde-lateral aspect of the quadratus lumborum muscle provides a safety mechanism to prevent intra-peritoneal injection. The close relationship between this approach and the original landmark based approach show how the landmark based technique was most probably a quadratus lumborum block for outset

Recent reviews [17, 18] have reported trending towards more prolonged analgesia with landmark based approaches compared with ultrasound guided TAP blocks. This prolonged analgesia is likely due to spread of LA into the paravertebral space as described in distribution studies [19]. There have been numerous studies [6, 15, 20–25] demonstrating analgesic benefit in patients who received ultrasound guided TAP blocks in both upper and lower abdominal surgery. Aveline et al. [24] reported that ultrasound guided TAP blocks conferred superior analgesia as compared with the IIN and IHN blocks for day-case open inguinal hernia repair, which has resulted in increased application for this surgery. Tanggaard et al. demonstrated reduced pain scores using the BD TAP following laparoscopic appendicectomy as compared to saline injection [13]. When compared to epidural analgesia [26] the TAP block demonstrated equivalent analgesia but the TAP block group used significantly more opioid, presumably to manage visceral pain. With all these studies it is important to note the site of LA deposition, as the more posterior the block is performed the better the analgesic effect.

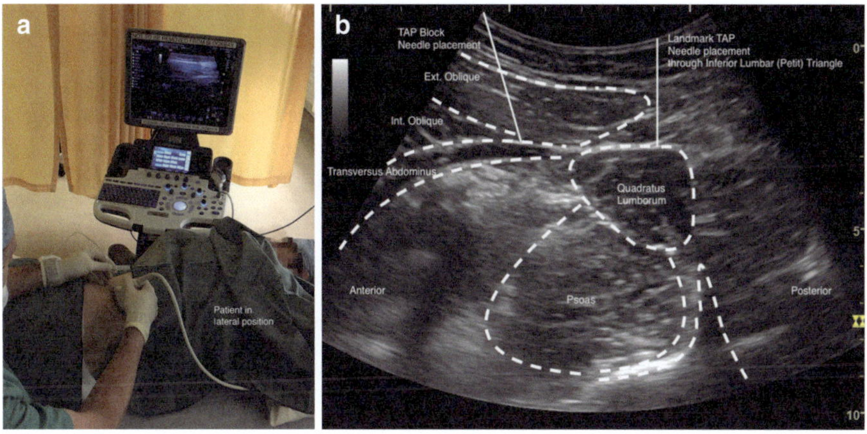

Fig. 11.4 (**a**) Posterior approach to the TAP block. The patient is placed in the lateral position with the ultrasound machine on the contralateral side to the anaesthetist. The probe is placed in the axial plane above the iliac crest. The relevant lateral abdominal musculature is identified prior to needle introduction in an anterior to posterior manner. For midline incisions the block needs to be repeated on the opposite side. (**b**) Posterior approach to the TAP block. Image obtained with a curved array probe in the axial plane above the iliac crest. The probe is moved in a craniocephalad manner to determine the L4 transverse process. This is the largest lumbar transverse process. Using the transverse process as a starting point the related musculature is delineated. The triangle of Petit is designated as the posterior aspect of the external oblique muscle and the point of needle entry for the landmark-based TAP block. The other lateral abdominal wall muscles can be clearly defined and their relationship to the quadratus lumborum muscle is the target area for the posterior approach to the TAP block

Derivation of the Tap Block: Transversalis Fascia Plane Block

Introduction

The TFP Block is a derivation of the TAP Block that specifically targets the branches of the L1 nerve root, that is to say the IHN and IIN. Superior spread of LA frequently covers the subcostal (T12) nerve. Hebbard et al. [27] and Chin et al. [28] have both described techniques for the TFP block that reliably blocks these nerves. The TFP Block differs from the TAP in that LA is deposited posterior to the TA muscle, it does not provide analgesia above the T12 dermatome and it more reliably covers the distribution of the L1 branches. It is indicated for analgesia following iliac crest bone grafting (ICBG) and can be considered for procedures on the lower abdominal wall such as inguinal hernia repair and open appendicectomy.

Technique

The TFP block has only being described using ultrasound guidance. The IHN and IIN are targeted for the TFP block at the point where they course between the fascia of the TA and the transversalis fascia. The TLF is a complex of several layers that separates the paraspinal muscles from the muscles of the posterior abdominal wall, the quadratus lumborum (QL) muscle and psoas major muscle. The oblique, transversus abdominis, QL and psoas major muscles originate from the hypaxial muscle compartment; and the erector spinae muscles from the epaxial myofascial compartments. The TLF contains the epaxial muscles and separates the two myofascial compartments [29].

With the patient in the supine or lateral decubitus position, an ultrasound probe is placed transversely over the abdomen between the iliac crest and the costal margin in the midaxillary line. The EO, IO, and TA muscles are identified and traced back to the point where the TA muscle and IO muscle taper into their common aponeurosis. The needle is then introduced in plane and the tip is positioned through the deep surface of the TA muscle. LA is then injected to separate the transversalis fascia from the TA muscle. If required, further LA can be injected into the TAP on withdrawal to achieve a more extensive block of the anterior branches of nerves above T12.

Evidence for Efficacy

The TFP block has as of yet little evidence to support its use. There is a lack of randomized controlled trials investigating the TFP block but preliminary evidence from smaller studies is encouraging. Most information stems from isolated case reports. An early pilot study by Chin et al. [28] demonstrated significant analgesic benefit with this block for ICBG. We are likely to see further clinical trials in the near future examining the clinical effectiveness of this block. Its use may be superceded by the development of newer blocks such as the quadratus lumborum block (QLB).

Ilio-Inguinal/Ilio-Hypogastric Nerve Blocks

Introduction

Blockade of the IIN and IHN provides analgesia to the inguinal region. This block has long been used as part of a multimodal analgesic approach to inguinal hernia repair. In some instances, IIN and IHN block has also been used to provide anaesthesia for this procedure with the caveat that supplemental LA must be infiltrated within the peritoneal sac by the surgeons as this has visceral innervation. Other indications include orchidopexy, varicocele or hydrocele repair and obstetric or gynaecological surgery.

Technique

The IIN/IHN block can be performed using either a landmark based or ultrasound guided technique.

Landmark-Based Technique

The patient lies in the supine position. The skin puncture point is 2 cm medial and 2 cm superior to the ASIS. A 35 mm 21 G needle is advanced at right angles to the skin in all planes. A characteristic "click" is felt on penetrating the EO at which point LA is injected to anaesthetize the IHN. Further advancement of the needle will result in a second characteristic "click" as the needle penetrates the IO. Further LA is injected at this point to anaesthetize the IIN. Redirection of the needle towards the ilium will permit subcutaneous injection of LA to block the lateral cutaneous branch of the subcostal nerve. A similar subcutaneous injection can be made towards the midline to block other branches of the subcostal nerve.

Ultrasound-Guided Technique

With the patient in the supine position, a linear transducer is placed along an oblique line between the ASIS and umbilicus. The nerves appear as hypoechoic fascicular structures with hyperechoic rims sandwiched between the TA and IO. The needle entry site is at the caudad border of the linear transducer. The needle is inserted in-plane and visualized along its entire path to the IIN and IHN. Accurate needle placement is indicated by fluid expansion in a space bounded by the hyperechoic fascial sheath of the IO and TA muscle layers (hydrodissection).

Caution needs to be exercised with this block for a number of reasons. Too deep an injection may result in an inadequate block and risks both inadvertent femoral nerve block and bowel perforation. The inferior epigastric vessels course close to the injection point and puncture of these has previously been described. Use of ultrasound may reduce the occurrence of these complications.

Evidence for Efficacy

IIN and IHN blocks have a long history of proven benefit to patients undergoing inguinal hernia repair in both the adult and paediatric populations. Early studies showed benefit to using this block in patients undergoing inguinal herniorrhaphy [29–32] with reduced opioid requirements and earlier mobilization. Previous studies also looked at its potential use after Caesarean delivery and although some benefit was demonstrated with this block for use with the Pfannenstiel incision, it has since, been superseded by newer blocks such as the TAP block. Using a landmark based approach the reported success rate with this block remains variable even in experienced hands, most probably due to anatomical variation and the operator not knowing the exact position of the needle tip [33]. When this block was performed using landmark techniques, only 14% of the LA solution was correctly placed in proximity to the nerves; the remaining 86% was administered into surrounding muscular structures [34]. The introduction of ultrasound has led to increased success rates for this particular block. Recent studies have looked at the ultrasound-guided approach to this block and its analgesic effect. Børglum et al. [35] recently conducted a randomized, controlled, double blind study of ultrasound guided IIN and IHN block in patients undergoing inguinal hernia repair. Their study concluded that ultrasound-guided blocks of the IIN and IHN resulted in a statistically significant and clinically relevant reduction in post-operative pain in the PACU, both at mobilization and at rest.

Pharmacological Considerations

Despite much research to help our understanding of truncal blocks in terms of landmark versus ultrasound guided blocks and optimal needle position for various blocks, there has being very little research into the pharmacokinetics and pharmacodynamics of the LA used. Regarding techniques that aim to block specific nerves, such as the Ilioinguinal and Iliohypogastric block, it is clear that enough LA is needed to bathe the nerves in order to produce optimal analgesia. There has been no research to date on using different volumes or substances with this block. Volume seems to be of critical importance for blocks involving multiple nerves. Many institutions that routinely perform truncal blocks will use between 0.3 mL/kg to 0.6 mL/kg of LA, in concentrations that do not exceed maximum allowable dose for that patient. In the case of the TAP block and QLB which have centrally mediated effects, the appropriate volume seems to be of importance in ensuring spread of LA into the paravertebral space. The results of a recent pilot study from Forero et al. [36] seems to suggest that increasing the volume of LA while maintaining the overall dose does not increase block height and may reduce duration of action when lower concentrations of LA are used. Further larger trials are awaited to confirm these findings.

With regards to adjuvants to LA used in truncal blocks there is very little evidence to support their use. One would assume adjuvants would confer beneficial effects to block quality and duration, as has been demonstrated in other regional anaesthetic techniques [37, 38]. Two recent small studies investigated the addition of dexamethasone [39] and dexmedetomidine [40] to the LA mixture. The authors found improved block quality and duration with the addition of dexamethasone. A separate study found that the addition of dexamethasone to the LA mixture prolonged block duration. Further larger, adequately powered randomized trials will be required before the addition of adjuvants to the LA mixture is routinely advocated.

Safety Considerations

Although truncal blocks are regarded as relatively safe, we must not become complacent about performing them due to the potential to cause harm. The introduction of ultrasound into routine clinical practice has reduced the incidence of complications, but even with the ability to visualize the needle complications still arise. The more technically advanced blocks, for example the QLB, should only be performed by those with adequate experience.

Along with the general complications associated with carrying out any invasive procedure such as introduction of infection, bleeding and patient discomfort, each block has its own associated complications specific to that block. A major complication associated with all truncal blocks is peritoneal and visceral puncture. This complication has been reported in the literature for all of the major truncal blocks, both landmark and ultrasound guided. Intraperitoneal injection has been reported in both adults and paediatric patients undergoing ilioinguinal and TAP block [41, 42]. Weintraud et al. [43] demonstrated a 2% incidence of intraperitoneal injection during ultrasound guided ilioinguinal block. Other rarely reported complications may include colonic or small bowel puncture and pelvic haematoma. Liver trauma has also being reported in the literature after TAP block [44]. Regarding rectus sheath blocks, peritoneal and visceral puncture have also being reported, as has inadvertent puncture of the inferior epigastric vessels, resulting in significant haemorrhage. Despite the use of ultrasound practitioners performing these blocks must be diligent, use an in-plane technique as much as possible, and visualize the needle through the entirety of performing the block.

Transient inadvertent femoral nerve block is another complication associated with truncal blocks, especially ilioinguinal blocks, TFP blocks and even TAP blocks. Transient femoral nerve block is a potential cause of delayed mobilisation and patient discharge, both of which are undesirable, and may have actually being the reason for avoiding neuraxial blockade in the first instance. If the nerve block is not recognised this may lead to further trauma to the patient if they fall.

LA toxicity must also be recognised as a potential complication while performing truncal blocks. Large volumes are generally used when performing these blocks to achieve optimal analgesia and clinicians must always be mindful of maximum allowable doses of LA while performing these procedures. Studies investigating plasma concentrations of LA after injection have been conducted in blocks where high volumes are used. Griffiths et al. [41] demonstrated toxic levels of plasma ropivacaine one hour after injection of 2.5 mg/kg of ropivacaine in 40% of subjects. With this in mind we must always be mindful of maximum allowable doses of LA when employing such blocks. Addition of epinephrine containing solutions has being shown to slow absorption following TAP block, but not with RSB [24].

Role Within Enhanced Recovery After Intestinal Surgery Program

TAP blocks are ideally suited to Enhanced Recovery After Intestinal Surgery, with the absence of motor block and hypotension easing early mobilization and the opiate sparing effect advantageous for early nutrition. The combination of different approaches allows selective blockade of just the lower abdominal wall, upper abdominal wall or the entire abdominal wall depending on the nature of the incision.

References

1. Moore K, Dalley A. Clinically oriented anatomy. 4th ed. Philadelphia, PA: Lippincott Williams and Watkins; 1999.
2. Rozen WM, Tran TMN, Ashton MW, Barrington MJ, Ivanusic JJ, Taylor GI. Refining the course of the thoracolumbar nerves: a new understanding of the innervation of the anterior abdominal wall. Clin Anat. 2008;21:325–33.
3. Van Schoor AN, Boon JM, Bosenberg AT, Abrahams PH, Meiring JH. Anatomical considerations of the pediatric ilioinguinal/iliohypogastric nerve block. Paediatr Anaesth. 2005;15:371–7.
4. Rafi AN. Abdominal field block: a new approach via the lumbar triangle. Anaesthesia. 2001;56:1024–6.
5. Loukas M, Tubbs RS, El-Sedfy A, Jester A, Polepalli S, Kinsela C, Wu S. The clinical anatomy of the triangle of Petit. Hernia. 2007;11:441–4.
6. McDonnell JG, Curley G, Carney J, Benton A, Costello J, Maharaj CH, Laffey JG. The analgesic efficacy of transversus abdominis plane block after caesarean delivery: a randomized controlled trial. Anesth Analg. 2008;106:186–91.
7. McDonnell JG, O'Donnell BD, Farrell T, Gough N, Tuite D, Power C, Laffey JG. Transversus abdominis plane block: a cadaveric and radiological evaluation. Reg Anesth Pain Med. 2007;32:399–404.
8. Blanco R. TAP block under ultrasound guidance: the description of a "no pops" technique. Reg Anesth Pain Med. 2007;32(S1):130.
9. Hebbard P. Subcostal transversus abdominis plane block under ultrasound. Anesth Analg. 2008;106(2):674–5.
10. Carney J, McDonnell JG, Bhinder R, Maharaja CH, Laffey JG. Ultrasound guided continuous transversus abdominis plane block for post-operative pain relief in abdominal surgery. Reg Anesth Pain Med. 2007;32(S1):24.
11. Walter EJ, Smith P, Albertyn R, Uncles DR. Ultrasound imaging for transversus abdominis blocks. Anaesthesia. 2008;63:211.
12. Børglum J, Maschmann C, Belhage B, Jensen K. Ultrasound-guided bilateral dual transversus abdominis plane block: a new four-point approach. Acta Anaesthesiol Scand. 2011;55:658–63.
13. Tanggaard K, Jensen K, Lenz K, Vazin M, Binzer J, Lindberg-Larsen VO, Niegsch M, Bendtsen TF, Jorgensen LN, Borglum J. A randomised controlled trial of bilateral dual transversus abdominis plane blockade for laparoscopic appendicectomy. Anaesthesia. 2015;70(12):1395–400.
14. McDonnell JG, O'Donnell B, Curley G, Heffernan A, Power C, Laffey JG. The analgesic efficacy of transversus abdominis plane block after abdominal surgery: a prospective randomized controlled trial. Anesth Analg. 2007;104:193–7.
15. Carney J, McDonnell JG, Ochana A, Bhinder R, Laffey JG. The transversus abdominis plane block provides effective postoperative analgesia in patients undergoing total abdominal hysterectomy. Anesth Analg. 2008;107:2056–60.
16. Carney J, Finnerty O, Rauf J, Curley G, McDonnell JG, Laffey JG. Ipsilateral transversus abdominis plane block provides effective analgesia after appendectomy in children: a randomized controlled trial. Anesth Analg. 2010;111:998–1003.
17. Peterse PL, Mathiesen O, Torup H, Dahl JB. The transversus abdominis plane block: a valuable option for postoperative analgesia? A topical review. Acta Anaesthesiol Scand. 2010;54:529–35.
18. Abdallah FW, Chan VW, Brull R. Transversus abdominis plane block: a systematic review. Reg Anesth Pain Med. 2012;37:193–209.
19. Carney J, Finnerty O, Rauf J, Bergin D, Laffey JG, Mc Donnell JG. Studies on the spread of local anesthetic solution in transversus abdominis plane blocks. Anaesthesia. 2011;66:1023–30.
20. Conaghan P, Maxwell-Armstrong C, Bedforth N, et al. Efficacy of transversus abdominis plane blocks in laparoscopic colorectal resections. Surg Endosc. 2010;24:2480–4.

21. El-Dawlatly AA, Turkistani A, Kettner SC, et al. Ultrasound-guided transversus abdominis plane block: description of a new technique and comparison with conventional systemic analgesia during laparoscopic cholecystectomy. Br J Anaesth. 2009;102:763–7.
22. Mukhtar K, Khattak I. Transversus abdominis plane block for renal transplant recipients. Br J Anaesth. 2010;104:663–4.
23. Niraj G, Searle A, Mathews M, Misra V, Baban M, Kiani S, Wong M. Analgesic efficacy of ultrasound-guided transversus abdominis plane block in patients undergoing open appendicectomy. Br J Anaesth. 2009;103:601–5.
24. Aveline C, Le Hetet H, Le Roux A, Vautier P, Cognet F, Vinet E, Tison C, Bonnet F. Comparison between ultrasound-guided transversus abdominis plane and conventional ilioinguinal/iliohypogastric nerve blocks for day-case open inguinal hernia repair. Br J Anaesth. 2011;106:380–6.
25. Araco A, Pooney J, Araco F, Gravante G. Transversus abdominis plane block reduces the analgesic requirements after abdominoplasty with flank liposuction. Ann Plast Surg. 2010;65:385–8.
26. Niraj G, Kelkar A, Jeyapalan I, Graff-Baker P, Williams O, Darbar A, Maheshwaran A, Powell R. Comparison of analgesic efficacy of subcostal transversus abdominis plane blocks with epidural analgesia following upper abdominal surgery. Anaesthesia. 2011;66(6):465–71.
27. Hebbard P. Transversalis fascia plane block, a novel ultrasound-guided abdominal wall nerve block. Can J Anesth. 2009;56:618–20.
28. Chin J, Hebbard P, Harris M. Ultrasound-guided transversalis fascia plane block provides analgesia for anterior iliac crest bone graft harvesting. Can J Anesth. 2012;59:122–3.
29. Willard FH, Vleeming A, Schuenke D, Danneels L, Schleip R. The thoracolumbar fascia: anatomy, function and clinical considerations. J Anat. 2012;221:507–36.
30. Ding Y, White PF. Post-herniorrhaphy pain in outpatients after preincision ilioinguinal-hypogastric nerve block during monitored anaesthesia care. Can J Anesth. 1995;42:12–5.
31. Harrison CA, Morris S, Harvey JS. Effect of ilioinguinal and iliohypogastric nerve block and wound infiltration with 0.5% bupivacaine on postoperative pain after hernia repair. Br J Anaesth. 1994;72:691–3.
32. Bugedo GJ, Carcamo CR, Mertens RA, Dagnino JA, Munoz HR. Preoperative percutaneous ilioinguinal and iliohypogastric nerve block with 0.5% bupivacaine for post-herniorrhaphy pain management in adults. Reg Anesth. 1990;15:130–3.
33. Toivonen J, Permi J, Rosenberg PH. Effect of preincisional ilioinguinal and iliohypogastric nerve block on postoperative analgesic requirement in day-surgery patients undergoing herniorrhaphy under spinal anaesthesia. Acta Anaesthesiol Scand. 2001;45:603–7.
34. Willschke H, Marhofer P, Bosenberg A, Johnston S, Wanzel O, Cox SG, Sitzwohl C, Kapral S. Ultrasonography for ilioinguinal/iliohypogastric nerve blocks in children. Br J Anesth. 2005;95:226–30.
35. Weintraud M, Marhofer P, Bosenberg A, Kapral S, Willschke H, Felfernig M, Kettner S. Ilioinguinal/ailiohypogastric blocks in children: where do we administer the local anesthetic without direct visualization? Anesth Analg. 2008;106:89–93.
36. Forero M, Heikkila A, Paul JE, Cheng J, Thabane L. Lumbar transversus abdominis plane block: the role of local anesthetic volume and concentration—a pilot, prospective, randomized, controlled trial. Pilot Feasibil Stud. 2015;1:10.
37. Choi S, Rodseth R, McCartney CJL. Effects of dexamethasone as a local anaesthetic adjuvant for brachial plexus block: a systematic review and meta-analysis of randomized trials. Br J Anaesth. 2014;112(3):427.
38. Abdallah FW, Brull R. Facilitatory effects of perineural dexmedetomidine on neuraxial and peripheral nerve block: a systematic review and meta-analysis. Br J Anaesth. 2013;110:915–25.
39. Ammar A, Mahmoud K. Effect of adding dexamethasone to bupivacaine on transversus abdominis plane block for abdominal hysterectomy: a prospective randomized controlled trial. Saudi J Anaesth. 2012;6(3):229–33.
40. Almarakbi W, Kaki A. Addition of dexmedetomidine to bupivacaine in transversus abdominis plane block potentiates post-operative pain relief among abdominal hysterectomy patients: a prospective randomized controlled trial. Saudi J Anaesth. 2014;8(2):161–6.

41. Griffiths JD, Le NV, Grant S, Bjorksten A, Hebbard P, Royse C. Symptomatic local anaesthetic toxicity and plasma ropivacaine concentrations after transversus abdominis plane block for Caesarean section. Br J Anaesth. 2009;105:853–6.
42. Jankovic Z, Ahmad N, Ravishankar N, Archer F. Transversus abdominis plane block: how safe is it? Anesth Analg. 2008;107(5):1758–9.
43. Weintraub M, Marhofer P, Bosenberg A, Kapral S, Willschke H, Felfernig M, Kettner S. Ilioinguinal/iliohypogastric blocks in children: where do we administer the local anesthetic without direct visualization? Anesth Analg. 2008;106:89–93.
44. Farooq M, Carey M. A case of liver trauma with a blunt regional anesthesia needle while performing transversus abdominis plane block. Reg Anesth Pain Med. 2008;33(3):274–5.

Recommended Reading

Abdallah FW, Laffey JG, Halpern SH, Brull R. Duration of analgesic effectiveness after the posterior and lateral transversus abdominis plane block techniques for transverse lower abdominal incisions: a meta-analysis. Br J Anaesth. 2013;111(5):721–35.

Bærentzen F, Maschmann C, Jensen K, Belhage B, Hensler M, Børglum J. Ultrasound-guided nerve block for inguinal hernia repair: a randomized, controlled, double-blind study. Reg Anesth Pain Med. 2012;37(5):502–7.

Finnerty O, Carney J, McDonnell JG. Trunk blocks for abdominal surgery. Anaesthesia. 2010;65(S1):76–83.

Husain NKA, Ravalia A. Ultrasound-guided ilioinguinal and rectus sheath nerve blocks [letter]. Anaesthesia. 2006;61:1126.

Smith BE, Suchak M, Siggins D, Challands J. Rectus sheath block for diagnostic laparoscopy. Anaesthesia. 1988;43:947–8.

Yentis SM, Hills-Wright P, Potparic O. Development and evaluation of combined rectus sheath and ilioinguinal blocks for abdominal gynaecological surgery. Anaesthesia. 1999;54:466–82.

Truncal Blocks: Rectus Sheath Catheters 12

Anton Krige and Mark Daugherty

Key Points

1. Rectus sheath catheters (RSC) provide selective dermatomal blockade of the abdominal wall to ensure good somatic analgesia for open major abdominal surgery requiring a median or paramedian incision.
2. RSC has minimal side effects, few contra-indications and a low failure rate. No motor block enables early mobilisation a key component of enhanced recovery programmes.
3. RSC blocks the abdominal wall component of pain so there is a requirement of additional analgesia (such as opiates) to manage the early visceral pain. This can be minimised by the use of transdermal fentanyl patches.
4. RSC can be placed under ultrasound guidance after induction of general anaesthesia and prior to the start of surgery, or surgically placed at the end of surgery. These techniques are easy to learn.
5. The block can be maintained by administering a manual or portable pump delivered bolus of local anaesthetic via both catheters every four to six hours. Alternatively, portable elastomeric pumps can be used to deliver a continuous infusion of local anaesthetic.

A. Krige (✉)
Department of Anaesthesia and Critical Care, Royal Blackburn Teaching Hospital, Blackburn, UK
e-mail: anton.krige@elht.nhs.uk

M. Daugherty
Department of Anaesthesia, Royal Devon and Exeter Hospitals, Exeter, UK

A. Krige, M. J. P. Scott (eds.), *Analgesia in Major Abdominal Surgery*,
https://doi.org/10.1007/978-3-319-94482-1_12

Introduction

The concept of fast track surgery promoted by Wilmore and Kehlet, using newer approaches to pain control and minimally invasive surgery [1], emerged from Denmark in 2001, and has evolved into Enhanced Recovery After Surgery (ERAS) protocols. Kehlet had originally developed the concept of using multimodal approaches to ameliorate the pathophysiological consequences of the surgical stress response in the 1990s, thus modifying the undesirable sequelae of major surgery. These combine various techniques to accelerate patient rehabilitation following surgery of which the provision of effective pain relief, alongside the use of minimally invasive surgery, is an essential pre-requisite [1].

Thoracic epidural analgesia (TEA) has been the commonest of several analgesic techniques used in clinical practice, and for some time considered the gold standard, particularly for major abdominal surgery. However, epidural analgesia is not without problems and risks and in recent years there has been a move to seek alternatives.

This chapter will explore in detail the re-emergence of bilateral rectus sheath blocks (RSB) maintained via rectus sheath catheters (RSC) as a novel analgesic approach and a viable alternative to thoracic epidural analgesia for midline open abdominal surgery.

The technique aims to block the ventral rami of the thoracolumbar spinal nerves T6–L1, that supply the rectus abdomini muscles and overlying skin. It is a compartment block achieved by injecting local anaesthetic into the potential space that exists between the rectus abdominus muscle and the posterior rectus sheath. By leaving a catheter in situ within this space, the block can be topped-up at regular intervals.

Historical Perspective

The RSB, which is an abdominal field block, was first described by Schleich in 1899, with the primary aim of providing muscle relaxation of the abdominal wall to assist surgery and also served as an analgesic adjunct [2]. The advent of neuromuscular blockers in the 1940s led to the decline in the use of RSB until a landmark study by Smith et al. in the late 1980s [3]. They established bilateral RSBs using a blind landmark technique, which significantly reduced post-operative pain and delayed the requirement for intramuscular analgesia for at least 10 h following diagnostic laparoscopy [3]. Initially RSB was largely confined to paediatric umbilical hernia repair and gynaecological laparoscopic surgery as it remained limited to single bolus injection, with limited duration of action, using a blind landmark technique, as described by Ferguson [4], which had a limited success rate and potential for complications [4–8]. It was not until 2006 that Willschkhe et al. [9] described ultrasound-guided placement of RSB. Shortly thereafter a Glasgow group [10] demonstrated the superiority of the ultrasound-guided approach over the landmark approach with novices achieving an 89% versus a 45% success rate.

Eventually descriptions emanated from Australasia [11, 12] of catheter placement in the rectus sheath space (RSS), thus providing the ability to prolong the block indefinitely. Surgical RSC placement, credited to Cornish and Deacon in 2007 [11], preceded ultrasound guided (USG) RSC placement, which was reported by Sandeman and Dilley in 2008 [12].

Subsequently blind landmark RSB has fallen away with all single shot RSB ultra-sound guided and RSC placement either surgically or ultra-sound guided.

Interestingly the positive trial reported by Watson et al. back in 1991 [13] utilising RSC for midline laparotomy seems to have gone unnoticed. It lacks any detailed description of how catheters were placed but as ultrasound RSB had not yet been reported it is assumed to been surgical placement.

Thus, the history of RSC is less than 10 years old and due to the widespread availability of small portable ultrasound machines coupled to disillusionment with alternatives implementation of these techniques is spreading in parallel with the spread in the enhanced recovery after surgery paradigm.

Evidence for Efficacy

Several blinded RCT comparing the efficacy (pain scores and opiate consumption) of single shot RSB injections using either LA or placebo following paediatric hernia repair or adult laparoscopic surgery have been published. The studies by Smith [3], Yentis [5] and Azemati [6] reporting in favour of RSB whilst the study by Isaac [7] reported no difference. Notably this latter study of paediatric hernia repair utilised landmark placed RSB, for which Dolan measured success rates as low as 48% [10]. Surprisingly Bashandy [14] reported benefit following single shot RSB following midline laparotomy compared to placebo for 48 h post-operatively, which is counter to the widely agreed maximum clinical duration of eight hours for a RSB.

Analgesia for major abdominal surgery, and in particular open midline (median or para-median incisions) surgery, is the niche of interest for RSC and where research is now focussed.

Several proof of concept RCT, where both groups receive a RSC, and then LA injection is compared to saline injection, following open midline abdominal surgery have been published. The outcomes are generally pain scores, opiate consumption (typically both groups will receive the same rescue analgesia, most commonly as morphine PCA), after the recovery profile and adverse events. These RCT have been contradictory, with the study by Watson [13] reporting efficacy for RSC whilst those by Su [8] and Padmanabhan [15] reported no efficacy. Importantly all three of these studies incorporated surgically placed RSC at the end of surgery and the study by Su did not include an adequate LA bolus at the outset and only a low dose continuous infusion. Observational data suggests a greater efficacy when the RSB is operational before the onset of surgery and that the failure rate of surgically placed RSC is greater than with ultrasound placement [16, 17].

Several case reports and case series have reported good quality analgesia following midline incisions with ultrasound-guided RSC [18–21].

There is acceptance that RSC, whether surgically placed or ultrasound-guided, provide good quality analgesia following midline laparotomy. Research is appropriately shifting to comparisons against thoracic epidural analgesia (TEA) and other techniques, for example TAP blocks and continuous wound infusion catheters (CWIC).

Several non-randomised comparisons of RSC to thoracic epidural analgesia have originated from the South West of England where this technique is very popular and implementation has been widespread. One of this chapter's authors works in one of these hospitals. The first was Parsons et al. [22] who compared ten patients who received USG RSC with ten patients who received TEA for open radical cystectomy surgery and found the analgesia to be equivalent with a lower rate of ileus and a shorter length of stay in the RSC group. Godden et al. [23] again compared RSC to TEA but this time for open midline colorectal surgery involving 85 in the TEA group and 24 in the RSC group. Again there was no difference in pain relief or complications but a higher incidence of hypotension in the TEA group. Two similar studies compared surgically placed RSC to TEA. Finch et al. [24] assessed 45 patients who had undergone open midline gynaecological oncological surgery and found low pain scores in both groups with better analgesia within the RSC group when placement was at the start of surgery compared to at the end. When Tudor et al. [25] compared 73 RSC cases to 22 TEA cases the analgesia was again equivalent, however the RSC group mobilised earlier with less hypotension. Finally, Dutton et al. [17] published a cohort study of 200 consecutive major urological surgery cases (106 radical prostatectomies and 94 open radical cystectomies) receiving RSC analgesia with a 100% success rate and no complications. Pain scores were universally low with half the patients requiring morphine PCA in the cystectomy group and none in the prostatectomy group after the first day. The total opiate consumed was modest and became minimal after 24 h. The RSC were used for an average of 3.6 days in the cystectomy group and only 6% were removed early. The mean length of stay for the cystectomy group over the course of 5 years from implementation of enhanced recovery, of which the introduction of RSC was a key feature, dropped from 17 to 10 days.

There has been a paucity of RCT comparing RSC to TEA but encouragingly all of the non-randomised and cohort studies above have reported equivalent analgesia but with other outcomes relating to hypotension and hospital stay in favour of RSC. In June 2017 Yassin et al. [26] published their RCT comparing the safety and efficacy of ultrasound guided RSC to TEA for midline upper abdominal surgery in 60 patients. The RSC group had greater opioid consumption and an earlier opioid requirement (resulting a greater early sedation), which is to be expected for visceral analgesia, whilst pain intensity at rest and coughing was similar, as was patient satisfaction. RSC had the advantage of earlier ambulation hence they concluded that RSC could be considered as an effective alternative to TEA for upper abdominal midline surgery.

Seidel et al. [27] published new data regarding RSC insertion technique to achieve optimal rectus sheath sensory blockage in July 2017, which will change this authors approach and can be considered an alternative to the insertion technique discussed later in this chapter. They performed six in-plane ultrasound guided dye injections to the rectus sheath space of three unfixed cadavers. All injections were with the linear transducer in the transverse plane with half the injections at the medial (in a lateral direction) and half at the lateral (in a medial direction) edge of the rectus abdominis muscle. They found that the dye injection at the medial edge did not reliably reach the target nerves and recommended that local anaesthetic should be injected at the lateral edge of the rectus sheath to achieve sufficient craniocaudal spread. This is probably because the anterior cutaneous branches of the thoracolumbar spinal nerves enter the rectus sheath at the lateral border and then leave the muscle after traversing a short distance ventrally.

Implementation of this new knowledge may change the outcome of future randomized trial comparisons with other techniques.

One of the authors of this chapter's team has completed, but not yet reported, a pilot RCT of RSC versus TEA for open abdominopelvic surgery, and the Dr. Krige is completing a similar study, the TERSC study, comprising 132 patients undergoing open midline surgery [28], which will be published in 2018. The TERSC study will also compare the relative magnitude of surgical stress response between ten patients in each group. This will add to our understanding of the relative impact on the surgical pathophysiology of these regional techniques, if any.

Recently Dowidar et al. [29] randomised sixty patients undergoing open midline colorectal surgery to RSC or continuous wound infusion catheters (CWIC). The RSC group had better pain scores at rest and on movement, required less rescue analgesia (6.6% vs 26%), lower opiate consumption and better patient satisfaction. There were no serious complications in either group. This was an important study as CWIC are being considered as the other major alternative to TEA for midline surgery.

A further interesting area of research regards the nature of the LA solutions. Shabana et al. [30] produced a blinded RCT whereby 50 patients for open midline colorectal surgery were randomised to receive either 0.25% bupivacaine only, or the same along with the addition of 100 μg/mL of morphine. The latter resulted in significantly better pain scores at multiple time points at both rest and on movement. Thus local anaesthetic/fentanyl mixtures, which are typically used for epidural infusions, could be considered for RSC to further increase efficacy.

Thus evidence is emerging which suggests that RSC can provide effective pain relief for all midline incisions, thus reducing post-operative opioids and allowing earlier mobilisation without complications.

Anatomy

Chapter 1 covers in detail the anatomy of the abdominal wall and cavity and the motor and sensory supply of nerves. Sensorimotor innervation of the anterior abdominal wall arises from the ventral rami of the thoracolumbar spinal nerves T7–L1. All the nerves innervating the anterior abdominal wall travel as multiple mixed segmental nerves, which branch and communicate widely within the

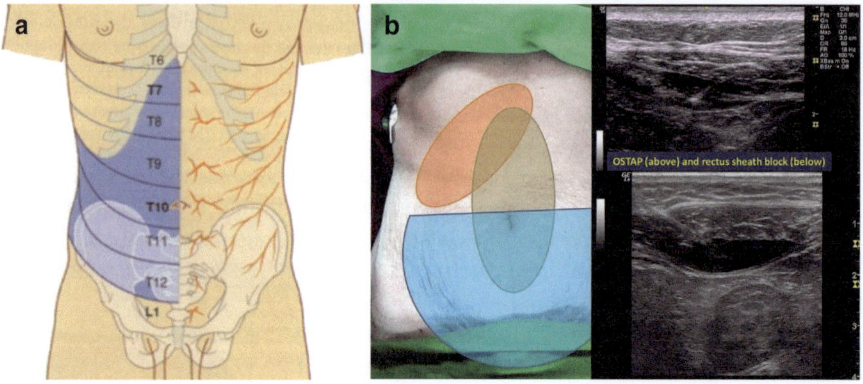

Fig. 12.1 Sensory innervation of the abdomen blocked by rectus sheath blockade. (**a**) Sensory dermatomes covered by rectus sheath blockade. (**b**) Comparative dermatomal cover of Subcostal TAP vs Posterolateral TAP vs RSB and associated Ultrasound images SCTAP above and RSB below [36]

transversus abdominal plane (TAP). These communications occur at multiple locations, including communications anterolaterally (intercostal plexus), and in plexuses that run with the deep circumflex artery (TAP plexus) and the deep inferior epigastric artery (rectus sheath plexus). Segments T7–T12 and L1 innervate the rectus abdominis muscle (Fig. 12.1a, b illustrate the dermatomes blocked by a RSB). A branch of T10 always innervates the umbilicus [31].

The thoracolumbar nerves course along the anterolateral wall within the TAP before entering the lateral aspect of the rectus sheath, where they enter the lateral aspect of the rectus muscle. Here they form a nerve plexus that runs cranio-caudally within the muscle in close relation to the lateral branch of the deep epigastric artery [31]. These nerves typically pierce the posterior border of the rectus muscle within 1.6–2.6 cm from the lateral edge. They provide muscular and cutaneous branches to innervate muscle fibres of the rectus muscle and the overlying skin. The branches do not cross the midline.

The skin and fascia of the anterior abdominal wall overlie the four muscles (rectus abdominis, external oblique, internal oblique and transversus abdominis). The rectus sheath is formed from the aponeuroses of the fascial sheaths of all three lateral abdominal muscles. The sheaths converge to form the lateral border of the rectus muscle, termed the linea semilunaris. The anterior and posterior sheaths of external oblique and the anterior sheath of internal oblique fuse together and continue medially over the anterior surface of rectus muscle to form the anterior rectus sheath. The posterior rectus sheath is formed by a combination of the posterior sheath of the internal oblique muscle, and the anterior and posterior sheaths of transversus abdominis muscle. At the medial border of the rectus muscle, the anterior and posterior rectus sheaths fuse with the fibres from the medial border of the contralateral rectus muscle forming the midline linea alba.

The anterior rectus sheath extends along the entire vertical length of the rectus muscle. In contrast the posterior rectus sheath extends only along the upper two thirds of the rectus muscle. In the lower one third the posterior rectus sheath stops midway between the umbilicus and the symphisis pubis. This transition point is known as the arcuate line and it is where the posterior rectus sheath aponeuroses courses over the anterior surface of the rectus muscle with the anterior rectus sheath. Below the arcuate line, only the transversalis fascia, a thin layer of connective tissue located deep to the posterior sheath, and the parietal peritoneum, lie posterior to the rectus muscle.

Anatomy and Landmarks Using Ultrasound

The following layers of the anterior abdominal wall, from superficial to deep, can be identified by positioning a high frequency linear array probe above, and lateral too, the umbilicus in a transverse plane (*see* Fig. 12.2a–c):

- Subcutaneous and adipose tissue layers that vary in depth depending on body habitus.
- The anterior rectus sheath, a bright hyperechoic linear structure extending from lateral to medial.
- The rectus abdominis muscle, which is relatively hypoechoic.
- The posterior rectus sheath, which also a bright hyperechoic structure.
- The deep superior (above the umbilicus) and inferior epigastric arteries may be seen in the deepest aspect of the rectus muscle, accentuated by colour flow doppler.
- The transversalis fascia is a hyperechoic linear structure found deep to the posterior rectus sheath and together they have the appearance of tramlines.
- Deep to posterior rectus sheath and transversalis fascia is the peritoneal cavity, identified by peristaltic movements of bowel loops.

The target site for LA solution is deep to the rectus muscle but superficial to the posterior rectus sheath. The ventral rami of the thoracoabdominal nerves are too small to be visualised as discrete structures, so the Rectus sheath block is actually a compartment block.

Placing the transducer in the midline above the umbilicus but below the Xiphisternum in a transverse position, allows visualisation of the Linea Alba. As the probe is moved laterally the bulk of the rectus muscle is observed covered by the anterior and posterior rectus sheaths, as well as the transversalis fascia, producing the tramlines. Moving more laterally the Linea Semiluminaris comes into view followed by the three lateral abdominal muscles (external oblique, internal oblique and transversus abdominis).

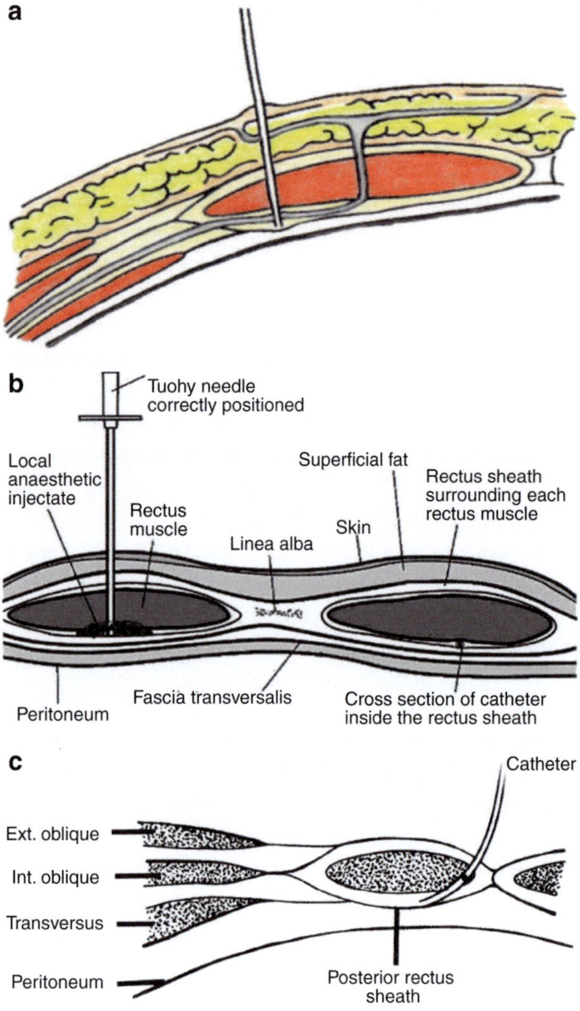

Fig. 12.2 Cross-sectional diagram of abdominal wall with needle and catheter placements. (**a**) Diagram of RSB needle target. (**b**) Transverse section of the anterior abdominal wall, with depiction of Tuohy needle position and location of local anaesthetic injectate for rectus sheath block Webster K (2010). (**c**) Schematic diagram rectus sheath catheter placement [15]

Catheter Insertion Techniques

The anaesthetist obtains consent from the patient during the pre-operative visit after explaining the procedure along with the risks and benefits. Specific risks of RSC placement discussed with the patient are failure of catheter placement, catheter related infection, iatrogenic haematoma, and the need for additional analgesia.

Figure 12.3 illustrates the positioning of needle insertion points immediately below each costal margin (the xiphisternum, costal margin above insertion point and umbilicus are marked for orientation) and the exit points of the tunnelled catheters above each costal margin.

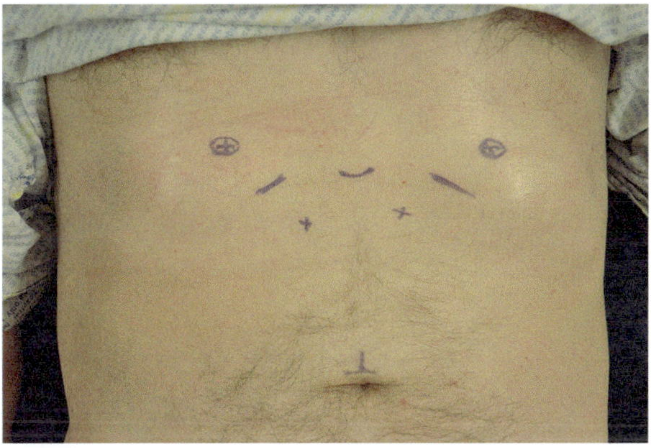

Fig. 12.3 Landmarks for needle insertion and exit points for tunneled catheters

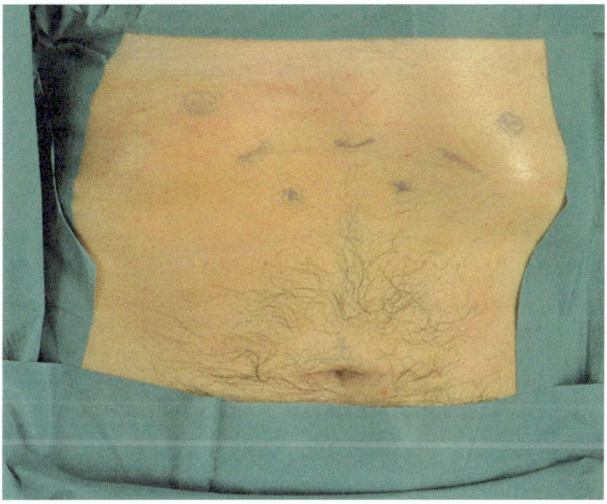

Fig. 12.4 Preparation of aseptic field

Rectus sheath blocks are usually performed after induction of general anaesthesia and intubation of the patient, in the anaesthetic room under strict aseptic conditions, using large sterile drapes with a large aperture for adequate ultrasound access to the upper abdomen (Fig. 12.4). The necessary equipment is placed on the sterile drape over the patient's chest in preparation for insertion. This will include the 16 G Tuohy needle, 10 mL of 0.9% saline, 20 mL of LA, catheter and the catheter clamp (Fig. 12.5).

Ultrasound-Guided Catheter Insertion

Using a portable ultrasound machine with a high frequency sheathed linear transducer probe, under real time direct ultrasound guidance, the Linea Alba is visualised in the middle of the epigastrium (Fig. 12.6). Still in the transverse plane, the probe

Fig. 12.5 Preparation of equipment

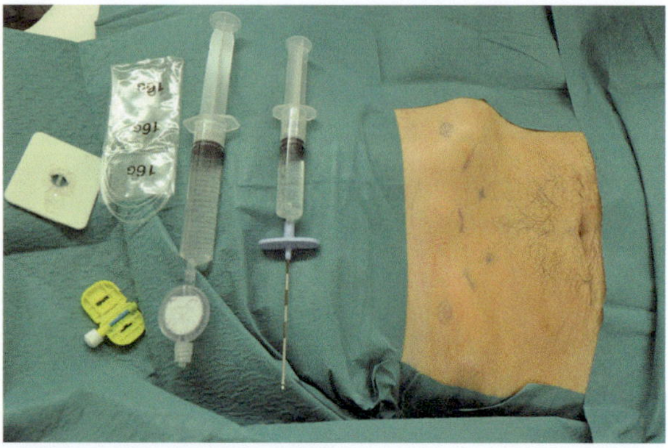

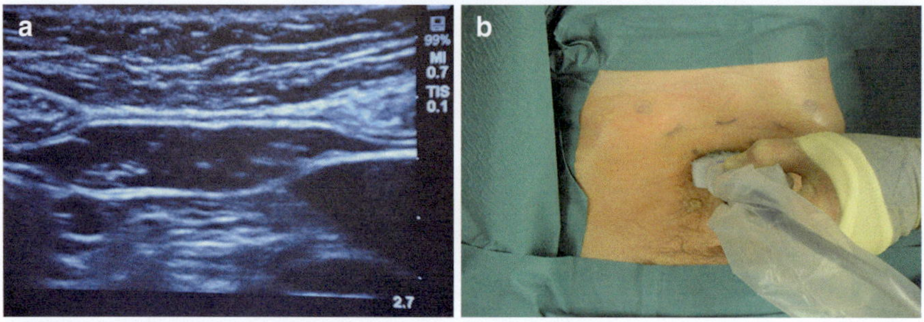

Fig. 12.6 Visualizing the linea alba. (**a**) Sonoanatomy of the linea alba. (**b**) Position of ultrasound probe position to identify the linea alba

is moved laterally to visualise the main body of the rectus abdominis muscle. The posterior rectus sheath and transversalis fascia are clearly visible as a set of tramlines posterior to the muscle. Within the potential space between the posterior aspect of the rectus muscle and the tramlines pass the ventral rami of the thoracolumbar spinal nerves, which supply the anterior abdominal wall. The ultrasound probe is then rotated 90 degrees in to the sagittal or longitudinal plane, approximately 3–5 cm from the midline. This allows an in-plane approach for the insertion of a 16 or 18 G Tuohy needle as high as possible in the abdomen, just below the costal margin (Fig. 12.7). The Tuohy needle is advanced in a caudal direction at approximately 45° until the tip lies on top or just anterior to the tramlines but posterior to the rectus muscle (Fig. 12.8a–c). The correct position is confirmed by injecting a bolus of normal saline to separate the planes and achieve hydro-dissection, indicated by the appearance of an anechoic fluid collection (Fig. 12.9a–c). A further 20 mL of LA is injected down the Tuohy needle which further opens up the potential space between posterior rectus sheath and rectus abdominis muscle and allows the epidural or rectus sheath catheters to be inserted relatively easily (Fig. 12.10a–e). The hydro-dissected space and catheters are easily visible on ultrasound and must be visualised to confirm correct position (Fig. 12.11a–b). The Tuohy needle is

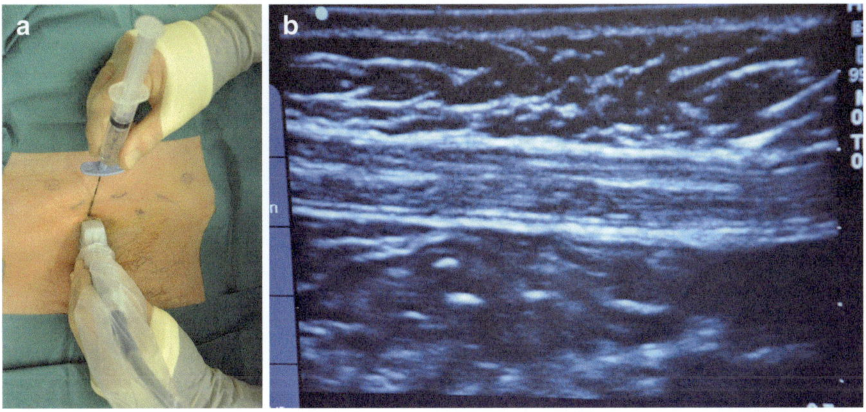

Fig. 12.7 Insertion Tuohy needle position. (**a**) Tuohy needle insertion point. (**b**) Sonoanatomy Tuohy needle insertion

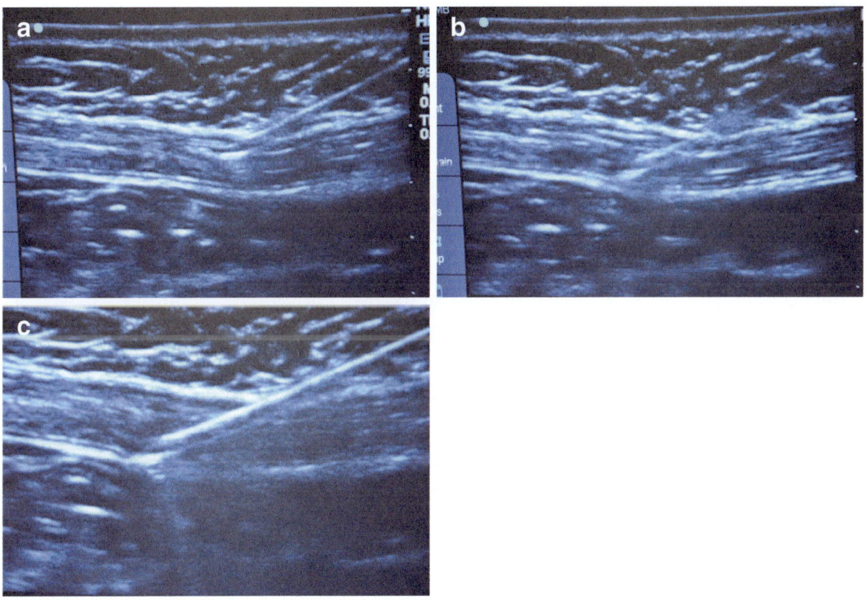

Fig. 12.8 Sonoanatomy of Tuohy needle advancement to target position. (**a**) Tuohy needle breaching anterior rectus sheath. (**b**) Tuohy needle reaching posterior rectus abdominus muscle. (**c**) Tuohy needle at interface between rectus muscle and posterior rectus sheath (tram lines visible are posterior rectus sheath followed by the peritoneum)

removed and the catheters can be tunnelled subcutaneously in a lateral-cephalad direction to above the costal margin and xiphisternum, keeping them clear of the surgical field (Fig. 12.12a–f). The procedure is repeated on the opposite side and it is best to secure the catheters at the skin with a dedicated catheter fixation device

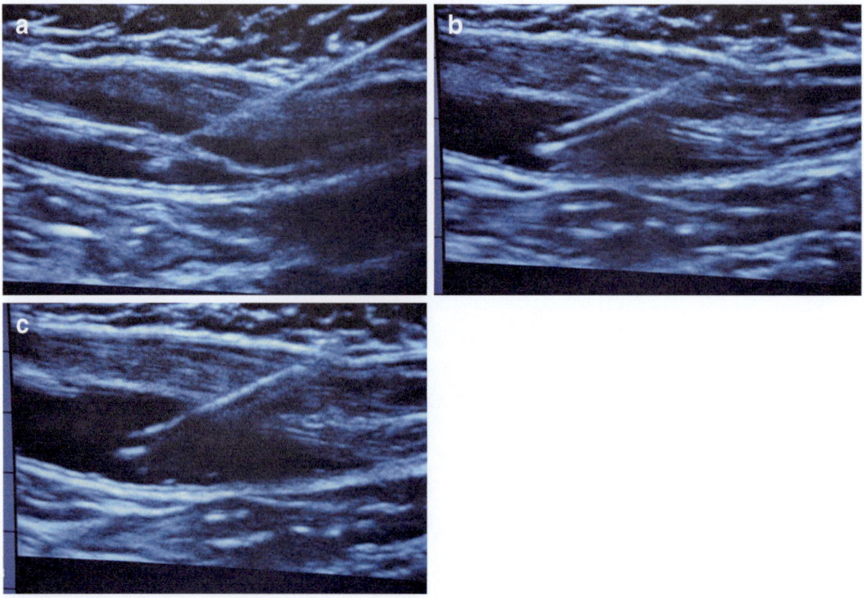

Fig. 12.9 (**a**–**c**) Hydro-dissection with progressive separation of rectus muscle from the posterior rectus sheath

(Fig. 12.13). The catheters are capped with luer lock filters and caps, and a clear sterile dressing is placed over each catheter (Fig. 12.14a–c). Approximately 6–8 cm of catheter is left in the rectus sheath compartment, thus following tunnelling the catheter reaches the skin at the 15 cm marking. The above technique is used as described at the authors' respective institutions for all major abdominal surgery where a midline or paramedian incision is used.

In urology the incisions are usually infra-umbilical extending above the umbilicus. In general surgery the incision may extend from pubis to xiphisternum particularly in emergency laparotomies, hence our technique in placing the RSC as high in the abdomen as possible allowing tunnelling to above the costal margins and out of the surgical field.

An alternative technique for ultrasound guided RSC placement has been described in which the probe is placed lateral to the rectus abdominis muscle and the needle advanced in plane from lateral to medial, penetrating through the lateral aspect of the linea semilunaris and entering the lateral aspect of the rectus muscle. The needle is advanced until it is positioned deep to the potential space between the posterior border of rectus muscle, but superficial to the posterior rectus sheath (tramlines), termed the posterior rectus sheath compartment. At this point injecting saline for hydro-dissection of rectus muscle away from posterior rectus sheath, indicated by an anechoic fluid collection, will confirm correct position of the needle tip. Further injection of 15–20 mL of local anaesthetic opens up the posterior rectus

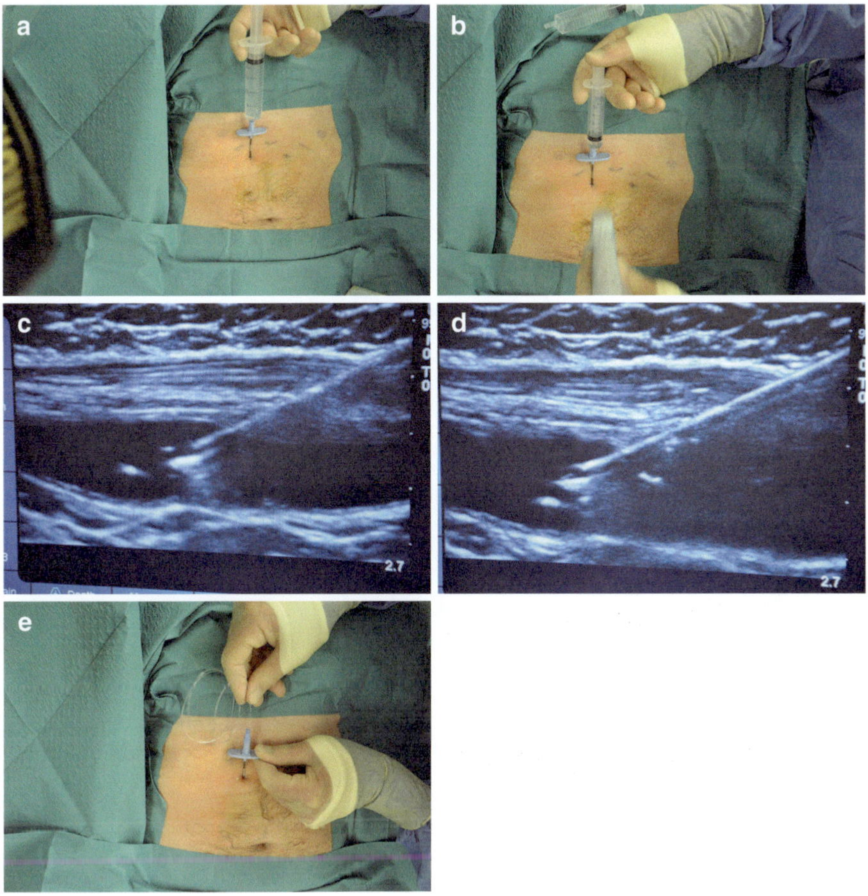

Fig. 12.10 (a–e) Initial bolus injection of local anaesthetic via the Tuohy needle and catheter insertion

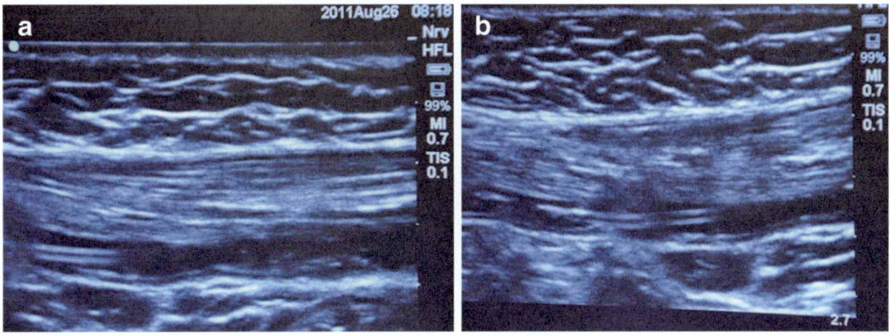

Fig. 12.11 (a, b) Ultrasound confirmation of catheter position

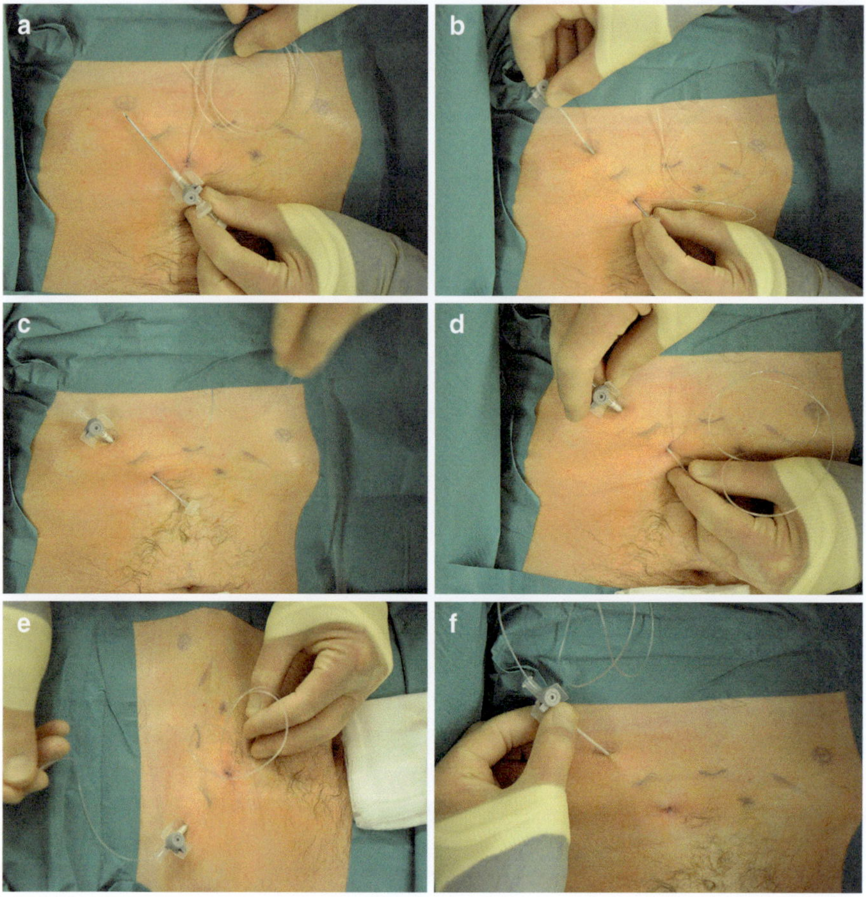

Fig. 12.12 (**a**–**f**) Tunneling of catheters from insertion point to the anterior chest wall

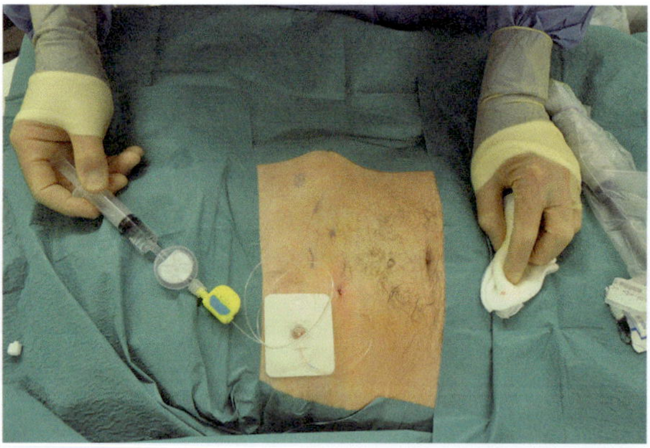

Fig. 12.13 Catheter fixation at the skin

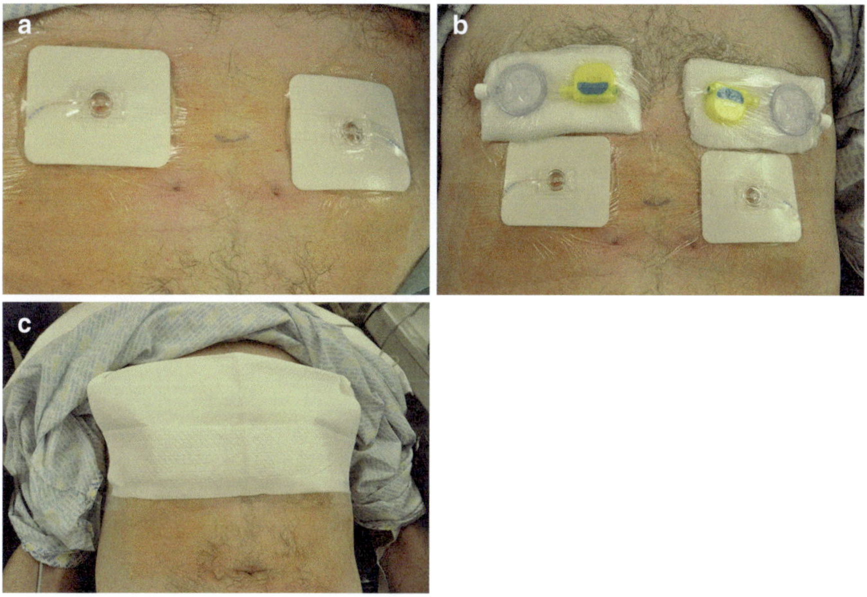

Fig. 12.14 (**a**–**c**) Covering and protection of catheters on the chest wall

sheath compartment allowing easier insertion of an epidural catheter leaving 4–6 cm in the compartment. Catheter tip is confirmed, the Tuohy needle is withdrawn and the catheter secured to the skin over the lateral abdomen. This lateral to medial technique follows the original description of a RSB for umbilical hernia repair and sites the catheter at approximately T10 or at the midpoint of an extended midline incision for laparotomy. The position of the catheters in the antero-lateral abdomen may encroach on the sterile surgical field.

Surgical Catheter Insertion

Some of the first descriptions of using RSCs were those placed under direct vision by a surgeon. In our institutions these are placed by our gynaecologists when performing radical open cancer surgery and by any surgeon operating via a midline incision when RSC placement under ultrasound guidance by the anaesthetist is not possible. These catheters can be placed at the start or end of the laparotomy and have been found to be safe and efficient. However, in urological pelvic surgery using an infra-umbilical incision, it is difficult for the surgeon to place the catheters above the umbilicus, so in all cases it is best for the anaesthetist to place them under ultrasound guidance before the start of surgery.

A description of surgically placed RSC was first published in 2007 [11], in which the surgeon makes a small incision in the posterior rectus sheath above the

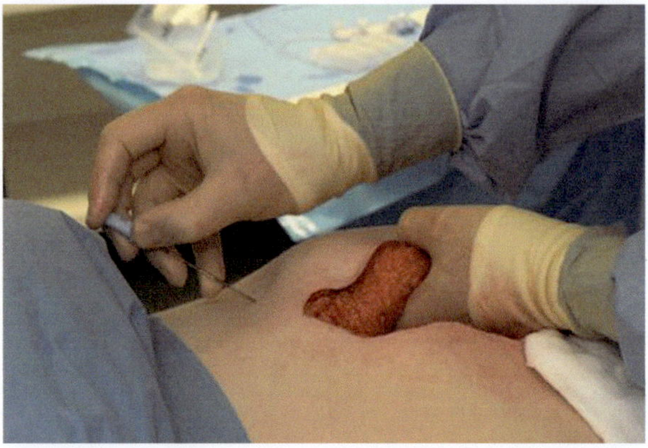

Fig. 12.15 Surgeon inserting Tuohy needle through the skin and fascia with one hand whilst palpating from inside the abdomen with the other hand

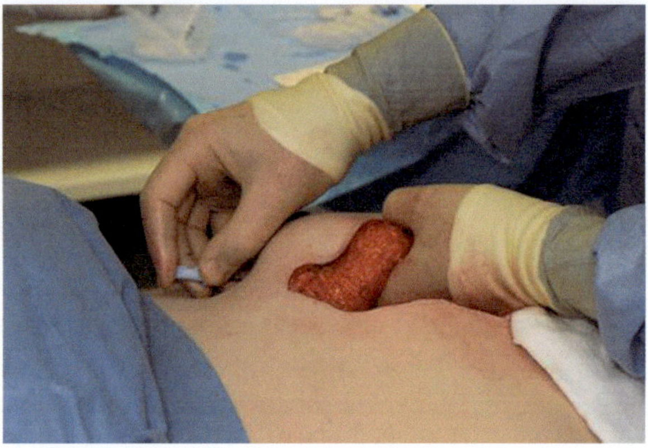

Fig. 12.16 Surgeon palpating needle tip once just superficial to the peritoneum—rectus muscle interface

umbilicus which is at their fingertips and then introduces the catheter clamped in small forceps between the sheath and the rectus muscle belly.

This technique has been adapted by the surgeons in the one author's institution whereby they place catheters bilaterally at the superior end of the laparotomy wound at the beginning of surgery after the peritoneum is first opened, or at the end of surgery just prior to closure [24]. The surgeon places one hand inside the abdomen and with the other hand inserts the Tuohy needle through the skin and fascia (Fig. 12.15). The surgeon palpates the needle tip when it is just superficial to the interface between the peritoneum and muscle layer (Fig. 12.16). As the inferior epigastric artery is palpable it can be avoided. The stylet is removed from the needle and the epidural catheter introduced until a 5 cm length is left in the peritoneum-muscle interface (Fig. 12.17). The surgeon holds on to the catheter tip while the needle is removed (Fig. 12.18). The catheter is secured at this point to avoid accidental removal. One can use an adhesive epidural catheter dressing or a suture. After connecting a bacterial filter the catheter is flushed with 20 mL of LA, which initiates a RSB. The procedure is repeated on the contralateral side. This initial bolus will block the thoracolumbar spinal nerves augmenting analgesia until the block is topped up by the next bolus 4–6 h later [32].

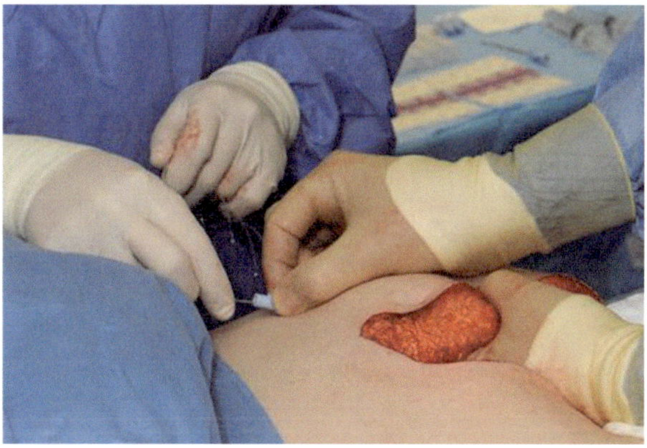

Fig. 12.17 Surgeon introducing catheter into the target space

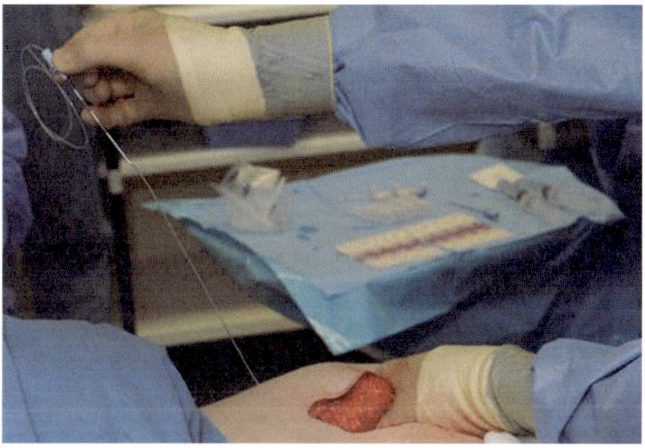

Fig. 12.18 Catheter tip being held intra-abdominally while removing the Tuohy needle

Management of the Rectus Sheath Catheter Block

A single shot RSB will last for 6–10 h. The advantage of inserting RSCs is that the block can be topped up, prolonging the use and benefits of the block to cover the somatic pain related to major midline abdominal surgery for up to 5 days.

When RSC were introduced at one of the authors' institutions, the standard operating procedures for their management received all the required clinical governance approvals allowing Nurses to be trained, assessed and authorised as competent to prepare the local anaesthetic (Levo-Bupivacaine) and then inject the prescribed amount into each rectus sheath catheter. Strict protocols were implemented regarding timing for each of these top ups, appropriate questions to ask the patient in order to detect signs of toxicity, and the minimum monitoring required during the top up and for 30 min afterwards. This has limited the introduction of RSC at other institutions across the UK, where these governance hurdles have been difficult to overcome.

To circumvent this problem, other methods have been tried and shown to be effective and safe. Ambulatory infusion pumps, of which there are several available, have been connected to the RSCs via a 'Y-connector' with settings to deliver 30–40 mL LA boluses every 4–6 h, with or without a background infusion.

Dr Krige employs such a technique in his institution. The RSC portable elastomeric pumps in a light-weight bag slung over the patient's shoulder is combined with transdermal fentanyl patches to treat the visceral pain component. Oral opiate is used for any further break though pain. This combination further eases mobility with the absence of an additional morphine PCA pump while avoiding any potential infection risk (although none have been reported) of repeated breaks in the line when employing manual RSC boluses.

Elastomeric infusion pumps have also been used to deliver 5mls/hr to each RSC, with good effect.

Safety

The placement and use of RSC are a relatively safe technique as compared to thoracic epidural analgesia with no reported serious critical incidents in the literature.

The theoretical risks during placement are needle injury to the superior epigastric vessels with an abdominal wall haematoma as a consequence or visceral organ puncture. The anatomical corridor for encountering the superior epigastric vessels is between 4 and 8 cm from the midline. The USG approach will allow visualisation of any vessels thereby avoiding them during needle insertion. USG will also allow accurate needle placement between rectus muscle and posterior rectus sheath while avoiding penetration of the peritoneum, which is clearly visible. During surgical placement as described the superior epigastric vessels are palpable by the surgeons guiding fingers against the peritoneum and easily avoided.

Possible problems during management are technique failure. The rate quoted in one large series is 6%, which is significantly lower than epidural failure rates (26). This may in turn lead to larger opiate requirements, as will cases with excessive visceral pain, with the concomitant opiate related side effects.

Catheter related wound infection is a possible late complication but none have been reported and neither author of this chapter has encountered any in their extensive RSC experience.

The catheters can become trapped within the wound closure sutures resulting in difficult removal. This has occurred in the institution of one of the chapter authors but only with surgically placed catheters and due to placement being too medial.

Systemic local anaesthetic toxicity is the potential complication with the gravest consequences.

There is little published literature regarding local anaesthetic toxicity and abdominal wall blocks with only one dose comparison study involving single bolus Rectus Sheath Blocks without catheter placement by Wada et al. [33] and two studies [26, 34] where local anaesthetic plasma concentrations were measured during use of TAP (transversus abdominis plane) catheters. The former was a dose comparison study and the latter two studies involved patients undergoing caesarean section and gynaecological surgery respectively. Although subcostal TAP catheters are also abdominal wall blocks placed in an adjacent location to RSC it is nevertheless a different anatomical space and results cannot be directly extrapolated. Therefore, there is no previously published data on the plasma levels of ropivacaine or bupivacaine during prolonged RSC use.

One of this chapter's authors has performed a yet unpublished sub-study of their comparison of RSC to thoracic epidural analgesia following radical cystectomy pilot RCT, in which they assessed plasma concentrations of laevobupivacaine in six patients following each dose. The protocol for their pilot RCT involved an initial bolus dose of 20 mL 0.375% levobupivacaine via each catheter at the end of surgery. This was followed by top up doses of 20 mL 0.25% levobupivacaine via each catheter every 4 h for the first 24 h whilst on ICU and then every 6 h on the ward. Levobupivacaine concentration levels increased with each top-up, never reached a plateau, and exceeded the toxic level of 2.5 μg/mL in all cases [26, 27, 33–35]. Although more than 2000 RSC had been performed in their hospital prior to this research without a single case of suspected LA toxicity in any patient, the prescription was altered by necessity following these results and further studies were delayed. The updated prescription is 20 mL of 0.25% levobubivacaine via each catheter on initial insertion of the catheters to establish the block, followed by top-ups of 20 mL of 0.125% levobupivacaine via each catheter every 6 h. They have not found a reduction in efficacy of the blocks, and their acute pain team continues to report excellent RSC analgesia using this dosing modification.

The other author of this chapter is undertaking a similar twenty patient sub-study of their main study, which compares RSC to epidural analgesia following midline laparotomy [28], to determine plasma concentrations of ropivacaine in the RSC group as well as plasma concentrations of bupivacaine in the epidural group. The dosing protocol for the RSC are 20 mL 0.2% ropivacaine via each catheter every four hours with this dosage halved for any patients less than 50 kg. This study will completed in January 2017.

Practical Considerations

It is important to remember that RSC blocks only provide somatic analgesia related to major abdominal surgery via a mid-line incision, and not the visceral pain related to the intra-peritoneal nociceptive insult. The RSB is part of a multimodal analgesia package, with visceral pain requiring some opiate analgesia. The visceral pain is short in duration (12–24 h) with opiate usually only required for 24–36 h. Multimodal analgesia is used for as long as required with the RSC being used for up to 7 days depending on the type of surgery.

Multimodal analgesia includes paracetamol, an NSAID (a COX2 or Ibuprofen), Tramadol or Codeine and a gabapentinoid (*see* Chap. 2). Opiates can be given orally, via a transdermal patch or using a PCA, depending on the extent of the abdominal surgery (see Chap. 3). An intra-operative bolus of ketamine is an additional non-opioid adjuvant to consider as part of this analgesic package (*see* Chap. 13).

As opiate is required for managing the early visceral pain component patients who are opiate tolerant, due to chronic pain treatment, are not well suited to this technique, or any other truncal block approach. Epidural analgesia would remain the ideal option for this group.

Extensive midline abdominal scarring may prevent spread of LA and establishment of a RSB and thus presents a relative contra-indication.

Typically a remifentanyl infusion or repeated boluses of other opiate are used intra-operatively as part of the GA technique, with morphine administered towards the end of the operation, in order to manage the visceral pain. An alternative approach would be to administer intrathecal opiate (*see* Chap. 3) prior to GA to provide the visceral analgesia intra-operatively and for the first 12–24 h post-operatively. Although no research exists regarding this hybrid alternative, based on evidence of the effectiveness of intrathecal opiate for managing the largely visceral pain from laparoscopic major abdominal surgery, this combination is likely to provide excellent analgesia, whilst maintaining all the mobility advantages and obviating the need for any other parenteral opiate post-operatively.

Audit data from the institution of one of this chapter's authors as well as the study by Finch et al. [24] suggests superior analgesia and reduced opiate requirements when the RSB is established prior to the surgical incision (USG insertion) compared to at the end of surgery. Possible reasons are the effect of pre-emptive analgesia and the nature of the different surgical placement techniques. Some describe incising the sheath and then introducing the catheter from the inside with forceps. This has the potential for leakage of LA and other techniques whereby the catheter placement may end up between posterior rectus sheath and the peritoneum rather than between the rectus muscle and the posterior rectus sheath. The former is essentially a continuous wound infusion and will not provide a RSB.

Rectus Sheath Catheters and Their Role in Enhanced Recovery Pathways

Rectus Sheath Catheters are an ideal analgesic component within an enhanced recovery pathway for major abdominal surgery requiring an open median or paramedian incision.

The combination of adequate analgesic efficacy allied to an absence of the other factors, which complicate early mobilisation and feeding. These are opiate sparing (minimises the side effects of high dose systemic opiate) hypotension, motor block, urinary catheters and large cumbersome infusion pumps attached to drip stands. The local anaesthesia to maintain the RSB can be administered by manual boluses or infused by portable pumps slung over the patient's shoulder.

A key aspect of successful Enhanced Recovery Programmes is standardisation of practice including analgesic techniques. The insertion technique needs to be easy to learn and the management easy to implement at large scale. RSC certainly fulfil these criteria with portable ultrasound present and ultrasound skills ubiquitous in modern anaesthetic departments. Where the ultrasound skill set or equipment is absent the surgical placement is an easy alternative.

In order to implement at scale the technique must be cost-effective. RSC consumables are only marginally more expensive than a single epidural set but will likely involve less healthcare worker management time and less time in higher care areas due to the difference in failure rates and side effects. RSC consumables are roughly half the cost of a continuous wound infusions wound soaker set—the other common alternative for these incisions.

Contra-indications are few and those that prevent neuraxial blockade do not apply. These neuraxial contraindications are particularly common during emergency abdominal surgery. RSC are particularly useful in this scenario and can even be inserted on the ICU before waking those patients kept ventilated and sedated following emergency laparotomy.

Finally as RSC are placed once the patient is already under GA their experience during insertion will be superior to neuraxial blocks as the latter are usually inserted awake.

References

1. Wilmore D, Kehlet H. Management of patients in fast track surgery. BMJ. 2001;322:473–6.
2. Schleich CL. Schmerzlose operationen. Berlin: Springer; 1899. p. 240–1.
3. Smith BE, Suchak M, Siggins D, Challands J. Rectus sheath block for diagnostic laparoscopy. Anaesthesia. 1988;43(11):947–8.
4. Ferguson S, Thomas V, Lewis I. The rectus sheath block in paediatric anaesthesia: new indications for an old technique? Paediatr Anaesth. 1996;6(6):463–6.
5. Yentis S, Hills-Wright P. Development and evaluation of combined rectus sheath and ilioinguinal blocks for abdominal gynaecological surgery. Anaesthesia. 1999;54:466–82.
6. Azemati S, Khosravi MB. An assessment of the value of rectus sheath block for postlaparoscopic pain in gynecologic surgery. J Minim Invasive Gynecol. 2005;12(1):12–5.
7. Isaac LA, McEwen J, Hayes JA, Crawford MW. A pilot study of the rectus sheath block for pain control after umbilical hernia repair. Pediatr Anesth. 2006;16:406–9.
8. Su S, Harris P. A randomised, placebo-controlled trial of continuous local anaesthetic rectus sheath infusion for pain management after major abdominal surgery [abstract]. ANZ J Surg. 2006;76:A16.
9. Willschke H, Bosenberg A, Marhofer P, Johnston S, Kettner SC, Wanzel O, et al. Ultrasonography-guided rectus sheath block in paediatric anaesthesia—a new approach to an old technique. Br J Anaesth. 2006;97(2):244–9.
10. Dolan J, Lucie P, Geary T, Smith M, Kenny G. The rectus sheath block for laparoscopic surgery in adults: a comparison between the loss of resistance and ultrasound guided techniques. Anaesthesia. 2007;62:302.
11. Cornish P, Deacon A. Rectus sheath catheters for continuous analgesia after upper abdominal surgery. ANZ J Surg. 2007;77(12):84.
12. Sandeman DJ, Dilley AV. Ultrasound-guided rectus sheath block and catheter placement. ANZ J Surg. 2008;78:621–3.
13. Watson D, Farquhar XX, Dennison A, Cole J, McAllister S. Postoperative analgesia by infusion of local anaesthetic into the rectus sheath. Br J Anaesth. 1991;67:656.
14. Bashandy GMN, Elkholy AHH. Guided rectus sheath block to multimodal analgesia for abdominal cancer surgery with midline incision. Anesth Pain Med. 2014;4(3):e18263.

15. Padmanabhan J, Rohatgi A, Niaz A, Chojnowska E, Baig K, Woods WGA. Does rectus sheath infusion of bupivacaine reduce postoperative opioid requirement? Ann R Coll Surg Engl. 2007;89:229–32.
16. Boyd N, Grice A, Jubb A. Audit of rectus sheath catheters at the Royal Devon and Exeter NHS Foundation Trust. Presented at the Society of Anaesthetists of the South Western Region meeting, Oct 2009.
17. Dutton TJ, McGrath JS, Daugherty MO. Use of rectus sheath catheters for pain relief in patients undergoing major pelvic urological surgery. Br J Urol Int. 2014;113(2):246–53.
18. Webster K, Hubble S. Rectus sheath analgesia in intensive care patients: technique description and case series [abstract]. Anaesth Intensive Care. 2009;37:855.
19. Shido A, Imamachi N, Doi K, Sakura S, Saito Y. Continuous local anesthetic infusion through ultrasound-guided rectus sheath catheters. Can J Anaesth. 2010;57(11):1046–7.
20. Malchow R, Jaeger L, Lam H. Rectus sheath catheters for continuous analgesia after laparotomy – without postoperative opioid use. Pain Med. 2011;12(7):1124–9.
21. Bakshi S, Mapari A, Paliwal R. Ultrasound-guided rectus sheath catheters: a feasible and effective, opioid-sparing, post-operative pain management technique: a case series. Indian J Anaesth. 2015;59(2):118–20.
22. Parsons B, Aning J, Daugherty M, et al. The use of rectus sheath catheters for patients undergoing radical cystectomy. BJU Int. 2011;4:24–30.
23. Godden AR, Marshall MJ, Grice AS, Daniels IR. Ultrasonography guided rectus sheath catheters versus epidural analgesia for open colorectal cancer surgery in a single centre. Ann R Coll Surg Engl. 2013;95(8):591–4.
24. Finch L, Phillips A, Acheson N, Dix P, Berry C. An evaluation of the effects of a service change from epidurals to rectus sheath catheters on postoperative pain. J Obstet Gynaecol. 2013;33(5):502–4.
25. Tudor ECG, Yang W, Brown R, Mackey PM. Rectus sheath catheters provide equivalent analgesia to epidurals following laparotomy for colorectal surgery. Ann R Coll Surg Engl. 2015;97(7):530–3.
26. Yassin HM, Elmoneim ATA, El Moutaz H. The analgesic efficiency of ultrasound-guided rectus sheath analgesia compared with low thoracic epidural analgesia after elective abdominal surgery with a midline incision: a prospective randomized controlled trial. Anesth Pain Med. 2017;7(3):e14244.
27. Seidel R, Wree A, Schulze M. Does the approach influence the success rate for ultrasound-guided rectus sheath blocks? An anatomical case series. Local Reg Anesth. 2017;10:61–5.
28. Wilkinson KM, Krige A, Brearley SG, Lane S, Scott M, Gordon AC, et al. Thoracic epidural analgesia versus rectus sheath catheters for open midline incisions in major abdominal surgery within an enhanced recovery programme (TERSC): study protocol for a randomised controlled trial. Trials J. 2014;15(1):1–12.
29. Dowidar AERM, Ezz HAA, Shama AAE, Eloraby MA. Postoperative analgesia of ultrasound guided rectus sheath catheters versus continuous wound catheters for colorectal surgery: a randomized clinical trial. Egypt J Anaesth. 2016;32(3):375–83.
30. Shabana A, Dar M, Ghanem MA. Surgically performed rectus sheath block – effect of morphine added to bupivacaine versus bupivacaine only: a prospective randomized controlled double blinded trial. Egypt J Anaesth. 2013;29:401–5.
31. Rozen WM, Tean TMN, Ashton MW, Barrington MJ IV, Anusic MJ, Taylor GI. Refining the course of the thoracolumbar nerves: a new understanding of the innervation of the anterior abdominal wall. Clin Anat. 2008;21:325–33.
32. McDermott F, Wilson L, Boorman P. Surgically placed rectus sheath catheters. Update Anaesth. 2010;26:9–11.
33. Wada M, Kitayama M, Hashimoto H, et al. Plasma ropivacaine concentrations after ultrasound-guided rectus sheath block in patients undergoing lower abdominal surgery. Anesth Analg. 2012;114:230–2.

34. Griffiths JD, Barron FA, Grant S, Bjorksten AR, Hebbard P, Royse CF. Plasma ropivacaine concentrations after ultrasound-guided transversus abdominis plane block. Br J Anaesth. 2010;105(6):853–6.
35. Griffiths JD, Le NV, Grant S, Bjorksten A, Hebbard P, Royse C. Symptomatic local anaesthetic toxicity and plasma ropivacaine concentrations after transversus abdominis plane block for Caesarean section. Br J Anaesth. 2013;110(6):996–1000.
36. Chakraborty A, Khemka R, Datta T. Ultrasound-guided truncal blocks: A new frontier in regional anaesthesia. Indian J Anaesth. 2016;60:703–11.

Recommended Reading

Webster K. Ultrasound guided rectus sheath block. Update Anaesth. 2010;26:12–7.

13 Continuous Wound Infiltration

Nicholas T. Ventham

Key Points

1. Local anaesthetic (LA) administered continuously to the operative site in the immediate post-operative period has demonstrable analgesic and opioid-sparing effects.
2. Sterile multi-holed fine bore catheters placed in the surgical wound site and connected to elastomeric pumps delivering a constant infusion for 24–48 h have extended the beneficial effects of LA beyond the first post-operative day.
3. Current evidence suggests an improved overall quality of recovery with earlier return of gut function and shorter hospital stay, probably due to the opioid sparing effect.
4. Several techniques have been described to enable use of continuous wound infusion (CWI) in a range of operative settings using different incisions. Wound catheters should be positioned pre-peritoneally in the subfascial or transversus abdominis plane to provide effective analgesia following abdominal surgery. Long acting LA with an adequate flow-rate is advocated to maintain adequate dispersion across the subfascial plane.
5. CWI is generally safe, and when used as part of a multimodal analgesic regimen can facilitate enhanced recovery after major abdominal surgery.

N. T. Ventham
Department of Colorectal Surgery, Western General Hospital, Edinburgh, UK

University of Edinburgh, Edinburgh, UK
e-mail: n.ventham@doctors.org.uk

A. Krige, M. J. P. Scott (eds.), *Analgesia in Major Abdominal Surgery*,
https://doi.org/10.1007/978-3-319-94482-1_13

Introduction

Subcutaneous infiltration of a short acting local anaesthetic (LA) around a surgical wound is widely performed despite little evidence supporting this practice [1]. Over the last two decades, novel LA techniques have been developed to improve either the efficacy and/or duration of action of LA [1, 2]. However the limited duration of action of 'single-shot' LA restricts the analgesic benefit to the first 24 h post-operatively. Placement of wound catheters can provide continuous or intermittent bolus administration of LA, thereby prolonging the duration of action beyond that of 'single-shot' administration of LA. The relative simplicity of placement under ultrasound guidance or under direct vision at the time of closure of the operative wound is an advantage, and may avoid some of the incumbent risks of landmark-guided placement of neuraxial techniques and nerve blocks.

Historical Perspective

The relatively simple technique of insertion of a multi-holed catheter (Figs. 13.1 and 13.2) into the surgical wound is not new. There are several reports of the post-operative infusion of LA via polythene tubes placed into abdominal surgical wounds at the time of operation from as early as the 1950s [4–6]. There were a number of randomised controlled trials (RCT) published in the 1980s [7, 8] and towards the end of that decade there was increased use of continuous infusion using syringe pumps [9]. From the 1990s onwards, single-use elastomeric pumps were increasingly used for the purposes of continuous wound infusion (see list of operations studied below). At the turn of the millennium, significant progress in demonstrating the efficacy of CWI of LA was made, with improved RCT trial design including sham catheter placement, placebo infusion of saline and appropriate blinding of participants and assessors. Some of the most notable trials used CWI in gynaecological surgery [10–15], the results of which have been extrapolated to other forms of abdominal surgery, and catalysed further RCTs in the context of elective ambulatory [16–19] and emergency [20] general surgical operations.

Continuous wound infusion of LA has also been used for non-abdominal surgical procedures including thoracic surgery [21–27] and orthopaedic surgery [28–30].

Mechanism of Action

The mechanism of action of local anaesthetic CWI is debated. The predominant analgesic effect is derived from sodium channel blockade of peripheral afferent pain fibres [31]. There is mounting evidence to suggest that LA may have significant anti-inflammatory properties [32]. Incision of the parietal peritoneum leads to a neural stress response via vagal and spinal afferents [33, 34]. It is thought that inhibition of these spinal afferents may be responsible for beneficial stress-response

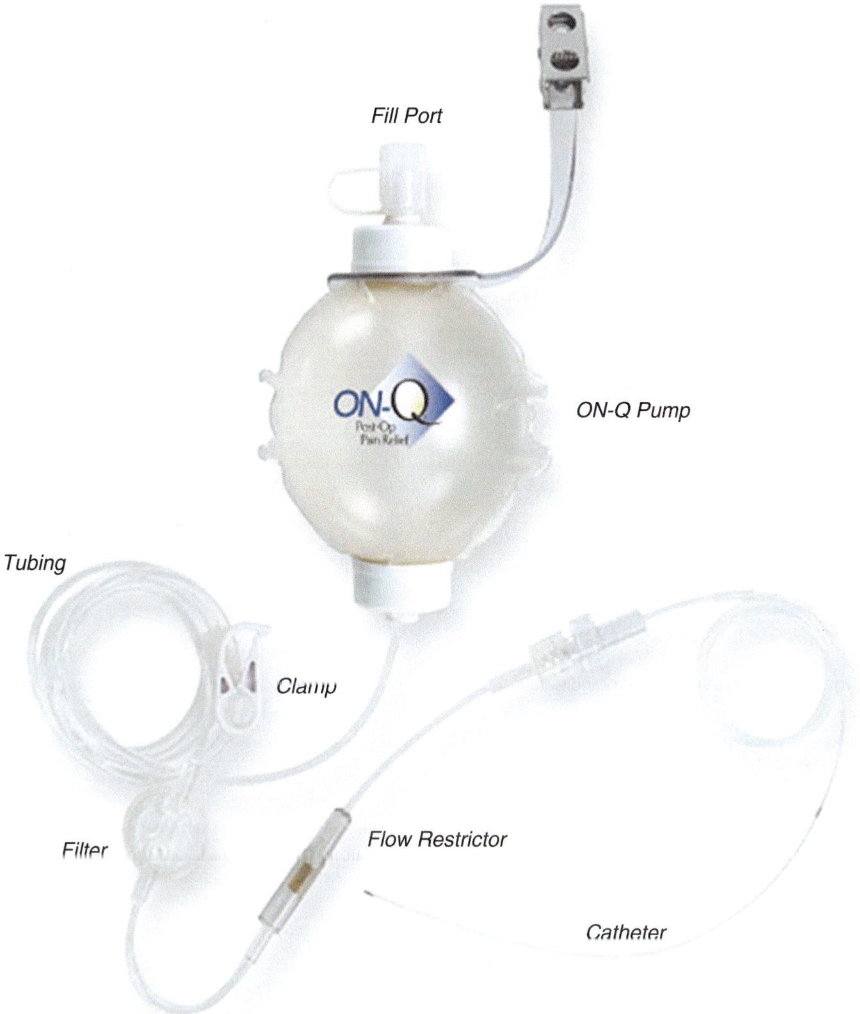

Fig. 13.1 An example of an elastomeric pump. Reprinted with permission from the original article Baig et al. Use of the ON-Q pain management system is associated with decreased postoperative analgesic requirement: double blind randomized placebo pilot study. Journal of the American College of Surgeons 2006:202(2):297–305 (Licence number 3750700323232) [3]

reduction following epidural anaesthesia. CWI may have the additional benefit of inhibiting both spinal and vagal afferents [35]. LA may also reduce 'hyperalgesia' following surgery as a result of LA acting on nociceptive afferents thereby reducing spinal dorsal horn sensitisation ('wind up') [36]. There is some evidence to suggest that at least some of the beneficial action of CWI may result from systemic absorption of LA [37–39]. This is especially pertinent given the increasing use of intravenous lidocaine [40] (see Chap. 6) in the peri-operative setting. CWI is unlikely to

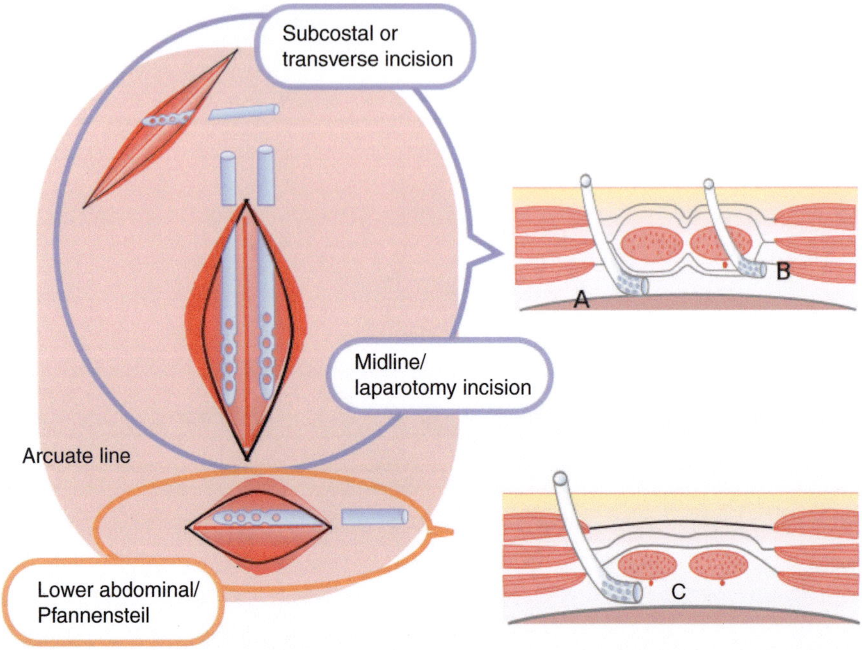

Fig. 13.2 Wound catheter placement according to incision type. *A* pre-peritoneal, *B* transversus abdominis plane, *C* pre-peritoneal for lower abdominal incisions. A horizontal dotted line approximately demarcates the arcuate line where the layers of fascia change from enveloping the recti to passing in front of the rectus muscles

provide complete analgesia following major abdominal surgery through the mechanisms described above, but as part of a multimodal analgesia regimen may help to reduce the overall pain stimulus.

Efficacy and Evidence Base

There is a strong evidence base that demonstrates the efficacy of CWI in the context of major abdominal surgery. CWI is known to reduce opioid requirements, often used as a surrogate marker for pain, and numerical pain rating scores when compared with placebo or routine treatment usually including morphine patient controlled analgesia (PCA) [35, 41, 42].

Two systematic reviews of RCTs have demonstrated a benefit of CWI over morphine PCA for pain on movement following colorectal surgery, suggesting a dynamic analgesic effect [42, 43]. The benefit of opioid reduction may extend up to 24 h after CWI catheter removal [41], perhaps as a result of reduced spinal dorsal horn sensitisation [36].

The effect of CWI on other indices of recovery including post-operative gastrointestinal function is less clear. CWI may reduce the time until resumption of oral diet and time until passage of first flatus and stool when compared to placebo. This is a clear benefit in colorectal and other major abdominal surgery where ileus is often a major barrier to enhanced recovery and early discharge [41–43]. This effect is likely to arise from an opioid reduction, and a subsequent reduction in opioid related side effects [44]. Systematic reviews also indicate that CWI as part of a multimodal analgesia programme and enhanced recovery may reduce the length of stay, [41–43, 45] although studying this outcome in meta-analyses is fraught due to the skewed nature of this type of data.

A significant test of any new method is in direct head-to-head comparison with the current 'gold standard'; thoracic epidural in the case of major abdominal surgery [46]. A systematic review of nine RCTs [12, 47–54] (505 patients) comparing CWI with thoracic epidural analgesia demonstrated no significant difference in pain scores at movement or rest at any time point after surgery [55]. This finding comes with the caveat that CWI was often supplemented with other forms of analgesia and comparisons demonstrated high statistical heterogeneity. A recent study has similarly demonstrated not only no difference in pain scores, but also no difference in biochemical markers of inflammatory response (Interleukins 6810, HMGB1 and tumour necrosis factor-α) between CWI and epidural in the context of liver surgery [45]. Common issues resulting from the sympathetic block that often accompanies neuraxial block including hypotension with resulting increased intravenous fluid and need of vasopressor administration [45] may be avoided with CWI. Patients receiving CWI have a significantly lower incidence of urinary retention, a known complication of epidural analgesia [54, 56, 57]. (Figs. 13.3 and 13.4).

CWI may allow earlier mobilisation when compared with epidural. This is likely to be multifactorial; less postural hypotension, a shorter time with urinary catheter in-situ, and the light elastomeric pumps used for CWI are less cumbersome than the equipment required for epidural (+/− intravenous fluid and/or vasopressor) infusion. The extremely rare, but potentially disastrous complications of epidural (epidural haematoma/abscess) are also avoided.

The use of epidural analgesia following major abdominal surgery is established; epidural provides excellent analgesia and may be cardioprotective in high-risk cases [58]. Whilst further evidence is required to demonstrate non-inferiority of CWI compared with epidural, wound catheters together with other analgesic adjuncts can be recommended as an alternative in those whom epidural is contra-indicated.

Operations Studied Using CWI

- Aortic aneurysm surgery [50]
- Colorectal resection [3, 35, 41, 48, 59, 60] (laparoscopic [49, 61, 62])
- Hepatic resection [45, 47, 54]
- Caesarean [12, 14, 53]
- Prostatectomy [51, 63]
- Other major abdominal surgery [52]
- Open Hernia [16–18]
- Appendectomy [20]
- Obesity surgery [64]
- Open nephrectomy [65]
- Hysterectomy [11]

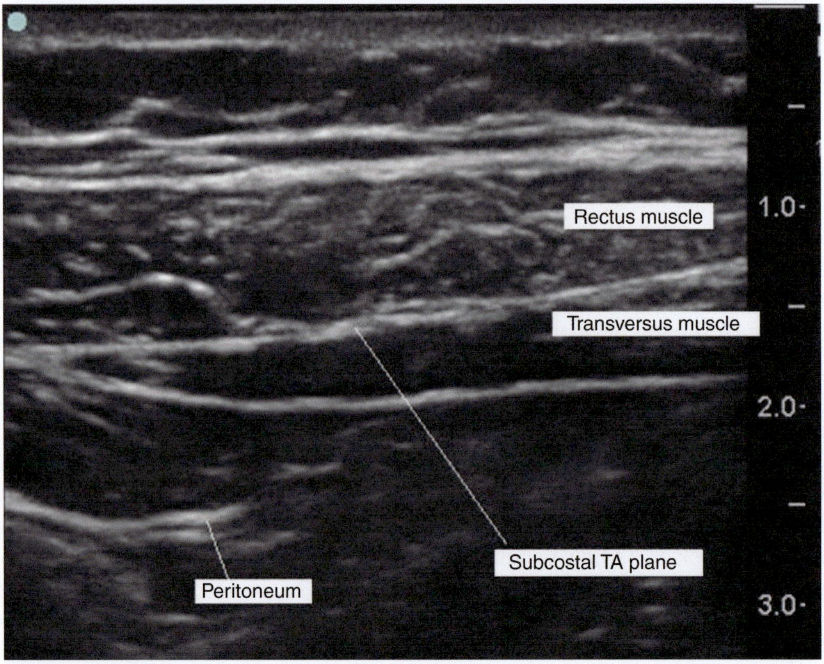

Fig. 13.3 Subcostal transversus abdominis plane under ultrasound visualisation. Reproduced with permission from Niraj G. et al. Comparison of analgesic efficacy of subcostal transversus abdominis plane blocks with epidural analgesia following upper abdominal surgery. Anaesthesia 2011:66(6);465–471. License number 3738370618406 [54]

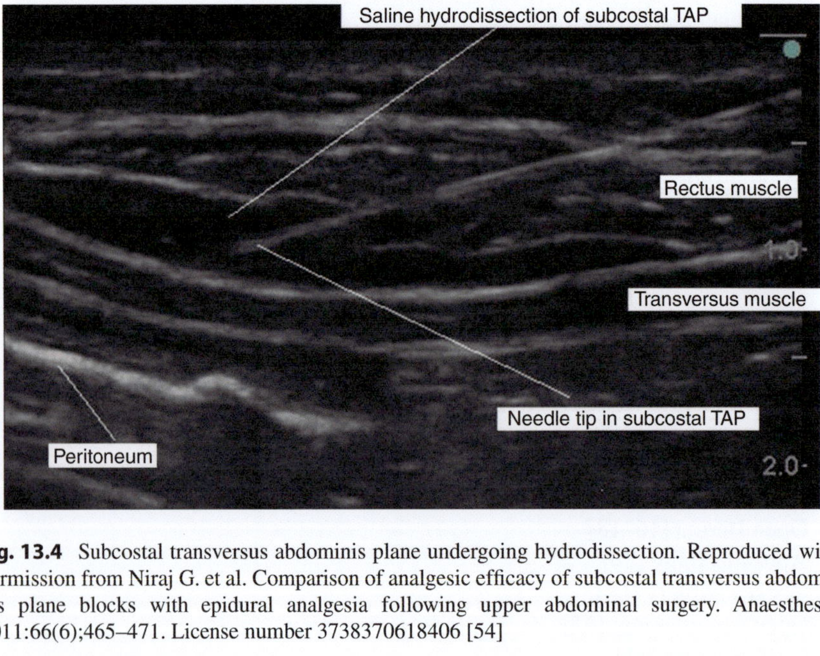

Fig. 13.4 Subcostal transversus abdominis plane undergoing hydrodissection. Reproduced with permission from Niraj G. et al. Comparison of analgesic efficacy of subcostal transversus abdominis plane blocks with epidural analgesia following upper abdominal surgery. Anaesthesia 2011:66(6);465–471. License number 3738370618406 [54]

Anatomical Considerations for CWI Placement

Wound catheters have been placed in several different locations within the abdominal wall. Early trials failed to show a clear therapeutic benefit for wound catheters in major abdominal surgery. Critically wound catheter placement in these trials was within the subcutaneous layers, thereby only providing LA to the most superficial layers of the abdomen [3, 10, 59, 60, 66]. Given that the anterior divisions of T6–11 thoracoabdominal intercostal nerves carrying pain afferent fibres targeted by CWI course through the subfascial/TAP plane intuitively this should be the most efficacious anatomical layer for wound catheters. In major abdominal surgery a large component of post-operative pain experienced is likely to derive from division of the parietal peritoneum and deep fascial layers. An early trial directly compared subfascial positioning of catheters compared to subcutaneous placement, and concluded the subfascial placement is more efficacious in terms of analgesic effect [67]. Later RCTs and subsequently meta-analyses have also demonstrated subfascial wound catheter placement to be consistently effective in reducing pain scores and morphine requirement compared to placebo/routine treatment [35, 43, 68, 69]. Figure 13.2 demonstrates the anatomical layers of the abdominal wall, and placement positions of catheters in various studies.

Safety Considerations

Meta-analyses of RCTs demonstrate CWI to be safe with a very low incidence of complications [43, 55, 70]. One of the main benefits of surgically placed CWI catheters is the avoidance of risks of some of the percutaneous transabdominal approaches, including neurovascular injury and inadvertent peritoneal entry where there is a possibility of visceral injury [71–73]. Initial concerns regarding an increased risk of wound infection have not been borne out by subsequent studies [74] or indeed meta-analyses [43]. One early report of cellulitis and tissue necrosis was related to the use of LA with adrenaline, and as such is not recommended for use in CWI [75].

A serious consideration should however be the risk of systemic toxicity from absorption of local anaesthetic into the blood stream. This has been studied in a number of trials as a secondary analysis. Beaussier used 0.2% Ropivacaine as CWI, delivered at a rate of 10 ml/h for 48 h and measured total plasma concentrations at 24, 48 and 60 h [41]. There was a decrease in plasma concentration between 23 and 48 h demonstrating a lack of accumulation. The maximum unbound concentration was 0.12 μg/ml at which one would expect mild CNS toxicity, although no patients in the trial demonstrated signs or symptoms of toxicity. Another study used 0.2% ropivacaine infusion for 96 h and measured levels at regular intervals [76]. Again the maximum unbound ropivacaine concentration was well below the toxicity threshold [76]. Chan et al. studied Ropivacaine levels following liver surgery [77]. Ropivacaine levels continued to rise whilst the infusion was on going (until 68 h). The authors advocated CWI use for up to 48 h following liver resection with a maximum concentration of 0.25% ropivacaine [77]. A study using 0.25%

laevobupivacaine at 15 ml/h reported safe levels throughout [11]. Clearly in practice, when using CWI, clinicians should be aware of the neurological and cardiac side effects of LA toxicity and have a low index of suspicion should the patient be demonstrating any such symptoms.

Surgically Placed Catheters

Surgically placed CWI catheters can be performed easily during closure of the abdominal incision. As this technique is performed under direct vision the possibility of iatrogenic injury (see safety considerations) are reduced and no specialised ultrasonography equipment is required. Multi-holed catheters with trocars/introducer needles are usually used for this technique. When the correct plane is identified (see Fig. 13.2) and developed as required, the trocar can be introduced with one hand from inside the abdominal wound and one hand bracing the skin (with care taken not to lance oneself). The trocar is used to penetrate the abdominal wall from inside the abdominal wound externally through the skin. Wound catheters should be tunnelled and externalised >3 cm away from the incision itself (they should not exit through the incision). Once the trocar has breached the skin it is important not to retract the 'external' part of the tubing back into the abdominal wall to limit the translocation of skin floral bacteria into the abdominal wall. The trocar can be removed and the internal part of the catheter can be adjusted so that >5 cm of the multi-holed section of the catheter lies in the appropriate plane. It is often helpful to lie the catheter along the length of the wound to ensure a wide and even spread of local anaesthetic. It is important to ensure the multi-holed component of the catheter is completely within the abdominal wall to stop leakage of local anaesthetic outwith the correct plane. There are several methods to fix the catheter tubing to the skin including using adhesive dressings with a locking system for the tubing or alternatively silk suture can be used, which can be removed at the same time as catheter removal. The catheter should be fitted with a bacterial filter and flushed to ensure patent tubing and correct placement. The catheter should be tested with 10 ml of 0.9% saline prior, followed by a loading dose of 10 ml of LA solution, before starting the elastomeric pump.

Midline Laparotomy Incision

Wound catheters should be placed in the pre-peritoneal plane following closure of the parietal peritoneum, and before closure of the fascia. The catheter therefore lies superior to the peritoneum and deep to the fascia. Catheters can be placed along the full length of the midline incision and be externalised inferiorly, [41] superiorly [35] and/or laterally to the skin incision. The rectus sheath is then closed with care taken not to include the catheter tubing into the closure (sliding the tube gently in-and-out 1–2 cm to ensure it is not caught). An alternative includes placement between the posterior rectus sheath and the rectus muscle itself. Care must be taken for the surgeon to identify the inferior epigastric artery to avoid damage to this structure. See also Chap. 12 on rectus sheath catheters.

Transverse Incision

The transvserse incision is ideal for the placement of CWI catheters as the transversus abdominis plane can be easily identified and developed by the surgeon by blunt dissection. The catheter can be placed in this plane under direct vision, and using a trocar, be brought out either superiorly or inferiorly to the wound. Several studies have used this method to good effect for subcostal wounds [47, 50, 77]. A similar musculofascial plane has also been used to good effect for the lumbar approach to open nephrectomy [65].

Lower Abdominal Incisions

Much of the research into CWI has been generated in the context of obstetrics and gynaecology [12, 53]. Below the arcuate line the fascia of the obliques and transversus abdominis muscle fuses and passes anteriorly to the rectus muscles. As a result the catheter should be sited between the fascial sheath and peritoneum.

Laparoscopic Surgery

CWI has also been used in laparoscopic surgery. Clearly when laparoscopic surgery is performed entirely through 5 and 10 mm ports CWI is unlikely to be the most appropriate form of analgesia. Several of the RCTs reporting this technique in laparoscopic colorectal surgery adopt similar principals to open surgery within the CWI catheter placed at the specimen extraction site [49, 61, 62]. In this context there has been limited benefit for CWI demonstrated, perhaps as a result of the reduced pain experienced overall in laparoscopic compared with open procedures or the smaller size and placement of the extraction site transversely below the umbilicus [62].

Intra-peritoneal Wound Catheter

Kahokehr et al. have published a RCT detailing the used of intra-peritoneal CWI following major open colorectal surgery [78]. The technique as described by the authors involves bathing the abdominal viscera in 50 ml of 0.9% saline containing 75 mg of ropivacaine following entry into the peritoneal cavity, but prior to the start of intra-abdominal dissection. Following completion of the abdominal dissection, two multi-holed catheters are placed in the respective paracolic gutters, and passed trans-abdominally laterally and distant from the midline wound. Following completion, 0.2% ropivacaine was infused for 68 h post-operatively using an elastomeric pump. Using this technique in an RCT including sixty patients, intraperitoneal CWI was associated with lower pain scores and opioid consumption, and lower levels of measured systemic cytokines compared with a placebo group. Intraperitoneal wound catheters have also been used in ambulatory procedures such as laparoscopic cholecystectomy, however given the low pain profile of these operations the value of CWI may be called into question [79].

Methods of Continuous Delivery of LA

Elastomeric pumps (Fig. 13.1) provide a continuous infusion simply by the sustained internal pressure of elastic recoil of an elastomeric reservoir containing the infusion LA solution. Such devices eliminate the need for an electrical pump thus allowing patients to be ambulatory [80]. Elastomeric pumps allow continuous infusion at a fixed rate over a period of between 24 h to 4 days. Alternatively spring powered pumps provide a similar effect. A study comparing pump types found that electric pumps remained the most accurate whilst both elastomeric and spring operated pumps initially infuse a higher rate than anticipated, and the rate gradually decreases over time [81].

Wound Catheters

Early examples of wound catheters involved the use of simple epidural catheters to deliver LA to the operative site [82]. More recently purpose designed flexible multichannelled perforated 'soaker' catheters (Fig. 13.1) have been developed to provide a more even spread of LA throughout the length of the operative wound [65]. Both types of catheter allow delivery of LA over large incisions [46]. Catheters are available in various sizes to suit different wound lengths and can be trimmed if required. Some catheters have a silver antimicrobial coating however there is little evidence to suggest that this type of catheter prevents infection.

Choice of Local Anaesthetic and Required Flow Rates

The optimum choice of LA and flow rate is currently not known. 0.25% [3, 10, 59] and 0.5% [59] Bupivacaine, 0.25% Levobupivicaine [11, 12, 35], 0.2% [41, 60, 64, 76] and 0.5% Ropivacaine [61, 65] have all been used for CWI. The maximum daily dose should be calculated according to the patients weight and not exceeded. Ropivacaine has been advocated by some authors due to a shorter elimination half life, thereby reducing the chance of systemic toxicity from accumulation of the drug [41]. Following hysterectomy, there was no difference in morphine rescue-analgesia when comparing 0.1% and 0.2% ropivacaine, however the wound catheter was sited in the less efficacious supra-fascial plane [83]. As previously mentioned compound solutions containing adrenaline should be avoided.

Flow rate of LA is important with rates of around 10 ml/h (infusion pressure = 10 psi/517 mmHg) [41] required to provide adequate volume to spread out along the desired plane to provide an analgesic effect [84]. Publications of lower flow rates (2 ml/h 0.5% bupivacaine) have been associated with negative results [63].

In the absence of a detailed head-to-head trial comparing LA types, pharmacokinetics, both 0.2% ropivacaine or 0.25% bupivacaine at a flow rate of 10 ml/h appears to be a reasonable starting point for centres wishing to establish CWI. Most commercially available CWI kits will have predetermined flow rates.

Post Procedure Care

Dedicated pain specialists are ideally placed to manage CWI, however all staff should be trained to recognise insufficient analgesia and be able institute alternatives and/or complementary analgesic modalities. Clear protocols should be widely available to instruct staff less familiar with managing CWI with alternatives in the event of failure and emergency procedures in the event of complications. Although CWI does not necessitate high level nursing care (unlike epidural in some centres), attending medical and nursing staff should be aware of the signs and symptoms of LA toxicity.

Ideally transparent dressings should be used to allow regular monitoring by healthcare staff. Checks of catheter sites and infusion volumes should take place regularly post-operatively. Wound catheters have been kept in situ for varying lengths of time in the literature including up to 4 days post-operatively [76]. Depending on the operative procedure performed, recovery time may be significantly less than this and usually 48–72 h post-operatively is sufficient for CWI to alleviate the period of most severe acute post-operative pain. CWI should not delay full mobilisation or any other part of an enhanced recovery programme.

Wound catheters should be carefully secured to the skin whilst still under general anaesthesia and following completion of the primary operative procedure. Data from a systemic review suggest a catheter displacement rate and/or pump mechanical failure of around 1.1% [85], although outside of the formal well-supervised RCT setting this figure is likely to be higher. Leakages around the catheter site are common and can lead to loosening of dressings. Precautions should be taken in order to limit the chance of accidental displacement. These include patient education (ideally pre-operatively), avoiding tension on tubing by supporting elastomeric pumps in drain bags or slings, and by using surgical tape and epidural-type dressings. In the event of displacement no attempt should be made to reintroduce the wound catheters. Alternative methods of analgesia should be employed in this eventuality.

Top-Tips

- Avoid passing catheters directly through surgical incisions. Tunnelling distant to the wound is recommended.
- Avoid LA with adrenaline in CWI.
- Subfascial/pre-peritoneal placement should be used.
- Flow rate appropriate to the size of the wound (usually 10 ml/h) to allow adequate volume for dispersion along the appropriate plane.
- Pre-operative patient education/awareness is critical to avoid inadvertent catheter dislodgement.
- CWI is unlikely to provide adequate analgesia in isolation, and should be complemented with other analgesic (this is usually multimodal analgesia including morphine PCA for visceral analgesia).

Cost Effectiveness

Few studies have assessed the health economic impact of CWI. One trial demonstrated a €15 cost reduction when using CWI compared with epidural as a result of lower medication costs [35]. A further secondary analysis in open nephrectomy demonstrated an approximate €273 saving associated with CWI, again as a result of a shorter hospital stay [65]. A US based study using CWI in bariatric surgery failed to show any cost benefit [64].

Tileul et al. evaluated the cost effectiveness (calculated taking into account procedural disposables costs, cost of time for insertion and maintenance and critical care/hospital length of stay) of CWI compared to epidural analgesia and morphine PCA after open abdominal surgery. They found the CWI to be equivalent to epidural, with both superior to morphine PCA, regarding analgesia whilst the CWI was more cost-effective than both (CWI arm €6460, Epidural analgesia €7500 and PCA €7273). This was largely due to the CWI group patients requiring less healthcare worker time to manage the intervention compared to the epidural group [83].

Conclusions

CWI extends the analgesic benefit of LA in a controlled way well into the postoperative period. When used in conjunction with other analgesic modalities it can reduce opioid requirements following major abdominal surgery. This opioid-sparing effect and reduction in related side effects is the likely reason for the improved quality of recovery after surgery. Current evidence clearly indicates that the position of the catheter is critical, with data suggesting TAP or subfascial plane placement to be optimal. CWI appears to be safe, although more research is required to better understand pharmacodynamics/kinetics and to avoid LA toxicity from systemic absorption. As elective major abdominal surgery moves towards fast-track enhanced recovery and less invasive approaches, further research is required to understand the position of CWI in this specific context.

Acknowledgements I would like to thank Consultant Anaesthetists Dr. Susan Nimmo and Dr. Craig Beattie, and fellow surgical trainee Mr. Michael J. Hughes for critically reviewing this book chapter.

References

1. Møiniche S, Jørgensen H, Wetterslev J, Dahl JB. Local anesthetic infiltration for postoperative pain relief after laparoscopy: a qualitative and quantitative systematic review of intraperitoneal, port-site infiltration and mesosalpinx block. Anesth Analg. 2000;90:899–912.
2. Barrington MJ, Watts SA, Gledhill SR, Thomas RD, Said SA, Snyder GL, et al. Preliminary results of the Australasian Regional Anaesthesia Collaboration: a prospective audit of more than 7000 peripheral nerve and plexus blocks for neurologic and other complications. Reg Anesth Pain Med. 2009;34:534–41.
3. Baig MK, Zmora O, Derdemezi J, Weiss EG, Nogueras JJ, Wexner SD. Use of the ON-Q pain management system is associated with decreased postoperative analgesic requirement: double blind randomized placebo pilot study. J Am Coll Surg. 2006;202:297–305.

4. Lewis DL, Thompson WAL. Reduction of post-operative pain. Br Med J. 1953;1:973–4.
5. Blades B, Ford WB. A method for control of postoperative pain. Surg Gynecol Obstet. 1950;91:524–6.
6. Gerwig WH, Thompson CW, Blades B. Pain control following upper abdominal operations. AMA Arch Surg. 1951;62:678–82.
7. Levack ID, Holmes JD, Robertson GS. Abdominal wound perfusion for the relief of postoperative pain. Br J Anaesth. 1986;58:615–9.
8. Gibbs P, Purushotham A, Auld C, Cuschieri RJ. Continuous wound perfusion with bupivacaine for postoperative wound pain. Br J Surg. 1988;75:923–4.
9. Chester JF, Ravindranath K, White BD, Shanahan D, Taylor RS, Lloyd-Williams K. Wound perfusion with bupivacaine: objective evidence for efficacy in postoperative pain relief. Ann R Coll Surg Engl. 1989;71:394–6.
10. Fredman B, Zohar E, Tarabykin A, Shapiro A, Mayo A, Klein E, Jedeikin R. Bupivacaine wound instillation via an electronic patient-controlled analgesia device and a double-catheter system does not decrease postoperative pain or opioid requirements after major abdominal surgery. Anesth Analg. 2001;92:189–93.
11. Gupta A, Perniola A, Axelsson K, Thörn SE, Crafoord K, Rawal N. Postoperative pain after abdominal hysterectomy: a double-blind comparison between placebo and local anesthetic infused intraperitoneally. Anesth Analg. 2004;99:1173–9.
12. Ranta PO, Ala-Kokko TI, Kukkonen JE, Ohtonen PP, Raudaskoski TH, Reponen PK, Rawal N. Incisional and epidural analgesia after caesarean delivery: a prospective, placebo-controlled, randomised clinical study. Int J Obstet Anesth. 2006;15:189–94.
13. Givens VA, Lipscomb GH, Meyer NL. A randomized trial of postoperative wound irrigation with local anesthetic for pain after cesarean delivery. Am J Obstet Gynecol. 2002;186:1188–91.
14. Mecklem DW, Humphrey MD, Hicks RW. Efficacy of bupivacaine delivered by wound catheter for post-Caesarean section analgesia. Aust N Z J Obstet Gynaecol. 1995;35:416–21.
15. Zohar E, Fredman B, Phillipov A, Jedeikin R, Shapiro A. The analgesic efficacy of patient-controlled bupivacaine wound instillation after total abdominal hysterectomy with bilateral salpingo-oophorectomy. Anesth Analg. 2001;93:482–7.
16. Lau H, Patil NG, Lee F. Randomized clinical trial of postoperative subfascial infusion with bupivacaine following ambulatory open mesh repair of inguinal hernia. Dig Surg. 2003;20:285–9.
17. Oakley MJ, Smith JS, Anderson JR, Fenton-Lee D. Randomized placebo-controlled trial of local anaesthetic infusion in day-case inguinal hernia repair. Br J Surg. 1998;85:797–9.
18. Sanchez B, Waxman K, Tatevossian R, Gamberdella M, Read B. Local anesthetic infusion pumps improve postoperative pain after inguinal hernia repair: a randomized trial. Am Surg. 2004;70:1002–6.
19. Schurr MJ, Gordon DB, Pellino TA, Scanlon TA. Continuous local anesthetic infusion for pain management after outpatient inguinal herniorrhaphy. Surgery. 2004;136:761–9.
20. Ansaloni L, Agnoletti V, Bettini D, Caira A, Calli M, Catena F, et al. The analgesic efficacy of continuous elastomeric pump ropivacaine wound instillation after appendectomy. J Clin Anesth. 2007;19:256–63.
21. Chan VW, Chung F, Cheng DC, Seyone C, Chung A, Kirby TJ. Analgesic and pulmonary effects of continuous intercostal nerve block following thoracotomy. Can J Anaesth. 1991;38:733–9.
22. Deneuville M, Bisserier A, Regnard JF, Chevalier M, Levasseur P, Hervé P. Continuous intercostal analgesia with 0.5% bupivacaine after thoracotomy: a randomized study. Ann Thorac Surg. 1993;55:381–5.
23. Dowling R, Thielmeier K, Ghaly A, Barber D, Boice T, Dine A. Improved pain control after cardiac surgery: results of a randomized, double-blind, clinical trial. J Thorac Cardiovasc Surg. 2003;126:1271–8.
24. Dryden CM, McMenemin I, Duthie DJ. Efficacy of continuous intercostal bupivacaine for pain relief after thoracotomy. Br J Anaesth. 1993;70:508–10.
25. François T, Blanloeil Y, Pillet F, Moren J, Mazoit X, Geay G, Douet MC. Effect of interpleural administration of bupivacaine or lidocaine on pain and morphine requirement after esophagectomy with thoracotomy: a randomized, double-blind and controlled study. Anesth Analg. 1995;80:718–23.

26. Karakaya D, Baris S, Ozkan F, Demircan S, Gök U, Ustün E, Tür A. Analgesic effects of interpleural bupivacaine with fentanyl for post-thoracotomy pain. J Cardiothorac Vasc Anesth. 2004;18:461–5.
27. White PF, Rawal S, Latham P, Markowitz S, Issioui T, Chi L, et al. Use of a continuous local anesthetic infusion for pain management after median sternotomy. Anesthesiology. 2003;99:918–23.
28. Bianconi M, Ferraro L, Traina GC, Zanoli G, Antonelli T, Guberti A, et al. Pharmacokinetics and efficacy of ropivacaine continuous wound instillation after joint replacement surgery. Br J Anaesth. 2003;91:830–5.
29. Gottschalk A, Burmeister M-A, Radtke P, Krieg M, Farokhzad F, Kreissl S, et al. Continuous wound infiltration with ropivacaine reduces pain and analgesic requirement after shoulder surgery. Anesth Analg. 2003;97:1086–91.
30. Solovyova O, Lewis CG, Abrams JH, Grady-Benson J, Joyce ME, Schutzer SF, et al. Local infiltration analgesia followed by continuous infusion of local anesthetic solution for total hip arthroplasty: a prospective, randomized, double-blind, placebo-controlled study. J Bone Joint Surg Am. 2003;95:1935–41.
31. Löfström B. Aspects of the pharmacology of local anaesthetic agents. Br J Anaesth. 1970;42:194–206.
32. Hollmann MW, Durieux ME. Local anesthetics and the inflammatory response: a new therapeutic indication? Anesthesiology. 2000;93:858–75.
33. Badia J, Whawell S, Scott-Coombes D, Abel PD, Williamson RC, Thompson JN. Peritoneal and systemic cytokine response to laparotomy. Br J Surg. 1996;83:347–8.
34. Sammour T, Kahokehr A, Soop M, Hill AG. Peritoneal damage: the inflammatory response and clinical implications of the neuro-immuno-humoral axis. World J Surg. 2010;34: 704–20.
35. Ozturk E, Yilmazlar A, Coskun F, Isik O, Yilmazlar T, et al. The beneficial effects of preperitoneal catheter analgesia following colon and rectal resections: a prospective, randomized, double-blind, placebo-controlled study. Tech Coloproctol. 2011;15:331–6.
36. Brennan TJ, Zahn PK, Pogatzki-Zahn EM. Mechanisms of incisional pain. Anesthesiol Clin North Am. 2005;23:1–20.
37. Groudine S. Transversus abdominis plane blocks and systemic absorption. Anesth Analg. 2014;119:1002.
38. Latzke D, Marhofer P, Kettner SC, Koppatz K, Turnheim K, Lackner E, et al. Pharmacokinetics of the local anesthetic ropivacaine after transversus abdominis plane block in healthy volunteers. Eur J Clin Pharmacol. 2012;68:419–25.
39. Griffiths JD, Barron FA, Grant S, Bjorksten AR, Hebbard P, Royse CF. Plasma ropivacaine concentrations after ultrasound-guided transversus abdominis plane block. Br J Anaesth. 2010;105:853–6.
40. Ventham NT, Kennedy ED, Brady RR, Paterson HM, Speake D, Foo I, Fearon KC. Efficacy of intravenous lidocaine for postoperative analgesia following laparoscopic surgery: a meta-analysis. World J Surg. 2015;39(9):2220–34.
41. Beaussier M, El'Ayoubi H, Schiffer E, Rollin M, Parc Y, Mazoit JX, et al. Continuous preperitoneal infusion of ropivacaine provides effective analgesia and accelerates recovery after colorectal surgery. Anesthesiology. 2007;107:461–8.
42. Karthikesalingam A. Continuous wound infusion of local anaesthetic agents following colorectal surgery: systematic review and meta-analysis. World J Gastroenterol. 2008;14:5301.
43. Ventham NT, O'Neill S, Johns N, Brady RR, Fearon KC. Evaluation of novel local anesthetic wound infiltration techniques for postoperative pain following colorectal resection surgery: a meta-analysis. Dis Colon Rectum. 2014;57:237–50.
44. Cali RL, Meade PG, Swanson MS, Freeman C. Effect of morphine and incision length on bowel function after colectomy. Dis Colon Rectum. 2000;43:163–8.
45. Hughes MJ, Harrison EM, Peel NJ, Stutchfield B, McNally S, Beattie C, Wigmore SJ. Randomized clinical trial of perioperative nerve block and continuous local anaesthetic infiltration via wound catheter versus epidural analgesia in open liver resection (LIVER 2 trial). Br J Surg. 2015;102(13):1619–28.

46. Thornton PC, Buggy DJ. Local anaesthetic wound infusion for acute postoperative pain: a viable option? Br J Anaesth. 2011;107:656–8.
47. Revie EJ, McKeown DW, Wilson JA, Garden OJ, Wigmore SJ. Randomized clinical trial of local infiltration plus patient-controlled opiate analgesia vs. epidural analgesia following liver resection surgery. HPB (Oxford). 2012;14:611–8.
48. Bertoglio S, Fabiani F, De Negri P, Corcione A, Merlo DF, Cafiero F, et al. The postoperative analgesic efficacy of preperitoneal continuous wound infusion compared to epidural continuous infusion with local anesthetics after colorectal cancer surgery: a randomized controlled multicenter study. Anesth Analg. 2012;115:1442–50.
49. Boulind CE, Ewings P, Bulley SH, Reid JM, Jenkins JT, Blazeby JM, Francis NK. Feasibility study of analgesia via epidural versus continuous wound infusion after laparoscopic colorectal resection. Br J Surg. 2013;100:395–402.
50. Renghi A, Gramaglia L, Casella F, Moniaci D, Gaboli K, Brustia P. Local versus epidural anesthesia in fast-track abdominal aortic surgery. J Cardiothorac Vasc Anesth. 2013;27(3):451–8.
51. Fant F, Axelsson K, Sandblom D, Magnuson A, Andersson SO, Gupta A. Thoracic epidural analgesia or patient-controlled local analgesia for radical retropubic prostatectomy: a randomized, double-blind study. Br J Anaesth. 2011;107:782–9.
52. De Almeida MCS, de Figueiredo LG, Gomes HP, Brunharo GM, Kauling AL. Postoperative analgesia: comparing continuous epidural catheter infusion of local anesthetic and opioid and continuous wound catheter infusion of local anesthetic. Rev Bras Anestesiol. 2011;61:293–303.
53. O'Neill P, Duarte F, Ribeiro I, Centeno MJ, Moreira J. Ropivacaine continuous wound infusion versus epidural morphine for postoperative analgesia after caesarean delivery: a randomized controlled trial. Anesth Analg. 2012;114:179–85.
54. Niraj G, Kelkar A, Jeyapalan I, Graff-Baker P, Williams O, Darbar A, et al. Comparison of analgesic efficacy of subcostal transversus abdominis plane blocks with epidural analgesia following upper abdominal surgery. Anaesthesia. 2011;66:465–71.
55. Ventham NT, Hughes M, O'Neill S, Johns N, Brady RR, Wigmore SJ. Systematic review and meta-analysis of continuous local anaesthetic wound infiltration versus epidural analgesia for postoperative pain following abdominal surgery. Br J Surg. 2013;100:1280–9.
56. Liang C-C, Chang S-D, Wong S-Y, Chang YL, Cheng PJ. Effects of postoperative analgesia on postpartum urinary retention in women undergoing cesarean delivery. J Obstet Gynaecol Res. 2010;36:991–5.
57. Marret E, Remy C, Bonnet F. Meta-analysis of epidural analgesia versus parenteral opioid analgesia after colorectal surgery. Br J Surg. 2007;94:665–73.
58. Rigg JR, Jamrozik K, Myles PS, Silbert BS, Peyton PJ, Parsons RW, et al. Epidural anaesthesia and analgesia and outcome of major surgery: a randomised trial. Lancet. 2002;359:1276–82.
59. Cheong WK, Seow-Choen F, Eu KW, Tang CL, Heah SM. Randomized clinical trial of local bupivacaine perfusion versus parenteral morphine infusion for pain relief after laparotomy. Br J Surg. 2001;88:357–9.
60. Polglase AL, McMurrick PJ, Simpson PJB, Wale RJ, Carne PW, Johnson W, et al. Continuous wound infusion of local anesthetic for the control of pain after elective abdominal colorectal surgery. Dis Colon Rectum. 2007;50:2158–67.
61. Moore SE, Reid KC, Draganic BD, Smith SR. Randomized clinical trial of ropivacaine wound infusion following laparoscopic colorectal surgery. Tech Coloproctol. 2012;16:431–6.
62. Fustran N, Dalmau A, Ferreres E, Camprubí I, Sanzol R, Redondo S. Postoperative analgesia with continuous wound infusion of local anaesthesia vs saline: a double-blind randomized, controlled trial in colorectal surgery. Color Dis. 2015;17:342–50.
63. Wu CL, Partin AW, Rowlingson AJ, et al. Efficacy of continuous local anesthetic infusion for postoperative pain after radical retropubic prostatectomy. Urology. 2005;66:366–70.
64. Medbery RL, Chiruvella A, Srinivasan J, et al. The value of continuous wound infusion systems for postoperative pain control following laparoscopic Roux-en-Y gastric bypass: an analysis of outcomes and cost. Obes Surg. 2014;24:541–8.
65. Forastiere E, Sofra M, Giannarelli D, Fabrizi L, Simone G. Effectiveness of continuous wound infusion of 0.5% ropivacaine by On-Q pain relief system for postoperative pain management after open nephrectomy. Br J Anaesth. 2008;101:841–7.

66. Kushner DM, Lagalbo R, Connor JP, Chappell R, Stewart SL, Hartenbach EM. Use of a bupivacaine continuous wound infusion system in gynecologic oncology: a randomized trial. Obstet Gynecol. 2005;106:227–33.
67. Yndgaard S, Holst P, Bjerre-Jepsen K, Thomsen CB, Struckmann J, Mogensen T. Subcutaneously versus subfascially administered lidocaine in pain treatment after inguinal herniotomy. Anesth Analg. 1994;79:324–7.
68. Rackelboom T, Le Strat S, Silvera S, Schmitz T, Bassot A, Goffinet F, et al. Improving continuous wound infusion effectiveness for postoperative analgesia after cesarean delivery. Obstet Gynaecol. 2010;116:893–900.
69. Gupta A, Favaios S, Perniola A, Magnuson A, Berggren L. A meta-analysis of the efficacy of wound catheters for post-operative pain management. Acta Anaesthesiol Scand. 2011;55:785–96.
70. Richman JM, Liu SS, Courpas G, Wong R, Rowlingson AJ, McGready J, et al. Does continuous peripheral nerve block provide superior pain control to opioids? A meta-analysis. Anesth Analg. 2006;102:248–57.
71. Jankovic Z, Ahmad N, Ravishankar N, Archer F. Transversus abdominis plane block: how safe is it? Anesth Analg. 2008;107:1758–9.
72. Farooq M, Carey M. A case of liver trauma with a blunt regional anesthesia needle while performing transversus abdominis plane block. Reg Anesth Pain Med. 2008;33:273–4.
73. Lancaster P, Chadwick M. Liver trauma secondary to ultrasound-guided transversus abdominis plane block. Br J Anaesth. 2010;104:508–9.
74. Claroni C, Marcelli ME, Sofra MC, Covotta M, Torregiani G, Giannarelli D, Forastiere E. Preperitoneal continuous infusion of local anesthetics: what is the impact on surgical wound infections in humans. Pain Med. 2016;17(3):582–9.
75. Brown L, Morrison A. Local anesthetic infusion pump systems adverse events reported to the food and drug administration. Anesthesiology. 2004;100:1305–12.
76. Corso OH, Morris RG, Hewett PJ, Karatassas A. Safety of 96-hour incision-site continuous infusion of ropivacaine for postoperative analgesia after bowel cancer resection. Ther Drug Monit. 2007;9:57–63.
77. Chan SK, Lai PB, Li PT, Wong J, Karmakar MK, Lee KF, Gin T. The analgesic efficacy of continuous wound instillation with ropivacaine after open hepatic surgery. Anesthesiology. 2010;65:1180–6.
78. Kahokehr A, Sammour T, Shoshtari KZ, Taylor M, Hill AG. Intraperitoneal local anesthetic improves recovery after colon resection: a double-blinded randomized controlled trial. Ann Surg. 2011;254:28–38.
79. Gupta A, Thörn SE, Axelsson K, Larsson LG, Agren G, Holmström B, Rawal N. Postoperative pain relief using intermittent injections of 0.5% ropivacaine through a catheter after laparoscopic cholecystectomy. Anesth Analg. 2002;95:450–6.
80. [No authors listed]. Elastomeric pain pumps. Health Devices 2010;39:366–375.
81. Ilfeld BM, Morey TE, Enneking FK. New portable infusion pumps: real advantages or just more of the same in a different package? Reg Anesth Pain Med. 2004;29:371–6.
82. Zohar E, Shapiro A, Phillipov A, et al. The postoperative analgesic efficacy of wound instillation with ropivacaine 0.1% versus ropivacaine 0.2%. J Clin Anesth. 2004;16:399–404.
83. Tilleul P, Aissou M, Bocquet F, Thiriat N, le Grelle O, Burke MJ, et al. Cost-effectiveness analysis comparing epidural, patient-controlled intravenous morphine, and continuous wound infiltration for postoperative pain management after open abdominal surgery. Br J Anaesth. 2012;108(6):998–1005.
84. Beaussier M, White P, Raeder J. Is a negative meta-analyses consisting of heterogenic studies on wound catheters sufficient to conclude that no additional studies are needed? Acta Anaesthesiol Scand. 2011;56:396–7.
85. Liu SS, Richman JM, Thirlby RC, Wu CL. Efficacy of continuous wound catheters delivering local anesthetic for postoperative analgesia: a quantitative and qualitative systematic review of randomized controlled trials. J Am Coll Surg. 2006;203:914–32.

The Psychological Management of Acute Pain After Abdominal Surgery

14

Mark Rockett

Key Points

1. Effects on pain after abdominal surgery are inferred from experimental pain models and various forms of surgery, particularly arthroplasty, which may involve differing mechanisms.
2. The perception of acute pain is a complex biopsychosocial phenomenon and may not be in proportion to the physiological nociceptive stimulus.
3. In order to assess the impact of non-pharmacological interventions, acute pain should be ideally measured using multivariate scales. As a minimum, two scales could be employed, one assessing intensity (sensory-discriminative) and one unpleasantness (affective-emotional). Psychological interventions tend to reduce the affective component more than the sensory component of pain thus making pain less unpleasant, but not necessarily less intense.
4. It seems likely that at least some psychological interventions act by increasing activity in descending inhibitory pathways.
5. Psychological disorders (anxiety or depression) or non-pathological psychological traits (related to ethnicity and culture, patient beliefs and attributions or expectation) may influence pain perception. Some characteristics of the noxious stimulus itself may impact on pain perception via psychological mechanisms.
6. There is evidence for the role of psychological factors in predicting the severity of pain after abdominal surgery.

M. Rockett
Department of Anaesthesia, Intensive Care and Pain Medicine,
Derriford Hospital, Plymouth, UK
e-mail: mark.rockett@nhs.net

A. Krige, M. J. P. Scott (eds.), *Analgesia in Major Abdominal Surgery*,
https://doi.org/10.1007/978-3-319-94482-1_14

7. Psychological interventions for acute pain may be divided into five broad categories. These are: information giving and expectation manipulation; anxiety reduction and relaxation; hypnosis and guided imagery; distraction or attentional focus; and cognitive-behavioural approaches. Combination approaches seem to be most effective.

Introduction

This chapter reviews the evidence for the psychological management of acute pain, outlining potential mechanisms. Much of the evidence presented is based on either experimental pain or pain in mixed surgical settings. Effects on pain after abdominal surgery must therefore be inferred. The majority of systematic reviews are based on studies of varied surgical populations and much of the clinical work in this field has focused on arthroplasty surgery. Although psychological interventions can be applied to pain of all types, it is clear that the characteristics and implications of pain after major abdominal surgery will be different to that of total knee replacement, for example. After abdominal surgery, coughing and deep breathing often exacerbates pain, whereas pain following arthroplasty relates to weight-bearing and mobilization. Patients expect joint surgery to be painful, and it is likely that this pain will have a relatively neutral or positive attribution, compared to continuous abdominal pain following a non-curative laparotomy for malignant disease.

When considering the impact of psychological interventions on acute pain, it is important to remember that it is a complex biopsychosocial phenomenon. This complexity is reflected in the 1994 International Association for the Study of Pain (IASP) definition: "Pain is an unpleasant sensory and emotional experience associated with actual or potential tissue damage, or described in terms of such damage" [1].

It is important not to confuse pain with nociception, which is the transduction of noxious stimuli into action potentials in the somatosensory nervous system. Without a thorough understanding of the psychological component of pain, it is difficult to predict or understand why a proportion of patients do not respond in the expected manner to pharmacological analgesic techniques.

Our understanding of the biological substrate for these psychological processes has leapt forward in the last few decades thanks largely to techniques such as functional magnetic resonance imaging (fMRI) [2]. The impact of psychological factors such as anxiety, depression and expectation on acute pain perception is now known to be mediated via cortical areas influencing descending inhibitory and excitatory pathways, originating in the midbrain and brainstem, and having a profound effect on nociceptive transmission at the spinal cord level [3].

The Neurobiology of Pain Originating in Abdominal Structures

Following abdominal surgery, nociceptive input reaches the spinal cord from multiple segmental levels and via two types of primary afferent fibres—visceral and somatic.

Nociceptive information from visceral structures is carried mostly in unmyelinated C fibres, running with visceral sympathetic nerves [4]. The majority of visceral afferents are peptidergic and respond to physiological as well as noxious stimuli. Visceral nociceptors respond to stretch, pressure and chemical stimuli such as inflammatory mediators. Inflammation results in peripheral sensitization and recruitment of silent nociceptors—greatly augmenting noxious input to the central nervous system after surgery. Pain from visceral structures tends to be diffuse, dull, and referred to somatic structures sharing the same segmental input. Visceral pain is also associated with autonomic reflexes such as nausea or sweating.

Both Aδ and C fibres innervate somatic abdominal wall structures. Somatic pain is by contrast well localized. Fibres from abdominal structures synapse in Rexed's laminae within the dorsal horn. Neurons synapsing in the superficial dorsal horn are largely peptidergic in nature and ascend via the spinoparabrachial tract to the parabrachial area. From here, connections are made with cortical areas such as the insula and anterior cingulate—thought to represent affective aspects of pain. Fibres from deeper laminae in the dorsal horn (lamina V) receive some input from superficial laminae and ascend via the spinothalamic tract, synapsing in the thalamus before terminating in the somatosensory and motor cortices—representing somatosensory aspects of pain. Somatic abdominal wall structures therefore transmit most of their nociceptive information via the spinothalamic pathway, whereas visceral pain is transmitted via the parabrachial pathway.

Functional imaging studies have revealed that large areas of the cortex are activated during noxious stimulation. The primary (S1) and secondary (S2) somatosensory cortex, the posterior insula and the thalamus are associated with sensory-discriminative processing. The anterior cingulate cortex (ACC), the amygdala, periaqueductal gray area, the anterior insula, and the nucleus accumbens are associated with affective-emotional processing. Frontal areas, including the ACC, are involved in the cognitive appraisal of pain [5].

These anatomically distinct pathways represent the affective-emotional and sensory-discriminative components of pain respectively. It would seem appropriate therefore to measure these components independently [6]. The concept of measuring pain using two scales; one for intensity (sensory-discriminative) and one for unpleasantness (affective-emotional), are relatively underused in acute pain medicine, but is well established in the psychological literature [7]. The importance of this is that psychological interventions tend to impact upon the affective component of pain more than the sensory component. In other words, they make pain less unpleasant, but not necessarily less intense. We could term the beneficial effects of psychological interventions on pain "psychoanalgesia".

The Modulation of Pain: Descending Inhibitory and Facilitatory Pathways

Cortical areas involved in pain perception are linked to descending pathways, which have a potent effect on nociceptive transmission from the spinal cord to brainstem and cortical structures. The major descending pathway begins in the hypothalamus and amygdala, passing to the rostroventromedial medulla and midbrain periaqueductal grey (PAG) [8]. The inhibitory pathway is continuously active, providing tonic inhibition of transmission of information from noxious stimulation. Endogenous analgesia may be increased by prior exposure to noxious stimuli (termed conditioned pain modulation), and the evidence suggests that patients with ineffective descending inhibition are more likely to suffer acute and chronic post-surgical pain [9]. It seems likely that at least some psychological interventions act by increasing activity in descending inhibitory pathways.

The excitatory descending pathway originates in the entorhinal cortex of the hippocampal formation. When anxiety was evoked in an experimental setting, pain intensity from a standardized stimulus was increased, associated with an increase in activity in the hippocampus, cingulate and mid-insula areas [10]. In contrast, the induction of a depressed state increased pain unpleasantness in response to a standard noxious stimulus. Activation in the inferior frontal gyrus and amygdala correlated with the degree of unpleasantness [11].

Despite our improved understanding of the neural substrates of pain and emotion, the concept that patterns of activity within certain brain areas, detected by functional neuroimaging, reflect the activity of a pain specific "neuromatrix" is now being challenged. Current evidence suggests that widespread cortical activation occurs in response to any stimulus which is of high salience, potentially challenging the integrity of the organism, pain being only one of several such stimuli [12, 13].

Psychological Concepts Relevant to Acute Pain

An individual's psychological state may influence their perception of pain in two main ways: via psychological disorders or via non-pathological psychological traits. Examples of the former include clinical anxiety or depression, which may co-exist with and impact upon pain perception. Psychological traits may be related to ethnicity and culture, patient beliefs and attributions or expectation [14]. It is also clear that some characteristics of the noxious stimulus itself may impact on pain perception via psychological mechanisms. The context of pain is a key example of this effect. It may be possible to manipulate some of these factors in the peri-operative period and improve pain outcomes.

Anxiety and Depression

Both anxiety and depression appear to be common in surgical in-patients. Surveys of hospital in-patients have revealed that 30–38% had clinically significant scores on the hospital anxiety and depression scale [15]. Up to 50% of patients demonstrated significant anxiety prior to major gynaecological surgery, but the prevalence of depression mirrored that of the general population. Patients who were anxious before surgery, tended to remain anxious after surgery and this correlated with higher pain scores. High levels of pain and anxiety occurred in roughly one third of patients, and this reached a peak on post-operative day four [16].

Post surgical pain tends to reduce day by day. If pain scores are plotted on the *Y* axis against time on the *X* axis, a pain trajectory with a gradient and intercept can be seen [17]. Interestingly, both depression and anxiety impact on this trajectory. Anxious patients report higher pain scores immediately after surgery, but this resolves more rapidly (steeper gradient). Contrastingly, patients with depression had lower initial pain scores, but pain resolved more slowly (shallower gradient). Both anxiety and depression were associated with increased rates of chronic post surgical pain at 6 months after surgery [18]. The majority of systematic reviews have demonstrated a link between depression and long-term pain and anxiety and acute pain after surgery [19–21].

The Interruptive Nature of Pain

Pain grabs attention, and interrupts other thought processes. The degree to which pain interrupts activity depends upon multiple factors including the emotional significance of the pain and patient factors such as catastrophic thinking [22]. The more patients attend to pain, the worse the interruptions [23]. Repeated pain interruptions may lead to a downward spiral of reduced activity and result in chronic pain (the fear-avoidance model) [24].

Abnormal Thoughts and Beliefs

Incorrect thoughts and beliefs about pain can have a marked effect on perception. In the clinical setting this results in increased post-operative acute and chronic pain. Some patients make unrealistic negative appraisals of internal and external stimuli and expect the worst possible outcome in all situations where pain may occur. This is termed pain catastrophizing and may result in hypervigilance to afferent input—wrongly interpreting innocuous sensations as pain. In addition to increasing perceived acute pain, persistent catastrophic thinking and fear-avoidance results in an increased incidence of chronic pain after surgery and trauma. Meta analysis of outcomes after mixed surgical procedures revealed that both anxiety and catastrophizing resulted in increased chronic post surgical pain [25].

Pain Learning and Memory

Memory for pain and learning from prior pain experiences also impact on the post-operative period. The effect of prior pain experience is dependent upon its context and meaning for the patient. Pain experienced in a positive situation, such as childbirth, is likely to be recalled as less severe than it was reported at the time. Equally, prior pain with a negative connotation, such as surgery for cancer, is recalled as more severe and may have a negative effect on current pain perception [26].

Maladaptive Behaviour

Learned mal-adaptive responses to acute pain, such as avoidance of certain situations due to fear of further pain, result in reduced activity, physical de-conditioning and potentially chronic pain. This is known as fear avoidance [24, 27]. For example: fear-avoidance of movement in the early post-operative period predicted worse functional outcome after spinal surgery six months later [28].

The Context of Pain

That the context of a painful stimulus affects its interpretation is intuitively sensible. However, this concept has not been thoroughly investigated. In an experimental pain study in 2007, the concept of the context of pain was divided into three components [29]. The perceived importance of a noxious stimulus, in terms of its ability to damage tissue, is the evaluative context (or meaning). The temporal context relates to the degree of warning before a stimulus is applied and finally, the attentional focus of the subject to the stimulus is taken into consideration. The noxious stimulus was standardized in all conditions.

When meaning was manipulated, the higher tissue injury condition resulted in pain being perceived as more intense and more unpleasant. For this condition, the pain was also more unpleasant when warning was given. Also, attention to the stimulus increased the intensity of the pain but not unpleasantness.

It would seem, therefore that different aspects of the context of a noxious stimulus have differential effects on the sensory/discriminative and affective/emotional aspects of pain. Some contextual aspects of pain perception, such as attention to pain, may be manipulated in a clinical setting.

Do Psychological Factors Predict Acute Pain After Surgery?

It might be expected that psychological factors will impact on acute and chronic pain after surgery, but the size of any effect is not immediately clear.

There is evidence for the role of psychological factors in predicting the severity of pain after abdominal surgery and, despite large numbers of patients included in meta-analyses, individual studies are often small and of variable quality. In a small sample of patients, both pain catastrophizing and anxiety score predicted acute pain and analgesic use after elective abdominal surgery [30].

The strongest predictors of pain on day 0–4 after mixed day case surgery was the presence of pain before surgery, and the prediction of the clinician for pain after surgery. However, patient expectation of significant pain after surgery and fear of the short-term consequences of the operation were also significant [31].

A systematic review of 48 studies (including 11 of gastrointestinal surgery), involving 23,000 patients revealed a number of significant risk factors for pain and analgesic consumption after surgery. Pre-operative pain, anxiety, age, and type of surgery were the key factors in determining post-operative pain. Post-operative opioid consumption correlated with age, type of surgery and psychological distress (anxiety or depression). Abdominal surgery was correlated with the highest pain scores and the highest opioid intake. However, when used to generate a predictive model, these factors explained only 45% of the variance in pain experience after surgery [21].

A more recent prospective study of 1500 patients undergoing mixed surgical procedures, revealed similar risk factors for moderate to severe pain up to 5 days post-operatively. The most important predictors of pain were pre-operative pain, expected pain, fear of surgery and pain catastrophizing [32].

It would seem that some psychological factors consistently predict moderate or severe acute pain after surgery. However, it is clear that these factors only account for a proportion of the variance in pain experience. Some psychological factors such as anxiety or incorrect expectation of pain may be addressed in the peri-operative period and appropriate management could reduce severe post-operative pain.

Psychological Strategies for Reducing Acute Pain After Abdominal Surgery

Psychological interventions for acute pain may be divided into five broad categories. These are: information giving and expectation manipulation; anxiety reduction and relaxation; hypnosis and guided imagery; distraction or attentional focus; and cognitive-behavioural approaches. In order for any of these approaches to be successful, the patient needs to have confidence in the credibility of the proposed intervention and therapist or mode of delivery [33]. Multiple strategies may be used together as part of a prehabilitation programme including exercise and lifestyle modification [34]. As might be expected in a mixed cohort of patients with differing coping strategies, combination approaches seem to be most effective. For example, a study of pain relief in children after scoliosis surgery (n = 109) found that teaching coping strategies plus information giving was more effective than each strategy alone, and resulted in a mean analgesic effect of 35% [35]

Information and Expectation Manipulation

It is clear that fear of surgery or unrealistic expectations for pain outcomes, correlate with worse post-surgical pain [32]. Prior experience of painful stimuli tends to increase perception of repeated painful stimuli [36]. However, memory for previous painful events depends on the context of that pain, with positive emotional experiences being remembered as less painful [26].

Providing accurate information about the procedure and the recovery period may help to correct abnormal expectations. Providing information about a surgical procedure (procedural information) reduces pre-operative anxiety on average, but seems to have little effect on pain or functional outcome [37].

It is also possible to provide information explaining how the patient may feel after surgery—this could be termed sensory information. A meta-analysis of the impact of several types of psychological intervention, including information giving, found little overall effect for sensory information, but positive effects on pain and analgesia use for procedural information and behavioural instruction [38]. Combining both types of information seems to have the most consistent positive effect, based on a meta analysis of 21 papers, conducted in 1989 [39].

The impact of expectation of treatment effect on pain and analgesia has been nicely demonstrated by a study using a concealed analgesic paradigm. Noxious stimuli were delivered to volunteers who were connected to a concealed infusion of opioid analgesic (remifentanil). Expectancy was controlled by telling the subject that the infusion was either on or off. In the positive expectancy condition, the analgesic infusion was on and the patient was informed that it was on. In the negative expectancy condition, the analgesic infusion was on but the subjects were informed that it was off.

Interestingly, in the positive expectancy condition, the analgesic effect of the infusion was doubled, and contemporaneous fMRI scanning revealed increased activity in the brain areas linked to the descending inhibitory pathway. Similar changes in cortical activity have been found in studies of placebo analgesia. In the negative expectancy condition, the analgesic effect of the infusion was abolished, with fMRI revealing increased activity in the hippocampal area [40].

The ability of endogenous analgesic mechanisms to either double or completely abolish the analgesic effect of a remifentanil infusion serves to highlight the potential impact of expectancy on pain outcomes after abdominal surgery.

Anxiety Reduction and Relaxation

Since anxiety, and in particular anxiety sensitivity, seem to be strongly correlated with severe acute pain and disability after surgery, it would seem likely that anxiety management might prove useful in reducing acute post-surgical pain [21, 41, 42]. Anxiety is defined as a feeling of worry, nervousness, or unease about something with an uncertain outcome. This varies from a normal response to a clinically relevant anxiety disorder. Several tools have been used to assess anxiety; from simple verbal or numerical rating scales to complex questionnaires. There are brief screening questionnaires, such as the GAD-7, for the commonest anxiety disorder (generalized anxiety disorder) [43]. These screening tools may be used clinically to identify patients suffering from significant anxiety.

There may be a concern that pre-operative education or relaxation training may worsen anxiety in anxious patients. However, there is evidence that relaxation training works for patients with different coping styles and therefore may be appropriate for patients with varying degrees of background anxiety [44].

Multiple pharmacological and non-pharmacological methods are available to reduce anxiety, all of which have demonstrated some efficacy in reducing pain unpleasantness (affective component) and/or pain intensity (sensory component), in the post-operative setting.

Pharmacological methods of reducing anxiety in the acute peri-operative period have been evaluated in a number of settings. Gabapentin as a single large preoperative dose had no effect prior to hip joint replacement, but was effective in reducing anxiety and pain catastrophizing in anxious patients undergoing major surgery [45, 46]. These findings question our current practice of avoiding sedative premedication in almost all patients. It is not clear whether gabapentinoid drugs are uniquely effective in this role, or whether alternatives such as benzodiazepines would work equally well.

Relaxation training is designed to induce a state of reduced muscle tension and anxiety. This may include focus on breathing or progressive muscle relaxation.

It may also include the use of relaxing imagery, music and elements of self-hypnosis or meditation [47]. Training may be administered face-to-face or using recorded or written materials. Web-based or application-based tools are ideally suited to this purpose in appropriate patient populations. Whatever techniques are used, they must be practiced by patients prior to surgery, to maximize any effect.

Evidence for the efficacy of relaxation techniques for post-operative pain is patchy and meta analysis limited by methodological shortcomings in many of the studies. There is no clear dose-response relationship for the analgesic effect of relaxation and it is not clear which patients might benefit most from these interventions. Systematic review in 2006 revealed 15 studies (n = 1269), eight of which found some positive results for relaxation. The most frequently effective techniques for post-operative pain were jaw relaxation and systematic relaxation. Progressive muscle relaxation also demonstrated some benefit [47].

The use of music during or after abdominal surgery has demonstrated a reduction in anxiety and/or pain. This effect was found in about 50% of 42 randomised controlled studies in a 2008 systematic review, although the quality of individual studies was poor [48]. Cochrane review and meta-analysis of 51 studies (n = 3663) showed some positive results for pain reduction after surgery using music [49]. Pain scores were 0.5 points lower in patients listening to music than in controls (0–10 scale). Additionally, participants listening to music had a 70% better chance of receiving 50% pain relief than controls, with an NNT of 5 (CI 95% [4; 13], four studies). Opioid requirements in the first 24 h post-operatively were also reduced in the music group (15.4% less morphine, four studies).

Hypnosis and Guided Imagery

When using hypnosis to reduce pain perception, the subject is guided by the hypnotist to respond to suggestions for changes in their subjective experience of pain. Self-hypnosis is also possible where a state of increased response to hypnotic suggestions is induced by the subject alone. It is unclear whether the hypnotic state represents a uniquely altered state of consciousness.

As with many psychological interventions, hypnosis may overlap with other treatments such as suggestion. The following meta-analysis restricted studies to those administering hypnosis pre- and/or post-operatively or during the procedure. Hypnosis had to be provided face to face or via a recording. This 2013 meta-analysis of hypnotic interventions for patients undergoing surgery or medical procedures included 34 RCTs, involving 2597 patients. Effect sizes were measured using Hedges' g parameter, which determines the number of standard deviations between two sample means. An effect size of 0.5 is a medium effect and an effect size of 0.8 is a large effect. Small to medium sized effects were seen for pain (g = 0.44, CI 95% [0.26; 0.61]), emotional distress (g = 0.53, CI 95% [0.37; 0.69]) and medication consumption (g = 0.38, CI 95% [0.2; 0.56]) [50].

Guided imagery in the peri-operative period involves directing the patient's imagination to focus on positive aspects of care. They might visualize the healing process or think positively about the skills of their healthcare team. It is designed to increase the patients' feelings of safety, confidence and empowerment [51].

In a randomized controlled study of patients undergoing elective colorectal surgery, the intervention group received guided imagery prior to surgery and the control group was usual care. Prior to surgery, anxiety scores increased in the control group but decreased in the imagery group. Post-operatively, worst pain, least pain, opioid use and time to bowel function were all significantly lower in the treatment group [52, 53].

Even brief guided imagery interventions seem to have some effect. In a study of day case surgery patients, the intervention was a half-hour CD of guided imagery listened to once prior to surgery. The control group received no guidance. This single blind study revealed lower anxiety and pain scores in the hours after surgery than the control group [54].

Distraction and Attentional Focus

Attention is largely a singular process—a little like a spotlight. We struggle to divide our attention between two tasks (although there is some cultural variation in this ability). Only items which are clearly illuminated by our attentional spotlight enter conscious perception. Pain grabs our attention, and interrupts us from carrying out other simultaneous tasks. It is a stimulus with high salience to the overall integrity of our bodies [12]. If we believe a noxious stimulus is highly salient and harmful, we perceive it as more painful. This process appears to be mediated by structures such as the anterior insula and midcingulate cortex, which are increasingly activated in high threat situations, when subjects are more likely to perceive stimuli as painful [13]. The degree to which painful stimuli monopolize our attention depends upon a number of factors, some related to the stimulus and some related to patient factors. The intensity of pain, its novelty and unpredictability are key stimulus factors. The degree to which we attend to bodily sensations, emotional arousal, pain catastrophizing, the emotional significance of the pain and the presence of distracting tasks are all patient factors which will impact on our attention to, and perception of, noxious stimuli.

If we are able to distract our attention away from a painful stimulus, it is perceived as less severe. Experimental pain studies have demonstrated that a more complex distracting task is more effective at reducing pain perception than a simple neutral task [55]. Virtual reality (VR) provides an interesting new option as a significant distracting stimulus. VR has demonstrated reductions in pain unpleasantness and an additive effect with opioid analgesia in an experimental heat pain model [56]. This approach has also shown analgesic effects in patients suffering from burns [57].

As an alternative to distracting away from pain, some techniques involve shifting attentional focus to the pain, but in a neutral non-judgmental way. This form of observation of sensation in the present moment without judgement is termed mindfulness. Mindfulness meditation involves neutral observation of sensations combined with breathing exercises [58]. Mindfulness and acceptance are currently popular therapies in chronic pain, but may also be applied to acute post-surgical pain [59]. Meta-analysis of mindfulness and acceptance strategies demonstrated superior effects on pain tolerance, but not pain intensity, than other psychological approaches for acute experimental pain (30 RCTs, n = 2085) [60].

Direct comparisons have been made between acceptance-based strategies, distraction and cognitive restructuring in an experimental acute pain study (n = 109) [33]. The variables measured were pain tolerance and pain intensity to a thermal noxious stimulus. Acceptance increased pain tolerance more than cognitive restructuring. Distraction reduced pain intensity more than acceptance. Cognitive restructuring did not differ from acceptance or distraction in its effect on pain intensity.

The mechanism of the analgesic effect of mindfulness is not yet clear but may involve increased sensory processing rather than activation of descending inhibitory pathways [61]. The lack of clinical trials of mindfulness or acceptance in patients undergoing abdominal surgery means we can only extrapolate the findings of experimental pain studies.

Cognitive-Behavioural Approaches

Cognitive-behavioural approaches to pain management are intended to change unhelpful thoughts and behaviours to improve coping with pain. The aim is to reduce the threat value of pain, reduce pain catastrophizing and therefore increase the patient's ability to cope with pain. It is unlikely that these approaches will dramatically reduce pain intensity but may impact upon unpleasantness and reduce pain-related disability in the acute setting.

We are familiar with the use of cognitive behavioural therapy (CBT) in chronic pain management. For chronic pain, CBT has a weak effect on pain severity. It has minimal effects on disability associated with chronic pain but is effective in altering mood outcomes, and there is some evidence that these changes are maintained long term [62]. Generally, CBT for chronic pain involves relatively lengthy sessions over several weeks. To date, no trials of longer term CBT interventions prior to surgery have been completed. However, at least two trials were underway in 2015 in patients prior to joint replacement (ISRCTN 80222865 and clinical trials.gov NCT01772329).

For acute pain management, an ideal CBT intervention could be provided by non-specialists in a brief time-frame. Evidence exists for the efficacy of such interventions in an experimental pain paradigm (heat pain). Subjects received a 5 min training session, when they were taught about the relationship between the sensory, cognitive and emotional responses to pain. They were trained to reduce their stress response to pain by reappraising their situation and focusing on the positive effects of their training. In this small study, pain unpleasantness to the noxious thermal stimulus reduced by 58% and intensity by 38% after CBT training as opposed to 31% and 28% in controls with no training (unpleasantness: $p < 0.05$, severity: non-significant) [63].

This study also provides insight into the potential mechanism of CBT induced analgesia. In the CBT group, secondary mechanical hyperalgesia (due to central sensitization) was reduced by 38% versus an 8% increase in the control group ($p < 0.05$). This finding suggests that central sensitization occurs to a lesser extent following CBT, possibly mediated by an altered balance in descending inhibition and excitation.

Conclusion

It is clear that psychological factors play a role in the perception of post-operative pain. Psychological illnesses, such as anxiety or depression, have an impact on acute pain and the development of chronic pain after surgery. Coping styles also modulate pain perception—in particular patients with high levels of pain catastrophizing are vulnerable to both severe acute and chronic pain after surgery and trauma.

Psychological interventions seem to have a positive effect on both intensity and unpleasantness components of post-surgical pain. However, the evidence is inconsistent despite some studies demonstrating large effect sizes. The use of the mean reduction in pain score as an outcome measure may not provide us with the most useful indicator of efficacy for these interventions. It is likely that some patients will respond to psycho-analgesic techniques and others will not [64]. More research is needed to highlight which patients will benefit most from these approaches. Future research should focus on specific surgical groups and operations, as the psychological impact of different interventions varies greatly.

If the behavioral changes brought about by psychological interventions continue into the post-operative period, it is possible that the development of maladaptive coping strategies such as fear-avoidance will be curtailed, reducing the prevalence of chronic pain after abdominal surgery [24, 65]. This important potential effect of psychological intervention requires further study.

With the growth in interest in peri-operative medicine and streamlining patient journeys through their surgery, pre-operative optimization is becoming standard practice in many centres. Pre-operative psychological assessment and the introduction of an appropriate combination of pain coping strategies including information giving, relaxation and possibly hypnosis and suggestion could be relatively easily integrated into prehabilitation programmes including exercise and lifestyle modification.

References

1. Merskey H, Bogduk N. Classification of chronic. Pain, IASP task force on taxonomy. 2nd ed. Seattle, WA: IASP Press; 1994.
2. Tracey I. Neuroimaging of pain mechanisms. Curr Opin Support Palliat Care. 2007;1(2):109–16.
3. Bee LA, Dickenson AH. The importance of the descending monoamine system for the pain experience and its treatment. F1000 Med Rep. 2009;1:83.
4. Sikandar S, Dickenson AH. Visceral pain: the ins and outs, the ups and downs. Curr Opin Support Palliat Care. 2012;6:17–26.
5. Flor H. Psychological pain interventions and neurophysiology: implications for a mechanism-based approach. Am Psychol. 2014;69(2):188–96.

6. Braz JM, et al. Parallel "pain" pathways arise from subpopulations of primary afferent nociceptor. Neuron. 2005;47(6):787–93.
7. Horn C, et al. Does pain necessarily have an affective component? Negative evidence from blink reflex experiments. Pain Res Manag. 2012;17(1):15–24.
8. Pertovaara A. Descending inhibitory systems. Handb Clin Neurol. 2006;81:179–92.
9. Yarnitsky D. Conditioned pain modulation (the diffuse noxious inhibitory control-like effect): its relevance for acute and chronic pain states. Curr Opin Anaesthesiol. 2010;23:611–5.
10. Ploghaus A, et al. Exacerbation of pain by anxiety is associated with activity in a hippocampal network. J Neurosci. 2001;21(24):9896–903.
11. Berna C, et al. Induction of depressed mood disrupts emotion regulation neurocircuitry and enhances pain unpleasantness. Biol Psychiatry. 2010;67(11):1083–90.
12. Legrain V, et al. The pain matrix reloaded: a salience detection system for the body. Prog Neurobiol. 2011;93(1):111–24.
13. Wiech K, et al. Anterior insula integrates information about salience into perceptual decisions about pain. J Neurosci. 2010;30(48):16324–31.
14. Eccleston C. Role of psychology in pain management. Br J Anaesth. 2001;87(1):144–52.
15. Rockett MP, et al. Characteristics of pain in hospitalized medical patients, surgical patients, and outpatients attending a pain management centre. Br J Anaesth. 2013;110(6):1017–23.
16. Carr EC, Nicky Thomas V, Wilson-Barnet J. Patient experiences of anxiety, depression and acute pain after surgery: a longitudinal perspective. Int J Nurs Stud. 2005;42(5):521–30.
17. Chapman CR, et al. Improving individual measurement of postoperative pain: the pain trajectory. J Pain. 2011;12:257–62.
18. Althaus A, Arranz Becker O, Neugebauer E. Distinguishing between pain intensity and pain resolution: using acute post-surgical pain trajectories to predict chronic post-surgical pain. Eur J Pain. 2014;18(4):513–21.
19. Hinrichs-Rocker A, et al. Psychosocial predictors and correlates for chronic post-surgical pain (CPSP) – a systematic review. Eur J Pain. 2009;13(7):719–30.
20. Phyomaung PP, et al. Are depression, anxiety and poor mental health risk factors for knee pain? A systematic review. BMC Musculoskelet Disord. 2014;15:10.
21. Ip HY, et al. Predictors of postoperative pain and analgesic consumption: a qualitative systematic review. Anesthesiology. 2009;111(3):657–77.
22. Schrooten MG, Karsdorp PA, Vlaeyen JW. Pain catastrophizing moderates the effects of pain-contingent task interruptions. Eur J Pain. 2013;17(7):1082–92.
23. McGowan N, et al. The effect of attentional re-training and threat expectancy in response to acute pain. Pain. 2009;142(1–2):101–7.
24. Crombez G, et al. Fear-avoidance model of chronic pain: the next generation. Clin J Pain. 2012;28(6):475–83.
25. Theunissen M, et al. Preoperative anxiety and catastrophizing: a systematic review and meta-analysis of the association with chronic postsurgical pain. Clin J Pain. 2012;28(9):819–41.
26. Babel P, Pieniazek L, Zarotynski D. The effect of the type of pain on the accuracy of memory of pain and affect. Eur J Pain. 2015;19(3):358–68.
27. Leeuw M, et al. The fear-avoidance model of musculoskeletal pain: current state of scientific evidence. J Behav Med. 2007;30(1):77–94.
28. Archer KR, et al. Early postoperative fear of movement predicts pain, disability, and physical health six months after spinal surgery for degenerative conditions. Spine J. 2014;14(5):759–67.
29. Moseley GL, Arntz A. The context of a noxious stimulus affects the pain it evokes. Pain. 2007;133(1–3):64–71.
30. Granot M, Ferber SG. The roles of pain catastrophizing and anxiety in the prediction of post-operative pain intensity: a prospective study. Clin J Pain. 2005;21(5):439–45.
31. Gramke HF, et al. Predictive factors of postoperative pain after day-case surgery. Clin J Pain. 2009;25(6):455–60.
32. Sommer M, et al. Predictors of acute postoperative pain after elective surgery. Clin J Pain. 2010;26(2):87–94.

33. Kohl A, Rief W, Glombiewski JA. Acceptance, cognitive restructuring, and distraction as coping strategies for acute pain. J Pain. 2013;14(3):305–15.
34. Berge DJ, et al. Pre-operative and post-operative effect of a pain management programme prior to total hip replacement: a randomized controlled trial. Pain. 2004;110(1–2):33–9.
35. LaMontagne LL, et al. Cognitive-behavioral intervention effects on adolescents' anxiety and pain following spinal fusion surgery. Nurs Res. 2003;52(3):183–90.
36. Galak J, Meyvis T. The pain was greater if it will happen again: the effect of anticipated continuation on retrospective discomfort. J Exp Psychol Gen. 2011;140(1):63–75.
37. Louw A, et al. Preoperative education addressing postoperative pain in total joint arthroplasty: review of content and educational delivery methods. Physiother Theory Pract. 2013;29(3):175–94.
38. Johnston M, Vogele C. Benefits of pscyhological preparation for surgery: a meta analysis. Ann Behav Med. 1993;15:245–56.
39. Suls J, Wan CK. Effects of sensory and procedural information on coping with stressful medical procedures and pain: a meta-analysis. J Consult Clin Psychol. 1989;57(3):372–9.
40. Bingel U, et al. The effect of treatment expectation on drug efficacy: imaging the analgesic benefit of the opioid remifentanil. Sci Transl Med. 2011;3(70):70ra14.
41. Keogh E, et al. Predicting pain and disability in patients with hand fractures: comparing pain anxiety, anxiety sensitivity and pain catastrophizing. Eur J Pain. 2010;14(4):446–51.
42. Payne LA, et al. Relationship of neuroticism and laboratory pain in healthy children: does anxiety sensitivity play a role? Pain. 2013;154(1):103–9.
43. Spitzer RL, et al. A brief measure for assessing generalized anxiety disorder: the GAD-7. Arch Intern Med. 2006;166(10):1092–7.
44. Miro J, Raich RM. Effects of a brief and economical intervention in preparing patients for surgery: does coping style matter? Pain. 1999;83(3):471–5.
45. Clarke H, et al. Gabapentin does not reduce preoperative anxiety when given prior to total hip arthroplasty. Pain Med. 2010;11(6):966–71.
46. Clarke H, et al. Gabapentin reduces preoperative anxiety and pain catastrophizing in highly anxious patients prior to major surgery: a blinded randomized placebo-controlled trial. Can J Anaesth. 2013;60(5):432–43.
47. Kwekkeboom KL, Gretarsdottir E. Systematic review of relaxation interventions for pain. J Nurs Scholarsh. 2006;38(3):269–77.
48. Nilsson U. The anxiety- and pain-reducing effects of music interventions: a systematic review. AORN J. 2008;87(4):780–807.
49. Cepeda MS, et al. Music for pain relief. Cochrane Database Syst Rev. 2006;2:CD004843.
50. Tefikow S, et al. Efficacy of hypnosis in adults undergoing surgery or medical procedures: a meta-analysis of randomized controlled trials. Clin Psychol Rev. 2013;33(5):623–36.
51. Nelson EA, et al. Systematic review of the efficacy of pre-surgical mind-body based therapies on post-operative outcome measures. Complement Ther Med. 2013;21:697–711.
52. Tusek DL, et al. Guided imagery: a significant advance in the care of patients undergoing elective colorectal surgery. Dis Colon Rectum. 1997;40(2):172–8.
53. Tusek DL, Cwynar RE. Strategies for implementing a guided imagery program to enhance patient experience. AACN Clin Issues. 2000;11(1):68–76.
54. Gonzales EA, et al. Effects of guided imagery on postoperative outcomes in patients undergoing same-day surgical procedures: a randomized, single-blind study. AANA J. 2010;78(3):181–8.
55. Bantick SJ, et al. Imaging how attention modulates pain in humans using functional MRI. Brain. 2002;125(Pt 2):310–9.
56. Hoffman HG, et al. The analgesic effects of opioids and immersive virtual reality distraction: evidence from subjective and functional brain imaging assessments. Anesth Analg. 2007;105(6):1776–83.
57. Hoffman HG, et al. Virtual reality as an adjunctive non-pharmacologic analgesic for acute burn pain during medical procedures. Ann Behav Med. 2011;41(2):183–91.
58. Chiesa A, Serretti A. A systematic review of neurobiological and clinical features of mindfulness meditations. Psychol Med. 2010;40(8):1239–52.

59. McCracken LM, Gauntlett-Gilbert J, Vowles KE. The role of mindfulness in a contextual cognitive-behavioral analysis of chronic pain-related suffering and disability. Pain. 2007;131(1–2):63–9.
60. Kohl A, Rief W, Glombiewski JA. How effective are acceptance strategies? A meta-analytic review of experimental results. J Behav Ther Exp Psychiatry. 2012;43(4):988–1001.
61. Gard T, et al. Pain attenuation through mindfulness is associated with decreased cognitive control and increased sensory processing in the brain. Cereb Cortex. 2012;22(11):2692–702.
62. Eccleston C, Williams AC, Morley S. Psychological therapies for the management of chronic pain (excluding headache) in adults. Cochrane Database Syst Rev. 2009;2:CD007407.
63. Salomons TV, et al. A brief cognitive-behavioural intervention for pain reduces secondary hyperalgesia. Pain. 2014;155(8):1446–52.
64. Moore A, et al. Expect analgesic failure; pursue analgesic success. BMJ. 2013;346:f2690.
65. Denison E, Åsenlöf P, Lindberg P. Self-efficacy, fear avoidance, and pain intensity as predictors of disability in subacute and chronic musculoskeletal pain patients in primary health care. Pain. 2004;111:245–52.

Chronic Pain: The Peri-operative Management of Chronic Pain Patients and Chronic Pain After Abdominal Surgery

15

Robert Searle and Nicholas Marshall

Key Points

1. Although the diagnostic criteria are not standardised the incidence of development of chronic postsurgical pain following abdominal surgery can be relatively high.
2. It is a serious complication with significant effects on quality of life and develops at variable time after surgery, often more than 6 months.
3. Management is aimed at preventing the development of new chronic postsurgical pain (correlated with the intensity of acute pain) by optimizing multimodal analgesia and optimally managing acute post-operative pain in existing chronic pain patients.
4. For the latter group this requires careful pre-operative planning between clinicians and acute pain teams to prevent withdrawal from any chronic opiate medication and effectively monitor and manage their acute post-operative pain.
5. Although evidence is lacking regarding the optimal analgesic techniques in this patient group it seems sensible to maximise the use of non-opioid analgesics and regional techniques due to their opiate tolerance.

Introduction

Chronic postsurgical pain is increasingly recognised as one of the most common and serious complications after surgery with significant impact for patients regarding their medication use, functional status, quality of life and healthcare utilization. Patients who undergo abdominal surgery are at risk of developing chronic pain as a result of surgery. Whilst it is often assumed the risk of developing chronic pain is restricted to those undergoing major procedures, it can be a problem even after

R. Searle · N. Marshall (✉)
Department of Anaesthesia, Royal Cornwall Hospital, Cornwall, UK
e-mail: nicholas.marshall@nhs.net

A. Krige, M. J. P. Scott (eds.), *Analgesia in Major Abdominal Surgery*,
https://doi.org/10.1007/978-3-319-94482-1_15

minor surgery. Chronic pain has been described as "the most serious long term problem after repair of an inguinal hernia" [1].

There is no universally agreed definition of chronic postsurgical pain, however the working definition proposed by Macrae and adopted by the International Association of the Study of Pain (IASP) has been commonly used [2, 3]. This defined chronic postsurgical pain as pain developing after a surgical procedure, of at least 2 months duration, and where other causes of pain have been excluded (such as on-going infection, malignancy or pain continuing from a pre-existing cause).

More recently, following improvements in the understanding of the pathophysiology and presentation of chronic postsurgical pain, an updated definition has been proposed [4].

Proposed Diagnostic Criteria for Chronic Postsurgical Pain [4]

- Pain develops after a surgical procedure or increases in intensity after the surgical procedure.
- Pain should be of at least 3–6 months duration and significantly affect the HR-QOL.
- Pain is either a continuation of acute post-surgical pain, or develops after an asymptomatic period.
- The pain is either localised to the surgical field, projected to the innervation territory of a nerve situated in a surgical field, or referred to a dermatome (after surgery in deep or visceral tissues).
- Other causes of the pain should be excluded (such as infection or malignancy).

Although it is likely that there will be a move towards more standardised outcome measures, it is important to realise that a lack of clarity in the definition of chronic postsurgical pain is likely to have contributed to the wide variations in the reported incidence of these problems. The incidence of chronic postsurgical pain following abdominal surgery is presented in Table 15.1 [5–10].

In one of the largest epidemiological studies of chronic postsurgical pain so far, using population based data from Norway, researchers found that the overall prevalence of postsurgical pain from abdominal and pelvic surgery was 20.3% [11]. The results for specific types of surgery were: Intestinal surgery 25%, Inguinal hernia repair 30% and gallbladder surgery 41%.

Table 15.1 The incidence of chronic postsurgical pain following abdominal surgery

Type of surgery	Incidence of chronic pain
Inguinal hernia repair	0–53% (5)
Cholecystectomy	5–50% (6)
Laparotomy	18–25% (7, 8)
Laparoscopic colorectal surgery	17% (9)
Donor nephrectomy	21% (10)

The natural history of chronic postsurgical pain following abdominal surgery is not well studied. There is some evidence that the natural course of chronic postsurgical pain improves with time, however it can take many years [12]. In one study of inguinal hernia repair, 65% of patients with chronic pain at 6 months were pain free after 5 years [13]. However, the study also found that a significant proportion (69%) of patients with pain at 5 years did not have pain at 6 months. This suggests that while for some patients chronic postsurgical pain represents a continuum of pain symptoms from the acute surgical insult into the chronic period, for others chronic pain develops after an initial pain free postsurgical period of 6 months or longer.

Risk Factors and Predictors for Chronic Postsurgical Pain After Abdominal Surgery

A number of risk factors and associations have been identified for the development of chronic postsurgical pain, and they can broadly be divided into pre-operative, intra-operative and post-operative factors.

Age has a variable effect on chronic pain after hernia surgery. In adults, increasing age reduces the risk of chronic pain, whereas children seem to have a lower incidence than adults [14–16]. Similar age related patterns are evident in other types of surgery (such as thoracic surgery). Female gender is another demographic factor associated with the development of chronic pain after abdominal surgery [7]. Pre operative pain at the surgical site seems to be a significant independent risk factor for some forms of abdominal surgery such as hernia repair [17]. Psychological traits seem to be important risk factors for some types of surgery, but not for others. Chronic pain after cholecystectomy is associated with premorbid depression, psychological vulnerability and anxiety, but these seem less important for procedures such as inguinal hernia repair [17, 18]. However, results are likely to be affected by factors such as the timing of the administered questionnaires and the implications of the surgery (e.g. cancer surgery compared to non-cancer procedures). Certainly there seems to be a pattern whereby psychological factors play a more important role when surgery is performed for more complex health problems. It may however be more helpful to consider an individuals typical emotional reaction to adversity rather than their immediate pre-operative emotional status. So, if an individual is prone to catastrophizing this may be more relevant than feelings of anxiety prior to an operation. Interestingly, for children, parent catastrophizing appears to be a risk factor for the development of chronic postsurgical pain [19].

Genetic factors almost certainly play a role in the development of chronic postsurgical pain although the picture is far from clear. There is some evidence that opioid receptor genotype is associated with the development of chronic pain after abdominal surgery, and that genetic polymorphism in some enzymes (such as catechol-O-methyltransferase) may influence the development of chronic pain states in other parts of the body, but not after abdominal surgery [20, 21]. However, disappointingly, attempts to identify reliable predictors for the development of chronic postsurgical pain in a cohort of hernia repair, hysterectomy and thoracotomy patients by studying 90 genetic markers failed to identify a genetic predisposition [22].

Whilst reliable genetic risk factors have yet to be fully identified, there are aspects of individual's pain phenotype that show some predictive qualities. We know that central nervous system descending pain pathways are important in modulating pain signals in the spinal cord. Some individuals seem to have more effective descending inhibitory pain pathways than others, and this can be tested in a laboratory setting using a Diffuse Noxious Inhibitory Control (DNIC) paradigm. Briefly, this tests pain thresholds (such as a heat stimulus to the forearm) before and after a conditioning painful stimulus to the other hand. The heat stimulus is applied to the forearm and pain intensity measured. This is then repeated following the conditioning stimulus. In patients with a well functioning descending inhibitory pathway, the painful conditioning stimulus triggers modulation of ascending pain pathways such that when the heat stimulus is reapplied to the forearm, the pain intensity generated is less. This is described as conditioned pain modulation, and there is evidence of a correlation between this innate ability to modulate pain signals and the development of chronic postsurgical pain. Yarnitsky et al. [23] showed that for each 10/100 reduction in test pain scores due to conditioning, the chance of acquiring chronic pain after thoracic surgery were halved.

Whilst testing the effectiveness of individuals pain physiology may not be practical in a clinical setting, if an individuals physiological make up means they are prone to developing pain problems, the presence of other chronic pain conditions may be a risk factor for the development of chronic postsurgical pain. Wylde et al. [24] showed that if patients had one or two pre-existing chronic pain problems, their odds of developing chronic postsurgical pain were raised (OR 2.6). If they had five or more chronic pain problems they were even more likely to develop chronic postsurgical pain (OR 14.8) [24].

Intra-operative surgical factors understandably influence the development of chronic postsurgical pain. As shown in Table 15.1, different types of surgery have different rates of persistent postsurgical pain. Surgery where there is a high risk of damaging major nerves appears to have a higher incidence of chronic pain. Examples include thoracic surgery (intercostal nerves), breast surgery (intercostobrachial nerves) and inguinal hernia repair (inguinal nerves). Nerves can become damaged both at the time of operation and also later in the healing process, either as part of an inflammatory mediated neuropathy or as part of the mechanical or fibrotic response to scar tissue formation. Surgical approaches that minimise trauma, such as laparoscopic techniques used for cholecystectomy and hernia repair may therefore reduce the risk of chronic pain developing [17]. Other surgical factors that may influence the development of chronic pain include the duration of operation (with longer operations having more risk) and the expertise of the surgeon [25]. The indication for surgery may also influence outcomes, with redo surgery for post-operative peritonitis and inflammatory bowel disease both identified as risk factors for the development of chronic pain after laparoscopic colorectal surgery [9].

Post-operative predictors of the development of chronic pain mainly seem to be related to the acute pain experience in the immediate post-operative period. The intensity of acute post-operative pain is consistently associated with the development of chronic pain problems. Patients who experience poorly controlled post-operative pain are more likely to develop chronic pain following a number of different types of surgery, including surgery on the abdomen [17]. It is likely that sensitization of both peripheral and central nervous system nociceptive pathways can be triggered by an intense and prolonged painful stimulus, such as poorly controlled post-operative pain. Acute pain descriptors have also been shown to be of some value in predicting those at risk of developing chronic pain. In particular, acute pain with features suggestive of a neuropathic element has been shown to be a risk factor for developing chronic pain from a number of different types of surgery, with positive scores from neuropathic screening tools such as the LANSS and DN4 having some predictive value [26, 27]. It might be assumed that as neuropathic pain descriptors in the post-operative period are predictive of chronic postsurgical pain, objective evidence of nerve damage may also be of value. However, quantitative sensory testing (QST) in the post-operative period does not appear to be as helpful. Indeed in the chronic pain setting, sensory changes elicited by QST are common, but in both those with chronic pain and those who are pain free.

Prevention of Chronic Pain After Abdominal Surgery

Having identified the extent to which chronic pain after surgery is a problem, attention has turned to developing interventions that prevent or reduce the risk of this problem occurring. Sadly, the only definitive way of preventing chronic pain developing is to not have surgery. Whilst this may not be an option for some, for those having surgery for non-life threatening conditions, or conditions that may be treated by other means, declining surgery is a possibility. For either group, the consent process should include a discussion of the risks and benefits of surgery, including the possibility of developing chronic pain and the impact this may have on quality of life. This may be particularly relevant for those elderly patients undergoing arthroplasty surgery for pain relief as opposed to poor function.

A variety of peri-operative interventions have been studied with the aim of preventing the development of chronic postsurgical pain, but in general, the evidence is conflicting, with small sample sizes and heterogenous study design making firm conclusions difficult.

In theory, regional anaesthetic techniques should offer the best hope of preventing some of the central nervous system changes thought to be involved in the development of chronic pain after surgery, such as wind-up and central sensitisation. Indeed, there is some evidence that both epidural and spinal anaesthetic techniques may help prevent chronic pain after abdominal surgery, although the picture is by no means conclusive. One study showed that patients undergoing colonic resection (for cancer) who received intra-operative epidural analgesia had less chronic postsurgical pain than those receiving either intravenous analgesia or post-operative epidural treatment [28]. Other studies of patients undergoing open abdominal surgery have shown that when compared to GA alone, GA and epidural analgesia roughly halved the incidence of post-operative pain at 6 months [29]. Spinal anaesthesia for patients having gynaecological surgery or Caesarean section also seems to reduce the risk of developing chronic postsurgical abdominal pain, when compared to general anaesthesia [30, 31].

Another avenue of investigation into preventing chronic postsurgical pain has been pharmacotherapy. Types of analgesic and anaesthetics have both been examined, with some evidence that both may influence the development of chronic pain.

Intense, repeated or sustained nociceptive input (such as one might expect with poorly controlled post-operative pain) results in activity dependent central nervous system sensitisation via the activation of NMDA receptors, which in turn contribute to the maintenance of this sensitised pain state. Therefore, NMDA receptor antagonists have been the target of chronic postsurgical pain investigation focused on prevention. The results of a meta-analysis of 14 studies evaluating ketamine given for a variety of surgical procedures suggests that it may have a preventive effect, although most studies were of small sample size, with differing doses and duration of treatment [32]. Nevertheless, the authors concluded that peri-operative ketamine, if given for more than 24 h, reduced the incidence of pain at 3 and 6 months following surgery, with a NNT of about 10 for preventing moderate to severe chronic pain at 6 months [32].

Nitrous Oxide is also an NMDA receptor antagonist, and a single centre sub-group analysis of patients recruited to the ENIGMA study found that the incidence of chronic pain in the group randomised to 70% intra-operative nitrous oxide was about half that of the nitrous oxide free group (a median of 4.5 years after surgery) [33]. Of note in this study was that the surgery performed was mainly abdominal. In contrast, the intra-operative use of remifentanil has demonstrated a dose dependent relationship with the development of chronic pain 1 year after sternotomy surgery where the risk of chronic pain was increased in proportion to the dose of remifentanil given [34].

The gabapentinoids, pregabalin and gabapentin, have also been widely studied. Although the mechanism of action is not completely understood for these drugs, they appear to bind to a subunit of voltage gated calcium channels in the central nervous system. These channels modulate the release of excitatory neurotransmitters involved in nociception and may also block new synaptic formation. Theoretically this might be one mechanism by which the incidence of chronic postsurgical pain is reduced. Despite these theoretical reasons why the gabapentinoids might be helpful, and positive results from some studies, metanalysis of available studies have failed to demonstrate clear effects on the development of chronic postsurgical pain [32, 35, 36]. Part of the difficulty in analysing the data is that different doses, timing and duration of therapy are used in studies, and investigations with negative outcomes have not always been published [35, 37].

As psychological factors are thought to be risk factors in developing chronic pain after surgery, interventions to modify anxiety, catastrophizing or other unhelpful psychological conditions pre-operatively may have a role in preventing chronic pain. There is a lack of research to support this, although studies investigating interventions such as mindfulness have been registered [38].

Peri-operative Management of Patients with Chronic Pain

Acute post-operative pain is multifactorial and due to activation of nociceptors from tissue injury, leading to inflammation and ischaemia of these tissues as part of an inflammatory cascade [39]. This means that if a patient has abdominal surgery then a multimodal approach to analgesia is required to treat the anatomical and physiological disturbance cause by surgery. Ensuring and choosing the most appropriate pain relief can be challenging, especially when there are a multitude of options available. This is especially challenging when treating those patients who already have chronic pain, and who may be having surgery as a result of their chronic pain complaint, or due to a separate pathology.

Additional Acute Pain Challenges in Chronic Pain Patients

Analgesic control after abdominal surgery presents extra challenges in chronic pain patients, who are not opiate naive, may be on a large list of medications, and have established psychological and emotional responses to painful stimuli. In the acute pain setting four main groups of opioid tolerant patients are encountered [40].

- Patients who have prescribed opiates for cancer pain. These patients may be in palliation, remission or receiving active treatment (for example abdominal surgery).
- Patients who have prescribed opiates for chronic non-cancer pain (CNCP).
- Patients with a substance use disorder. This can be illicit drug use or those on an opioid maintenance treatment programme.
- Patients who have developed acute or subacute opioid tolerance due to peri operative or post-operative opioid administration.

Patients who are on long term opioids usually have significantly higher post-operative requirements than those who are opioid naïve [41]. This is in part due to tolerance, where the dose response curve for opioids has shifted to the right, with increased doses needed to achieve a desired response or effect. There is also evidence for a phenomenon known as opioid-induced hyperalgesia (OIH) [42], where there is an amplified response to normal painful stimulus as a result of taking opioids. This has also been described as a state of nociceptive sensitization caused by exposure to opioids. The evidence for clinical OIH is limited, one reason being that increases in pain in patients on long term opioids, for example those with cancer, could be due to disease progression or indeed tolerance. There is evidence that OIH can develop acutely due to high dose intra-operative fentanyl or remifentanil [42]; however, it is often difficult to tease apart whether the results indicate OIH, or tolerance, or a combination of both. The contribution played by tolerance and OIH to increased pain experienced by this group of patients is unknown. However, it is clear that opioid tolerant patients will often not respond to intra-operative opioids as expected. This may lead to the situation where it is challenging for a health care professional to decide whether a patient needs increased doses of opioids (tolerance) or will actually respond better to dose reductions (OIH).

Opioid tolerant patients not only require higher doses of opioids but they report higher pain scores and require input from acute pain teams for longer [41]. Post-operative pain takes longer to resolve and they have longer lengths of stay in hospital and higher rates of readmission [43].

Principles

Management of patients with chronic pain having abdominal surgery should begin as early as possible in the surgical pathway. Ideally they should be identified at a pre-operative assessment clinic followed by a collaborative approach involving the acute pain, anaesthesia and surgical teams ensuring continuity of care. The goals of peri-operative management are to aim for adequate peri-operative analgesia, prevent drug withdrawal syndromes and support any social, psychiatric and behavioral issues the patient may present with. In-patient admissions can be challenging for both the patient and staff, and the wider pain team can offer reassurance and set realistic treatment goals and expectations for patients that may be on a complicated combination of pain relieving medication.

Pre-operative Management

It is vital to carry out a full pre-operative assessment paying particular attention to the correct doses of current medication, previous operations and their pain management, as well as the patient's current expectations. Occasionally it may only become apparent that a patient is opioid tolerant in the post-operative period when surgical pain is difficult to manage. It may be difficult to verify the doses of particular drugs but if possible the GP or pharmacist should be contacted or a prescription visualised. Occasionally medication may be prescribed by a third party (homeless shelter with GP access or drug treatment centre) and contacting them may not be easy, especially if information is needed out of hours. If a patient presents out of hours, or as an emergency, it is important to give enough opioid to avoid the risk of withdrawal (the dose required to prevent this is normally 25% of their daily dose and is known as the detoxification dose) [44]. If the dose is not known one method is to give the reported daily dose in up to four divided doses whilst monitoring the patients conscious level and respiratory rate [40].

In order to prevent withdrawal after elective or routine surgery it is important that regular opioids and other pain medication are prescribed and given on the day of surgery. Alternatively substitution of one opioid with another, or the same opioid by an alternative route of administration, should be prescribed. There may be reasons why certain drugs are omitted but this should be the exception and not the rule. Those patients on opioid replacement programmes may need to be given their daily dose prior to surgery so that they can take it pre-operatively in hospital. Those patients on opioid replacement programmes (methadone or buprenorphine) pose particular challenges, where the choice of management may depend on the dose of medication the patient is taking, the proposed surgery and period of nil by mouth [45].

Methadone Management

Methadone is a long acting opioid agonist, usually prescribed once daily with a dose range of 50–120 mg. It is used in patients with opioid addiction and in the doses described is sufficient to suppress the symptoms of opioid withdrawal. The drug does have an analgesic action, however, this effect is much shorter than that of withdrawal suppression [45]. Therefore, if given in divided doses (twice or three times a day) there may be a better analgesic effect.

If a patient admitted for surgery is taking methadone then this should be continued if possible. When the surgery precludes taking the methadone orally then conversion to parenteral methadone or another opioid will be required. Parenteral methadone doses have been calculated to be 0.7 of the oral dose [46]. Dosing regimes are also available for SC, IM and continuous infusions [45, 47].

Buprenorphine Management

Buprenorphine is a partial opioid agonist. It is usually prescribed in sublingual doses of 8–32 mg for the treatment of opioid addiction [48]. With a terminal half-life of 28 h it is sufficient to give once a day, or even every second day, to prevent the symptoms of withdrawal. It is also prescribed (as patches) in the treatment of chronic pain conditions.

Pharmacologically there are two approaches that could be taken in the peri-operative management of those taking buprenoprhine. Taking into account the neuropharmacology and the dose that the patient is taking, the first is to stop the drug, and the second is to continue it [49].

Patients taking low dose buprenorphine (200–400 μg) for the management of chronic pain has some opioid receptors that are not occupied, therefore, higher doses of full agonists could be used for analgesia.

In those taking high dose buprenorphine (16–32 mg) for substitution therapy there will be full receptor occupancy, and full agonists will not be able to easily achieve analgesia. In this situation, if elective surgery were planned, then it would seem appropriate that the buprenorphine should be withheld and substituted with an alternative opioid (e.g. methadone). However, recent evidence supports continuing the drug and managing as any other opioid tolerant patient [50].

Intra-operative Management

The appropriate amount of intra-operative opioid may be very difficult to judge but it is likely that requirements will be much higher than anticipated [41]. The same approach of titrating opioids to respiratory rate that is used in opioid naive patients for spontaneously breathing techniques can still be used. Likewise when a patient has required paralysis for ventilation aiming for a respiratory rate of 8–10 at the end of the operation is a good starting point. The use of multimodal techniques (adjuvant drugs and regional techniques) should be considered where appropriate and these will be discussed later [47].

Post-operative Management

Treatment of acute pain in the post-operative period is often the most challenging time for opioid tolerant patients. It requires a structured approach and reassurance of both the patient and staff. Standard drug protocols may not be sufficient, and multimodal strategies and polypharmacy may be required to establish adequate pain management. This may lead to the need for higher levels of monitoring than anticipated. Post-operative pain scores are likely to be higher and difficult to interpret, therefore, assessment of dynamic measures of pain (coughing, deep inspiration) become even more important [51]. Priority should be given to those analgesic techniques that are known to be opioid sparing.

Non-opioid Adjuvants

The following selection of drugs have been used in acute pain and studied in many different types of operations. This heterogeneity and the fact that few studies have been carried out in the chronic pain population makes drawing conclusions difficult. However, many of the drugs have shown benefit in certain patient groups and show promise for future research and further development.

- Simple analgesics: regular simple analgesics (paracetamol, NSAIDS) should be prescribed unless contra-indicated.
- Ketamine (see Chap. 5) is an NMDA antagonist that is known to improve pain relief after surgery in opioid tolerant patients [52]. It has benefits in both the intra- and post-operative periods. The NMDA receptor is thought to have a role in tolerance and OIH and a reduction in the incidence, associated with intra-operative remifentanil use, has been shown [53]. Intra-operative boluses (up to 0.5 mg/kg) followed by low dose infusions of 0.1 mg/kg/h seem to offer opioid sparing effects with a reduction in hallucinations and dysphoria. The effect of ketamine in opioid tolerant patients undergoing a variety of surgeries has been studied, concluding that particular benefit was observed in painful procedures, including upper abdominal, thoracic, and major orthopaedic surgeries [54]. A Cochrane review (that has subsequently been withdrawn due to being outdated) concluded that peri-operative ketamine reduced 24-h morphine consumption and PONV [55]. However, a new review with the objectives to evaluate the efficacy and tolerability of ketamine administered intravenously during general anaesthesia or peri-operatively for the treatment or prevention of acute post-operative pain in adult patients is underway. One study showed that intra-operative ketamine (bolus plus infusion) reduced pain scores and opioid requirements in the first 48 h and at 6 weeks. Ketamine related adverse effects were mild or absent [56].

The general conclusion is that peri-operative ketamine use in opioid tolerant patients results in a reduction in pain scores. This may or may not lead to a reduction in opioid requirements.

- Gabapentinoids (see Chap. 4) are commonly used in chronic pain clinics in the treatment of neuropathic pain. The rationale for their peri-operative use includes possible anti-hyperalgesic, anti-allodynic and anti-tolerance effects [47]. Some studies have also shown that they can reduce post-operative opioid consumption and improve pain relief in opioid naive patients [57]. These drugs can lead to sedation, therefore the drugs are often given as tolerated, and titrated to effect. They may have an opioid sparing effect but dosing regimes vary widely and there is little consensus on appropriate dosing, and therefore establishing the correct dose can be challenging. The use of gabapentinoids in opioid tolerant patients undergoing abdominal surgery has not been studied.
- IV Lidocaine (see Chap. 6): Lidocaine has analgesic, anti-inflammatory and anti-hyperalgesic properties. Analgesic effects are due to inhibition of Na channels, NMDA and G-protein linked receptors, causing suppression of impulses from injured nerve fibres and the proximal dorsal root ganglion. The use of IV lidocaine has been studied in open and laparoscopic abdominal surgery, tonsillectomy, orthopaedic, cardiac and ambulatory surgery. The peri-operative administration of IV lidocaine seems to have particular benefits in abdominal surgery (but not specifically in opioid tolerant patients) and this may be because IV lidocaine confers specific benefit to visceral pain. McCarthy, Marret, Sun and Vigneault have all conducted meta-analyses that have suggested benefit, with research showing that it significantly reduced anaesthetic and opioid requirements intra-operatively [58–61]. Studies have shown that it reduces rest and dynamic pain intensity as well as the duration of post-operative ileus. There is no clear consensus on what dose should be given and when, but some studies have used a bolus of 100 mg or 1.5–2 mg/kg half an hour before surgical incision. This is then followed by infusions ranging in dose from 1.5 to 3 mg/kg/h, which in some cases are continued for up to 24 h post-operatively. The studies have not reported complications due to local anaesthetic toxicity but patients would need monitoring in a level 1 area for the duration of the infusion and further studies are required to establish the safety of IV lidocaine. Some studies have shown continued analgesic effect once the infusion has stopped, and one study found a preventative effect on post-operative pain after abdominal surgery for up to 72 h.
- Alpha-2 adrenoreceptor antagonists: De Kock et al. compared intra-operative administration of IV clonidine to control in patients undergoing major abdominal surgery [62]. A clonidine dose of 4 μg/kg was given over 30 min followed by an infusion of 2 μg/kg/h until the peritoneum was closed. Clonidine reduced pain scores and morphine consumption in the 12 h following surgery. The study also compared intravenous to epidural administration of clonidine and found that epidural administration had more benefit.

Opioid Analgesia (See Chap. 3)

It is widely accepted that the post-operative doses of opioid required for those patients that are opioid tolerant will be substantially higher than in opioid naive patients [47, 63]. Research has shown that PCA usage can be up to three times greater in the opioid tolerant group. This is an important consideration for those clinicians that take part in acute pain ward rounds [41]. Use of PCAs should be encouraged, whilst ensuring that sufficient background requirements are provided (if normal route of administration is not possible), as well as larger bolus doses. This group are also likely to report higher pain scores and remain in hospital longer under the observation from an acute pain team [43], due to the fact that post-operative pain takes longer to resolve than in opioid naive patients.

Epidural Analgesia (See Chap. 8)

For many years epidural anaesthesia was seen as gold standard management for abdominal surgery. One meta-analysis found that overall mortality was reduced by about a third and reduced the odds of deep vein thrombosis by 44%, pulmonary embolus by 55%, transfusion requirements by 50%, pneumonia by 39% and respiratory depression by 59% [64]. The study concluded that these findings supported more widespread use of neuraxial blockade, and for the early part of this century epidural use was commonplace. These findings were challenged by the MASTER trial which concluded that adverse outcomes in high risk patients undergoing major abdominal surgery were not reduced by the use of combined epidural and general anaesthesia and post-operative epidural anaesthesia [65]. There were, however, improvements in analgesia and a reduction in respiratory failure in the epidural group. Editorials followed in 2012 adding to the debate. Rawal agreed that newer, evidence-based outcome data cast doubt over the benefits of epidural anaesthesia that had previously been claimed and that the number of indications for their use was on the decline [66]. Another editorial by Wildsmith cautioned on the weaknesses of the earlier studies, stating that 'the implication is that good patient outcome is as much about quality of care as it is the method of care [67].

A recent meta-analysis by Popping et al. has swung the debate in favour of epidurals once again, finding that epidurals reduce mortality (3.1% versus 4.9%) and significantly decreased the risk of supra ventricular tachycardia, atrial fibrillation, deep vein thrombosis, respiratory depression, atelectasis, pneumonia, ileus and post-operative nausea and vomiting [68]. The study was designed to look at outcomes other than analgesia. There are multiple meta-analyses that show, despite different level of epidural, analgesic agent used or type of pain assessment, that epidurals provide superior analgesia to that of parenteral opioids. Despite all this controversy the evidence suggests that epidurals do offer better pain relief in the immediate post-operative period, and in chronic pain patients this may mean that an epidural should still be considered.

No discussions about epidurals can occur without considering the risk they pose. These range from relatively minor such as hypotension, incomplete pain relief and pruritis through to epidural abscess and haematoma potentially leading to cord ischaemia. The third National audit project (NAP 3) performed by the Royal College of Anaesthetists involved a year long survey to capture all major complications of central neuraxial blockade (CNB) in the UK National Health Service [69]. The complications included vertebral canal abscess or haematoma, meningitis, nerve injury, spinal cord ischaemia, fatal cardiovascular collapse and wrong route errors. The survey established a denominator (via a 2 week national census) of 707,455 CNB with 84 major complications reported over a 1 year period. After being reviewed, 52 of these met the inclusion criteria for the survey. They reported that the incidence of permanent nerve injury was pessimistically 4.2 per 100,000 cases and optimistically 2.0 per 100,000 cases. The conclusion they drew was that the data was reassuring and the CNB had a low incidence of major complications, many of which resolve within 6 months. Although the survey was not looking at pain relief as an outcome, the data is important as it allows the clinician and patient to have an informed discussion about the risks posed by CNB in a group of patients that are very likely to benefit from it.

Currently there are no randomised controlled trials comparing epidurals to other forms of pain relief in chronic pain patients undergoing abdominal surgery, so drawing peer-reviewed conclusions is not possible. There has been recent interest in other regional anaesthetic techniques that include transverse abdominus plane blocks and rectus sheaths blocks and catheters. The interest in these blocks has in part been growing due to the discussion of the risk-benefit of epidurals. These alternatives are now widely used but an evidence base in opioid tolerant patients does not exist, and in fact the evidence in opioid naive patients is similarly lacking. However, there is a study in progress comparing rectus sheath catheters to epidurals for abdominal surgery, which may help to support the use of this promising technique [70].

Laparoscopic Versus Open Colonic Resection

Laparoscopic colonic resection has been shown to have less complications, improved pain scores and reduced length of stay when compared with open surgery. There is evidence that intrathecal morphine in combination with bupivacaine in patients having laparoscopic bowel resections, leads to improved pain scores and less post-operative opioid consumption when compared to morphine PCA [71]. This research is not specific to chronic pain patients; however, this finding should be considered when planning surgery in opioid tolerant patients.

Conclusions

The research on this specific group of patients is limited and much of the discussion has focused on the general principles of treating acute pain in the opioid tolerant population. The advice that exists for these patients remains based on case series, case reports, expert opinion and personal experience [40]. It is important to identify opioid tolerant patients prior to having surgery so that options and expectations can be discussed, as well as having a strategy to avoid a withdrawal syndrome. Epidurals have been shown to have improved pain scores in the general surgical population and it seems a pragmatic approach to consider offering one to appropriately selected patients who do not have any contraindications. The use of a multimodal analgesic strategy should be considered in all patients, and consideration as to what combination of drugs would be best suited to a particular individual. It is also important to accept that treating pain in these individuals can be immensely challenging and multi-disciplinary discussions and repeated patient consultations may be required, over a longer than normal time frame, to reach an acceptable level of pain management.

References

1. Jenkins JT, O'Dwyer PJ. Inguinal hernias. BMJ. 2008;336(7638):269–72.
2. Macrae WA. Chronic pain after surgery. Br J Anaesth. 2001;87(1):88–98.
3. Crombie IK, Croft PR, Linton SJ, Leresche L, Korff MV, editors. Epidemiology of pain: a report of the task force on epidemiology of the international association for the study of pain. Seattle, WA: IASP Press; 1999.
4. Werner MU, Kongsgaard UE. I. Defining persistent post-surgical pain: is an update required? Br J Anaesth. 2014;113(1):1–4.
5. Poobalan AS, Bruce J, Smith WC, King PM, Krukowski ZH, Chambers WA. A review of chronic pain after inguinal herniorrhaphy. Clin J Pain. 2003;19(1):48–54.
6. Macrae WA. Chronic post-surgical pain: 10 years on. Br J Anaesth. 2008;101(1):77–86.
7. Bruce J, Krukowski ZH. Quality of life and chronic pain four years after gastrointestinal surgery. Dis Colon Rectum. 2006;49(9):1362–70.
8. Ramos PA, Vilchez AL, Beltrán de Heredia S, Bernedo GC, Sardà SM. Incidence of chronic post-surgical pain after midline laparotomy: 14AP9–11. Eur J Anaesth. 2010;27(47):217.
9. Joris JL, Georges MJ, Medjahed K, Ledoux D, Damilot G, Ramquet CC, et al. Prevalence, characteristics and risk factors of chronic postsurgical pain after laparoscopic colorectal surgery: Retrospective analysis. Eur J Anaesthesiol. 2015;32(10):712–7.
10. Owen M, Lorgelly P, Serpell M. Chronic pain following donor nephrectomy: a study of the incidence, nature and impact of chronic post-nephrectomy pain. Eur J Pain. 2010;14(7):732–4.
11. Johansen A, Romundstad L, Nielsen CS, Schirmer H, Stubhaug A. Persistent postsurgical pain in a general population: prevalence and predictors in the Tromso study. Pain. 2012;153(7):1390–6.
12. Sandblom G. Is chronic post-herniorrhaphy pain always chronic? A literature review. J Pain Res. 2015;8:241–5.
13. Reinpold WM, Nehls J, Eggert A. Nerve management and chronic pain after open inguinal hernia repair: a prospective two phase study. Ann Surg. 2011;254(1):163–8.
14. Poobalan AS, Bruce J, King PM, Chambers WA, Krukowski ZH, Smith WC. Chronic pain and quality of life following open inguinal hernia repair. Br J Surg. 2001;88(8):1122–6.
15. Aasvang EK, Kehlet H. Chronic pain after childhood groin hernia repair. J Pediatr Surg. 2007;42(8):1403–8.

16. Kristensen AD, Ahlburg P, Lauridsen MC, Jensen TS, Nikolajsen L. Chronic pain after inguinal hernia repair in children. Br J Anaesth. 2012;109(4):603–8.
17. Aasvang EK, Gmaehle E, Hansen JB, Gmaehle B, Forman JL, Schwarz J, et al. Predictive risk factors for persistent postherniotomy pain. Anesthesiology. 2010;112(4):957–69.
18. Hinrichs-Rocker A, Schulz K, Jarvinen I, Lefering R, Simanski C, Neugebauer EA. Psychosocial predictors and correlates for chronic post-surgical pain (CPSP) – a systematic review. Eur J Pain. 2009;13(7):719–30.
19. Page MG, Campbell F, Isaac L, Stinson J, Katz J. Parental risk factors for the development of pediatric acute and chronic postsurgical pain: a longitudinal study. J Pain Res. 2013;6:727–41.
20. Kolesnikov Y, Gabovits B, Levin A, Veske A, Qin L, Dai F, et al. Chronic pain after lower abdominal surgery: do catechol-O-methyl transferase/opioid receptor mu-1 polymorphisms contribute? Mol Pain. 2013;9:19.
21. Nackley AG, Tan KS, Fecho K, Flood P, Diatchenko L, Maixner W. Catechol-O-methyltransferase inhibition increases pain sensitivity through activation of both beta2- and beta3-adrenergic receptors. Pain. 2007;128(3):199–208.
22. Montes A, Roca G, Sabate S, Lao JI, Navarro A, Cantillo J, et al. Genetic and clinical factors associated with chronic postsurgical pain after hernia repair, hysterectomy, and thoracotomy: a two-year multicenter cohort study. Anesthesiology. 2015;122(5):1123–41.
23. Yarnitsky D, Crispel Y, Eisenberg E, Granovsky Y, Ben-Nun A, Sprecher E, et al. Prediction of chronic post-operative pain: pre-operative DNIC testing identifies patients at risk. Pain. 2008;138(1):22–8.
24. Wylde V, Hewlett S, Learmonth ID, Dieppe P. Persistent pain after joint replacement: prevalence, sensory qualities, and postoperative determinants. Pain. 2011;152(3):566–72.
25. Lange JF, Meyer VM, Voropai DA, Keus E, Wijsmuller AR, Ploeg RJ, et al. The role of surgical expertise with regard to chronic postoperative inguinal pain (CPIP) after Lichtenstein correction of inguinal hernia: a systematic review. Hernia. 2016;20(3):349–56.
26. Searle RD, Simpson MP, Simpson KH, Milton R, Bennett MI. Can chronic neuropathic pain following thoracic surgery be predicted during the postoperative period? Interact Cardiovasc Thorac Surg. 2009;9(6):999–1002.
27. Martinez V, Ben Ammar S, Judet T, Bouhassira D, Chauvin M, Fletcher D. Risk factors predictive of chronic postsurgical neuropathic pain: the value of the iliac crest bone harvest model. Pain. 2012;153(7):1478–83.
28. Lavand'homme P, De Kock M, Waterloos H. Intraoperative epidural analgesia combined with ketamine provides effective preventive analgesia in patients undergoing major digestive surgery. Anesthesiology. 2005;103(4):813–20.
29. Bouman EA, Theunissen M, Bons SA, van Mook WN, Gramke HF, van Kleef M, et al. Reduced incidence of chronic postsurgical pain after epidural analgesia for abdominal surgery. Pain Pract. 2014;14(2):E76–84.
30. Nikolajsen L, Sorensen HC, Jensen TS, Kehlet H. Chronic pain following Caesarean section. Acta Anaesthesiol Scand. 2004;48(1):111–6.
31. Brandsborg B, Nikolajsen L, Hansen CT, Kehlet H, Jensen TS. Risk factors for chronic pain after hysterectomy: a nationwide questionnaire and database study. Anesthesiology. 2007;106(5):1003–12.
32. Chaparro LE, Smith SA, Moore RA, Wiffen PJ, Gilron I. Pharmacotherapy for the prevention of chronic pain after surgery in adults. Cochrane Database Syst Rev. 2013;7:CD008307.
33. Chan MT, Wan AC, Gin T, Leslie K, Myles PS. Chronic postsurgical pain after nitrous oxide anesthesia. Pain. 2011;152(11):2514–20.
34. van Gulik L, Ahlers SJ, van de Garde EM, Bruins P, van Boven WJ, Tibboel D, et al. Remifentanil during cardiac surgery is associated with chronic thoracic pain 1 yr after sternotomy. Br J Anaesth. 2012;109(4):616–22.
35. Clarke H, Wijeysundera DN, Bonin RP, Orser B, Englesakis M, Katz J. Pregabalin effective for the prevention of chronic postsurgical pain: really? Reply. Anesth Analg. 2013;116(2):508–9.

36. Clarke H, Bonin RP, Orser BA, Englesakis M, Wijeysundera DN, Katz J. The prevention of chronic postsurgical pain using gabapentin and pregabalin: a combined systematic review and meta-analysis. Anesth Analg. 2012;115(2):428–42.
37. Vedula SS, Bero L, Scherer RW, Dickersin K. Outcome reporting in industry-sponsored trials of gabapentin for off-label use. N Engl J Med. 2009;361(20):1963–71.
38. Dowsey MM, Castle DJ, Knowles SR, Monshat K, Salzberg MR, Choong PF. The effect of mindfulness training prior to total joint arthroplasty on post-operative pain and physical function: study protocol for a randomised controlled trial. Trials. 2014;15:208.
39. Loeser JD, Melzack R. Pain: an overview. Lancet. 1999;353(9164):1607–9.
40. PG SSA, Scott DA, Halliwell R, Trinca J, editors. Acute pain management: scientific evidence. Melbourne: ANZCA; 2015.
41. Rapp SE, Ready LB, Nessly ML. Acute pain management in patients with prior opioid consumption: a case-controlled retrospective review. Pain. 1995;61(2):195–201.
42. Fletcher D, Martinez V. Opioid-induced hyperalgesia in patients after surgery: a systematic review and a meta-analysis. Br J Anaesth. 2014;112(6):991–1004.
43. Gulur P, Williams L, Chaudhary S, Koury K, Jaff M. Opioid tolerance--a predictor of increased length of stay and higher readmission rates. Pain Physician. 2014;17(4):E503–7.
44. Inturrisi CE. Clinical pharmacology of opioids for pain. Clin J Pain. 2002;18(4 Suppl):S3–13.
45. Alford DP, Compton P, Samet JH. Acute pain management for patients receiving maintenance methadone or buprenorphine therapy. Ann Intern Med. 2006;144(2):127–34.
46. Gonzalez-Barboteo J, Porta-Sales J, Sanchez D, Tuca A, Gomez-Batiste X. Conversion from parenteral to oral methadone. J Pain Palliat Care Pharmacother. 2008;22(3):200–5.
47. Huxtable CA, Roberts LJ, Somogyi AA, MacIntyre PE. Acute pain management in opioid-tolerant patients: a growing challenge. Anaesth Intensive Care. 2011;39(5):804–23.
48. Mattick RP, Breen C, Kimber J, Davoli M. Buprenorphine maintenance versus placebo or methadone maintenance for opioid dependence. Cochrane Database Syst Rev. 2014;2:CD002207.
49. Greenwald MK, Johanson CE, Moody DE, Woods JH, Kilbourn MR, Koeppe RA, et al. Effects of buprenorphine maintenance dose on mu-opioid receptor availability, plasma concentrations, and antagonist blockade in heroin-dependent volunteers. Neuropsychopharmacology. 2003;28(11):2000–9.
50. Macintyre PE, Russell RA, Usher KA, Gaughwin M, Huxtable CA. Pain relief and opioid requirements in the first 24 hours after surgery in patients taking buprenorphine and methadone opioid substitution therapy. Anaesth Intensive Care. 2013;41(2):222–30.
51. Rapp SE, Wild LM, Egan KJ, Ready LB. Acute pain management of the chronic pain patient on opiates: a survey of caregivers at University of Washington Medical Center. Clin J Pain. 1994;10(2):133–8.
52. Barreveld AM, Correll DJ, Liu X, Max B, McGowan JA, Shovel L, et al. Ketamine decreases postoperative pain scores in patients taking opioids for chronic pain: results of a prospective, randomized, double-blind study. Pain Med. 2013;14(6):925–34.
53. Wu L, Huang X, Sun L. The efficacy of N-methyl-D-aspartate receptor antagonists on improving the postoperative pain intensity and satisfaction after remifentanil-based anesthesia in adults: a meta-analysis. J Clin Anesth. 2015;27(4):311–24.
54. Laskowski K, Stirling A, McKay WP, Lim HJ. A systematic review of intravenous ketamine for postoperative analgesia. Can J Anaesth. 2011;58(10):911–23.
55. Bell RF, Dahl JB, Moore RA, Kalso E. Perioperative ketamine for acute postoperative pain. Cochrane Database Syst Rev. 2006;1:CD004603.
56. Loftus RW, Yeager MP, Clark JA, Brown JR, Abdu WA, Sengupta DK, et al. Intraoperative ketamine reduces perioperative opiate consumption in opiate-dependent patients with chronic back pain undergoing back surgery. Anesthesiology. 2010;113(3):639–46.
57. Lam DM, Choi SW, Wong SS, Irwin MG, Cheung CW. Efficacy of pregabalin in acute postoperative pain under different surgical categories: a meta-analysis. Medicine. 2015;94(46):e1944.
58. Marret E, Rolin M, Beaussier M, Bonnet F. Meta-analysis of intravenous lidocaine and postoperative recovery after abdominal surgery. Br J Surg. 2008;95(11):1331–8.

59. McCarthy GC, Megalla SA, Habib AS. Impact of intravenous lidocaine infusion on postoperative analgesia and recovery from surgery: a systematic review of randomized controlled trials. Drugs. 2010;70(9):1149–63.
60. Sun Y, Li T, Wang N, Yun Y, Gan TJ. Perioperative systemic lidocaine for postoperative analgesia and recovery after abdominal surgery: a meta-analysis of randomized controlled trials. Dis Colon Rectum. 2012;55(11):1183–94.
61. Vigneault L, Turgeon AF, Cote D, Lauzier F, Zarychanski R, Moore L, et al. Perioperative intravenous lidocaine infusion for postoperative pain control: a meta-analysis of randomized controlled trials. Can J Anaesth. 2011;58(1):22–37.
62. De Kock M, Crochet B, Morimont C, Scholtes JL. Intravenous or epidural clonidine for intra- and postoperative analgesia. Anesthesiology. 1993;79(3):525–31.
63. Mitra S, Sinatra RS. Perioperative management of acute pain in the opioid-dependent patient. Anesthesiology. 2004;101(1):212–27.
64. Rodgers A, Walker N, Schug S, McKee A, Kehlet H, van Zundert A, et al. Reduction of postoperative mortality and morbidity with epidural or spinal anaesthesia: results from overview of randomised trials. BMJ. 2000;321(7275):1493.
65. Rigg JR, Jamrozik K, Myles PS, Silbert BS, Peyton PJ, Parsons RW, et al. Epidural anaesthesia and analgesia and outcome of major surgery: a randomised trial. Lancet. 2002;359(9314):1276–82.
66. Rawal N. Epidural technique for postoperative pain: gold standard no more? Reg Anesth Pain Med. 2012;37(3):310–7.
67. Wildsmith JA. Continuous thoracic epidural block for surgery: gold standard or debased currency? Br J Anaesth. 2012;109(1):9–12.
68. Popping DM, Elia N, Van Aken HK, Marret E, Schug SA, Kranke P, et al. Impact of epidural analgesia on mortality and morbidity after surgery: systematic review and meta-analysis of randomized controlled trials. Ann Surg. 2014;259(6):1056–67.
69. Cook TM, Counsell D, Wildsmith JA. Royal College of Anaesthetists Third National Audit P. Major complications of central neuraxial block: report on the Third National Audit Project of the Royal College of Anaesthetists. Br J Anaesth. 2009;102(2):179–90.
70. Wilkinson KM, Krige A, Brearley SG, Lane S, Scott M, Gordon AC, et al. Thoracic epidural analgesia versus rectus sheath catheters for open midline incisions in major abdominal surgery within an enhanced recovery programme (TERSC): study protocol for a randomised controlled trial. Trials. 2014;15:400.
71. Wongyingsinn M, Baldini G, Stein B, Charlebois P, Liberman S, Carli F. Spinal analgesia for laparoscopic colonic resection using an enhanced recovery after surgery programme: better analgesia, but no benefits on postoperative recovery: a randomized controlled trial. Br J Anaesth. 2012;108(5):850–6.

Index

A. Krige, M. J. P. Scott (eds.), *Analgesia in Major Abdominal Surgery*,
https://doi.org/10.1007/978-3-319-94482-1

MIX
Papier aus verantwortungsvollen Quellen
Paper from responsible sources
FSC® C105338

If you have any concerns about our products,
you can contact us on
ProductSafety@springernature.com

In case Publisher is established outside the EU,
the EU authorized representative is:
Springer Nature Customer Service Center GmbH
Europaplatz 3, 69115 Heidelberg, Germany

Printed by Libri Plureos GmbH
in Hamburg, Germany